BRADY

BTLS: BASIC TRAUMA LIFE SUPPORT

for the EMT-B and First Responder

Second Edition

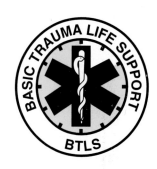

EDITED BY

John Emory Campbell

M.D., F.A.C.E.P

Basic Trauma Life Support International, Inc.

BRADY
Prentice Hall
Upper Saddle River, New Jersey 07458

Library of Congress Cataloging-in-Publication Data
BTLS: basic trauma life support for the EMT-B and first responder /
  edited by John Emory Campbell . — 2nd ed.
      p.   cm.
    Rev. ed. of: BTLS / John Emory Campbell. c1988.
    Includes index.
    ISBN 0-8359-4988-5·
      1. Emergency medicine.   2. Wounds and injuries.
  3. Emergency medical technicians.   I. Campbell, John E., 1943–   .
  II. Campbell, John E., 1943–   BTLS
    [DNLM: 1. Emergency Medical Services—United States.
  2. Emergencies. 3. Wounds and Injuries.   WX 215
  B916 1996]
  RC86.7.C342   1996
  617.1'026—dc20
  DNLM/DLC   95-36632
  for Library of Congress   CIP

Publisher: Susan Katz
Editorial/Production Supervision and Electronic
  Composition: Cathy O'Connell
Director of Manufacturing & Production: Bruce Johnson
Managing Editor: Patrick Walsh
Development Editor: Nancy Brandwein
Art Director: Marianne Frasco
Cover Design: Miguel Ortiz
Photography Manager: Michal Heron
Assistant Photography Editor: Maura McGloin
Photographer: George Dodson
Technical Advisor: Dave O. Colburn, Jr.
Cover Photographer: Michal Heron
Interior Design: Greene Communications Design, Inc.
Manufacturing Buyer: Ilene Sanford
Marketing Manager: Judy Streger
Editorial Assistant: Carol Sobel
Color Separator: Carlisle Communications, Ltd.

> This book is dedicated to the teachers of
> trauma care. In a world preoccupied with
> selfishness and greed, you are the exception.
> I consider it an honor to be counted among
> you.

Printed in the United States of America

10 9 8 7 6 5 4 3 2 1

ISBN: 0-8359-4988-5

Prentice-Hall International (UK) Limited, *London*
Prentice-Hall of Australia Pty. Limited, *Sydney*
Prentice-Hall Canada Inc., *Toronto*
Prentice-Hall Hispanoamericana, S.A., *Mexico*
Prentice-Hall of India Private Limited, *New Delhi*
Prentice-Hall of Japan, Inc., *Tokyo*
Simon & Schuster Asia Pte. Ltd., *Singapore*

NOTICE ON CARE PROCEDURES

It is the intent of the authors and publisher that this
textbook be used as part of an education program
taught by qualified instructors and supervised by a
licensed physician. The procedures described in this
textbook are based upon consultation with paramedics, nurses, and physicians. The authors and
publisher have taken care to make certain that these
procedures reflect currently accepted clinical practice; however, they cannot be considered absolute
recommendations.

The material in this textbook contains the most
current information available at the time of publica-
tion. However, federal, state, and local guidelines
concerning clinical practices, including, without lim-
itation, those governing infection control and universal precautions, change rapidly. The reader
should note, therefore, that new regulations may
require changes in some procedures.

It is the responsibility of the reader to familiarize
himself or herself with the policies and procedures
set by federal, state, and local agencies as well as the
institution or agency where the reader is employed.
The authors and the publisher of this textbook and
the supplements written to accompany it disclaim
any liability, loss, or risk resulting directly or indi-
rectly from the suggested procedures and theory,
from any undetected errors, or from the reader's
misunderstanding of the text. It is the reader's
responsibility to stay informed of any new changes
or recommendations made by any federal, state, and
local agency as well as by his or her employing institution or agency.

NOTICE ON GENDER USAGE

The English language has historically given prefer-
ence to the male gender. Among many words, the
pronouns, "he" and "his" are commonly used to
describe both genders. Society evolves faster than
language, and the male pronouns still predominate
our speech. The authors have made great effort to
treat the two genders equally, recognizing that a significant percentage of EMS Providers are female.
However, in some instances, male pronouns may be
used to describe both males and females solely for
the purpose of brevity. This is not intended to offend
any readers of the female gender.

Contents

Authors

BTLS For the EMT-B and First Responder

Gail V. Anderson, Jr., M.D., M.B.A.,
F.A.C.E.P.
Vice President, Medical Affairs
Grady Health System
Associate Professor
Department of Surgery
Division of Emergency Medicine
Emory University School of Medicine
Atlanta, Georgia

James J. Augustine, M.D., F.A.C.E.P.
Associate Director of Emergency
    Department
Miami Valley Hospital
Dayton, Ohio
Assistant Clinical Professor
Department of Emergency Medicine
Wright State University

Jere F. Baldwin, M.D., F.A.C.E.P.
Chief, Department of Emergency
    and Ambulatory Services
Mercy Hospital
Port Huron, MI

Russell Bieniek, M.D., F.A.C.E.P.
Medical Director of Emergency
    Services
Saint Vincent Health Center
Erie, Pennsylvania

John E. Campbell, M.D., F.A.C.E.P.

James H. Creel, Jr., M.D., F.A.C.E.P.

Ray Fowler, M.D., F.A.C.E.P.
Chairman, Department of Emergency
    Medicine
Parkway Medical Center
Lithia Springs, Georgia

Stephen W. Hargarten, M.D., M.P.H.
Assistant Professor
Vice Chairman
Department of Emergency Medicine
Medical College of Wisconsin

Donna Hastings, EMT-P
Grant MacEwan Community College
Edmonton, Alberta, Canada

Leah J. Heimbach, R.N., NREMT-P

Carden Johnston, M.D., F.A.A.P., F.A.C.E.P.
Professor of Pediatrics
University of Alabama at Birmingham

Ron Lee, M.D., F.A.C.E.P.
Assistant Professor of Medicine
Loyola University

Roger J. Lewis, M.D., Ph.D., F.A.C.E.P.
Director of Research
Department of Emergency Medicine
Harbor-UCLA Medical Center
Assistant Professor of Medicine
UCLA School of Medicine

Richard N. Nelson, M.D., F.A.C.E.P.
Associate Professor of Clinical Emergency
    Medicine
The Ohio State University
College of Medicine
Medical Director
Emergency Department
The Ohio State University Medical Center

Jonathan G. Newman, REMT-P

Paul Paris, M.D., F.A.C.E.P.
Associate Professor and Chief
Division of Emergency Medicine
University of Pittsburgh School of Medicine
Chief Medical Officer
Center for Emergency Medicine of
    Western Pennsylvania
Medical Director, City of Pittsburgh
Department of Public Safety

Andrew B. Peitzman, M.D.
Director, Trauma Services and Surgical
    Critical Care
University of Pittsburgh Medical
    Center

Paul E. Pepe, M.D., F.A.C.E.P., F.C.C.M.
Associate Professor
Department of Medicine, Surgery, &
    Pediatrics
Baylor College of Medicine
Director, City of Houston
Emergency Medical Services

Lisa Santer, M.D., F.A.A.P.
Assistant Professor of Pediatrics
University of Alabama at Birmingham

Cory Slovis, M.D, F.A.C.P., F.A.C.E.P.
Professor of Emergency Medicine and
    Medicine
Chairman, Department of Emergency
    Medicine
Vanderbilt University School of
    Medicine
Associate Medical Director,
Metropolitan Nashville
Emergency Medical Services

Walt A. Stoy, PhD., EMT-P
Director of Educational Programs
Center for Emergency Medicine
Research Assistant Professor of Medicine
University of Pittsburgh
Division of Emergency Medicine

Richard C. Treat, M.D.
Chief, Section of Trauma
Department of Surgery
University of Alabama at Birmingham

Howard Werman, M.D., F.A.C.E.P.
Associate Professor of Clinical Emergency
    Medicine
The Ohio State University
College of Medicine
Medical Director, Skymed
Mifflin Township EMS
City of Granview EMS

Janet M. Williams, M.D.
Assistant Professor
Dept. of Emergency Medicine
Research Director
Center for Rural Emergency Medicine
West Virginia University
Morgantown, WV

Arlo Weltge, M.D., F.A.C.E.P.
Assistant Professor
Emergency Medicine
UT - Houston Medical School
Medical Director
Houston Community College System
Program in EMS
Medical Director
P & S and Ambulance Service

**Arthur H. Yancy, II, M.D., M.P.H.,
F.A.C.E.P.**
Assistant Professor
Department of Surgery
Division of Emergency Medicine
Emory University School of Medicine
Atlanta, Georgia

Introduction

The first prehospital trauma course ever developed, *Basic Trauma Life Support* was introduced for Paramedics and Advanced EMS Providers in August of 1982. BTLS began as a local project of the Alabama Chapter of the American College of Emergency Physicians. Because of a similar need for trauma training for Basic EMTs, *Basic Trauma Life Support for Basic EMTs and First Responders* was offered in 1988. This second edition not only updates changes in prehospital trauma care, but also encorporates many suggestions to improve the course itself. The original BTLS course was modeled after the *Advanced Trauma Life Support* course (for physicians) so that the surgeon, emergency physician, trauma nurse, and EMT would think and act along similar lines. The courses differ in many respects because the prehospital situation differs markedly from the hospital.

Basic Trauma Life Support is endorsed by the American College of Emergency Physicians and the National Association of EMS Physicians. The National Registry of Emergency Medical Technicians recognizes the course for 16 hours credit for continuing education for all levels of EMTs. More than this, BTLS has become an international organization of instructors of prehospital trauma care. Each local chapter is represented at the international meetings. The purpose of the organization is to foster trauma training and maintain up-to-date high standards for the BTLS course.

Basic Trauma Life Support International, with the experience of training thousands of students over the last thirteen years, is responsible for the second edition of *BTLS: Basic Trauma Life Support for the EMT-B and First Responder*. Authors include distinguished trauma surgeons, emergency physicians, emergency nurses, and paramedics. The authors are balanced between those in academics and "field providers." We have attempted to make changes that are more practical to the real environment of the prehospital situation. Because EMS varies widely over the world, we have added some optional skill stations. There are several new chapters that are pertinent to trauma care but are not included in the course itself.

This course is designed for the EMT-A or First Responder who must initially evaluate and stabilize the trauma patient. Since this is a critical time in the management of these patients, this course is intended to teach the skills necessary for rapid assessment, resuscitation, packaging, and transport. It also stresses those conditions which cannot be stabilized in the field and thus require immediate transport. It is recognized that there is more than one acceptable way to manage most situations, and the procedures described here may be modified by your medical director. You should have your Medical Direction physician go over the material and give you advice as to how the procedures are to be done in your area. Modification of technique is allowed in the teaching of this course.

The primary objectives of the course are to teach you the correct sequence of evaluation and the techniques of resuscitation and packaging of the patient. You will be given enough practical training to perform these drills rapidly and efficiently, thus giving your patient the greatest chance of arriving at the emergency department in time for definitive care to be lifesaving.

Acknowledgments

Special thanks to these BTLS instructors who provided invaluable assistance with ideas, reviews, and corrections of the text.

Roy L. Alson, Ph.D., M.D., F.A.C.E.P.
H. Gibbs Andrews, M.D., F.A.C.S.
George Angus Jr., EMT-P
Ernest J. Baringer, III, B.A., EMT
Scott Bolleter, NREMT-P
Jackie Campbell, R.N.
Connie Clemmons, R.N., B.S.N.
Ann Dietrich, M.D.
Rick Harrington, EMT-P
John M. Kirkley Jr., NREMT-P
Brian D. Mahoney, M.D., F.A.C.E.P.
Michael Proctor, M.D., F.A.C.E.P.
Lee B. Smith, M.D.

Notes for Teachers

Though suitable as a reference text about prehospital trauma care, this book is designed to be part of an organized hands-on course for Basic EMTs and First Responders. An Instructor Guide and slides are available to be used in teaching the BTLS course. This course is monitored and certified in each area by the local chapter of Basic Trauma Life Support International, Inc. If you wish to arrange a certified course in your area but do not know the address of your local Chapter Coordinator, you may write or call:

Virginia Kennedy Palys
Executive Director
Basic Trauma Life Support International, Inc.
1 South 280 Summit Avenue
Court B
Oakbrook Terrace, Illinois 60181
Phone: 1-800-495-2857

Notes for Students

The BTLS course is an intensive, demanding experience that requires preparation in advance of the actual course. You should begin studying the book no less than two weeks before the course. The actual course is designed not to tell you, but rather to show you and allow you to practice managing trauma patients. If properly prepared, you will find this course to be the most enjoyable you have ever taken.

The first 20 chapters are essential and should be studied thoroughly in the weeks preceding the course. You will be tested on this material. The appendix contains important chapters, but due to time constraints they are not included in the course. You will *not* be tested on the chapters in the appendix.

The appendix contains some optional skills. If any optional skills are to be taught in the course, you will be notified in advance so that you may study them.

For information about BTLS call 1-800-495-BTLS

If you would like to place an order for textbooks, call 1-800-638-0220

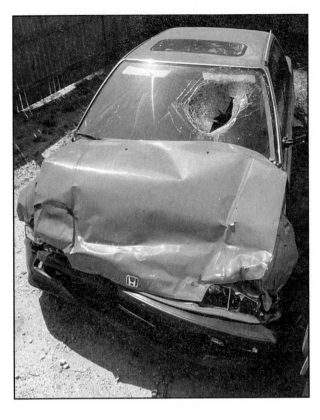

Mechanisms of Injuries Due to Motion

(High-Energy Events)

James H. Creel, Jr., M.D., F.A.C.E.P.

OBJECTIVES

Upon completion of this chapter, you should be able to:

1. List three basic mechanisms of motion injury.

2. Discuss mechanisms and settings for blunt versus penetrating trauma.

3. Identify the three collisions associated with a motor vehicle crash (MVC) and relate potential victim injuries to deformity of the vehicle, interior structures, and body structures.

4. Name the four common forms of MVCs.

5. Describe potential injuries associated with proper and improper use of seat restraints, head rests, and air bags in a head-on collision.

6. Differentiate lateral-impact collision from head-on collision based on the three collisions associated with an MVC.

7. Describe potential injuries from rear-end collisions.

8. Explain why the mortality rate is higher for victims ejected from vehicles in MVCs.

9. Describe the three assessment criteria for rapid vertical deceleration and relate them to anticipated injuries.

10. Identify the two most common forms of penetration injuries and discuss associated mechanisms and extent of injury.

11. Relate three factors involved in blast injuries to patient assessment.

Trauma, the medical term for injury, continues to be our most expensive health problem. The fourth leading cause of death for all ages, trauma is the leading cause of death for children and adults under the age of 45 years. For every fatality, there are ten more admitted to hospitals and hundreds more treated in emergency departments. The cost of injury is estimated to be over $180 billion annually. This represents a cost twice that of cardiovascular disease and cancer combined. The price of trauma, in both physical and fiscal resources, mandates that we learn more about this disease to treat its effects and decrease its incidence.

Injury is a disease process that is noted to have seasonal variations, epidemic episodes, long-term trends, and demographic distributions. Injuries can be described as interactions of the host (victim) and the agent (energy) in a given environment. The transmission of the energy to the host creates an injury. The agent, energy, comes in five basic forms: (1) mechanical or kinetic, (2) thermal, (3) chemical, (4) electrical, and (5) radiating. Mechanical energy (motion) remains the most common agent of injury and is the agent of vehicle crashes, falls, penetrating injuries, and blast injuries.

Energy transmission follows the laws of physics; therefore, injuries present in predictable patterns. Knowledge and appreciation of the mechanism of injury allows you to maintain a high index of suspicion to aid in the search for injuries. Missed or overlooked injuries may be catastrophic, especially when they become known only when the compensatory mechanisms are exhausted. Remember that patients who are involved in a high-energy event are at risk for severe injury. Five to 15 percent of these patients, despite normal vital signs and no apparent anatomic injury on the first survey, will later exhibit severe injuries that are discovered on repeat examinations. Therefore, a high-energy event signifies a large release of uncontrolled energy, and you should consider the patient injured until you have proven otherwise.

Factors to be considered are direction and speed of impact, patient kinetics and physical size, and the signs of energy release (e.g., major vehicle damage). There is a strong correlation between injury severity and automobile velocity changes as measured by the amount of vehicle damage. It is important that you consider these two questions:

1. What happened?

2. How was the patient injured?

Without an understanding of the mechanism of injury, you will be unable to predict what injuries may exist. This is a ticket to disaster: your first suspicion that an injury is present may be when the patient "crashes." Mechanism of injury is also an important triage tool and is information that must always be reported to the emergency physician or trauma surgeon. Severity of vehicle damage has also been suggested as a nonphysiologic triage tool.

Motion (mechanical) injuries are by and large responsible for the majority of the mortality from trauma in the United States. This chapter will review the most common mechanisms of motion injuries and will stress the potential injuries that may be associated with these mechanisms. It is essential to develop an awareness of mechanisms of injury and thus have a high index of suspicion for occult injuries. Always consider the potential injury to be present until it is ruled out in a hospital setting.

There are three basic mechanisms of motion injury:

1. Rapid forward deceleration

2. Rapid vertical deceleration
3. Projectile penetration

MOTOR VEHICLE COLLISIONS

Various injury patterns will be discussed in the following examples, which include automobiles, motorcycles, all-terrain vehicles (ATVs), and tractors. The important concept to appreciate is that the kinetic energy of motion must be absorbed and the absorption of energy is the basic component in producing injury. Motion injury may be blunt or penetrating. Generally, blunt trauma is more common in the rural setting, and penetrating trauma is more common in the urban setting. Rapid forward deceleration is usually blunt but may be penetrating. The most common example of rapid forward deceleration is the motor vehicle crash (MVC). You should consider all MVCs as occurring in three separate events (see Figure 1-1):

1. The machine collision
2. The body collision
3. The organ collision

Consider approaching an MVC in which an automobile has hit a tree head-on at 40 miles per hour. Appreciation of the rapid forward decelerating mechanism coupled with a high index of suspicion should make you concerned that the victim may have possible head injury, cervical spine injury, myocardial contusion, any of the "deadly dozen" chest injuries, intra-abdominal injuries, and musculoskeletal injuries (especially fracture or dislocation of the hip). To explain the forces involved here, you must consider Sir Isaac Newton's second law of motion: "a body in motion remains in motion in a straight line unless acted upon by an outside force." This law is well exemplified in the automobile crash. The kinetic energy of the vehicle's forward motion is absorbed as each part of the vehicle is brought to a sudden halt by the impact. Remember the body of the occupant is also traveling at 40 mph until impacted by some structure within the car such as the windshield, steering wheel, or dashboard. With awareness of this mechanism, one can see the multitude of potential injuries that may occur. The clues you should be aware of are

1. Deformity of the vehicle (indication of forces involved)
2. Deformity of interior structures (indication of where the victim impacted)
3. Deformity (injury patterns) of the victim (indication of what parts of the body may have impacted)

Motor vehicle crashes occur in several forms and each form is associated with certain patterns of injury. The four common forms of motor vehicle crashes are

1. The head-on collision
2. The T-bone or lateral-impact collision
3. The rear-end collision
4. The rollover collision

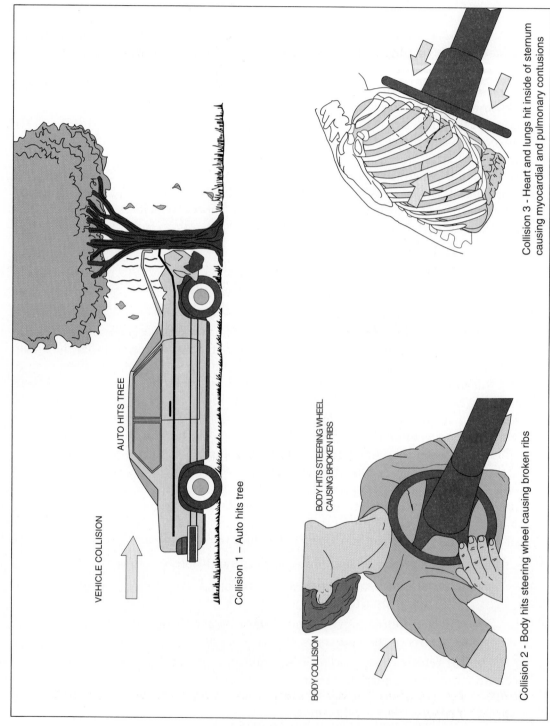

VEHICLE COLLISION

AUTO HITS TREE

Collision 1 – Auto hits tree

BODY COLLISION

BODY HITS STEERING WHEEL
CAUSING BROKEN RIBS

Collision 2 - Body hits steering wheel causing broken ribs

Collision 3 - Heart and lungs hit inside of sternum causing myocardial and pulmonary contusions

Figure 1-1 *The three collisions of an MVC.*

HEAD-ON COLLISION

In this type of MVC, an unrestrained body is brought to a sudden halt and the energy transfer is capable of producing multiple injuries.

Windshield injuries occur in the rapid forward decelerating type of events, where the unrestrained occupant impacts forcefully with the windshield (see Figure 1-2). The possibility for injuries is great under these conditions. Of utmost concern is the potential for airway and serious cervical spine (C-spine) injury. Remembering the three separate collision events, note the following:

Machine collision: deformed front end

Body collision: spider web pattern of windshield

Organ collision: coup/contracoup brain, soft tissue injury
 (scalp, face, neck), hyperextension/flexion of C-spine

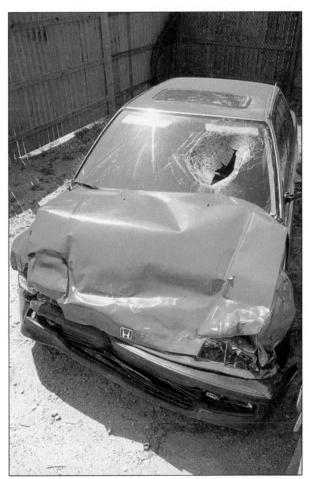

Figure 1-2 *Head-on Collision. Most injuries inflicted by: windshield, steering wheel, and dashboard.*

From the spider web appearance of the windshield and appreciation of mechanism of injury, you should maintain a high index of suspicion for possible occult injuries of the C-spine. The head usually strikes the windshield resulting in direct trauma to that structure. External signs of trauma include cuts, abrasions, and contusions. These may be quite dramatic in appearance; however, the key concern is airway maintenance with C-spine immobilization and evaluation of level of consciousness.

Steering wheel injuries most often occur to an unrestrained driver of a vehicle in a head-on collision. The driver may subsequently also impact with the windshield. The steering wheel is the vehicle's most lethal weapon for the unrestrained driver, and any degree of steering wheel deformity (check under collapsed air bags) must be treated with a high index of suspicion for face, neck, thoracic, or abdominal injury. The two components of this weapon are the ring and column (see Figure 1-3). The ring is a semirigid plastic-covered metal ring attached to a fixed inflexible post—a twentieth-century battering ram. Utilizing the three-collision concept, check for the presence of the following:

Machine collision: front-end deformity

Body collision: ring fracture/deformity, column
   normal/displaced

Organ collision: traumatic tattooing of skin

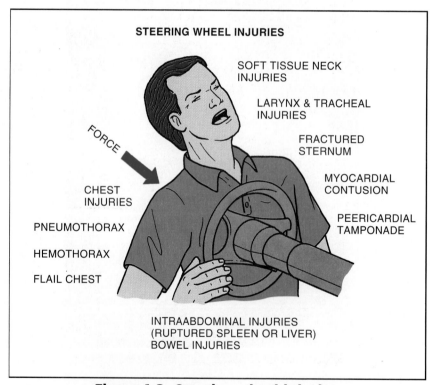

Figure 1-3 *Steering wheel injuries.*

The head-on collision is entirely dependent upon the area of the body that impacts with the steering wheel. These may be readily visible with direct trauma such as lacerations of mouth and chin, contusion/bruises of the anterior neck, traumatic tattoos of the chest wall and bruising of the abdomen. These external signs may be subtle or dramatic in appearance, but more important, they may represent the tip of the iceberg. Deeper structures and organs may harbor occult injuries due to shearing forces, compression forces, and displacement of kinetic energy. Organs that are susceptible to shearing injuries due to their ligamentous attachments are the aortic arch, liver, spleen, kidneys, and bowel. With the exception of small-bowel tears, these injuries are sources for occult bleeds and hemorrhagic shock. Compression injuries are common with lung, heart, diaphragm, and urinary bladder. An important sign is respiratory distress, which may be due to pulmonary contusions, pneumothorax,

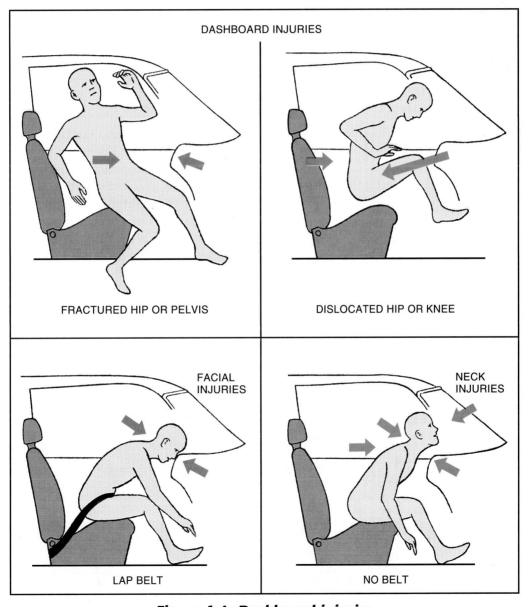

Figure 1-4 *Dashboard injuries.*

diaphragmatic hernia (bowel sounds in chest), or flail chest. Consider a bruised chest wall as a myocardial contusion that requires electrocardiogram monitoring.

In short, the steering wheel is a very lethal weapon that is capable of producing devastating injuries, many of which are occult. Steering wheel deformity is a cause for alarm and must heighten your index of suspicion. You must also relay this information to the receiving physician.

Dashboard injuries occur most often to an unrestrained passenger. The dashboard has the capability of producing a variety of injuries, depending upon the area of the body that strikes the dashboard. Most frequently, injuries involve the face and knees; however, many types of injuries have been described (see Figure 1-4).

Applying the three-event concept of collision you will note

> Machine collision: deformity of the car
>
> Body collision: fracture/deformity of the dash
>
> Organ collision: facial trauma, coup/contracoup brain, hyperextension/flexion C-spine, knee trauma

Facial, brain, and C-spine injuries have already been discussed. Like chest contusion, knee trauma may represent only the tip of the iceberg. Knees commonly impact with the dashboard. This may range from the simple contusion noted about the patella to the severe compound fracture of the patella. Frank dislocation of the knees can occur. In addition, this kinetic energy may be transmitted proximally and result in fracture of the femur or fractured/dislocated hip. On occasion the pelvis can impact with the dash, resulting in acetabulum fractures as well as pelvic fractures. These injuries are associated with hemorrhage that may lead to shock. Maintain a high index of suspicion and always palpate the femurs as well as gently rocking the pelvis and palpating the symphysis pubis.

Miscellaneous weapons involved in MVCs typically include unrestrained objects in the vehicle such as luggage, groceries, books, and most important, passengers. These objects may become deadly missiles in a rapid forward decelerating type of event.

T-BONE OR LATERAL-IMPACT COLLISION

The mechanism of the T-bone collision is similar to that of the head-on collision, with the addition of lateral energy displacement (see Figure 1-5). Using the three-collision concept, look for the presence of the following:

> Machine collision: primary deformity of the car, check the impact side (driver/passenger)
>
> Body collision: degree of door deformity (e.g., arm rest bent, outward or inward bowing of door)
>
> Organ collision: includes multiple possibilities

The most common injuries to look for are

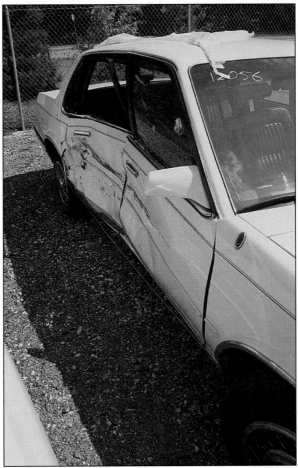

Figure 1-5 *Lateral-impact collision. Most injuries inflicted by: intrusion of door, arm rests, side window, or door post.*

Head: coup/contracoup due to lateral displacement

Neck: lateral displacement injuries range from cervical muscle strain to subluxation with neurological deficit

Upper arm and shoulder injuries on the side of the impact

Thorax/abdomen: injury due to direct force either from inward bowing of door on the side of the impact or unrestrained passenger being propelled across seat

Pelvis/legs: occupants on the side of the impact are likely to have pelvic, hip, or femur fractures

Injuries of the thorax vary from soft tissue to flail chest, lung contusion, pneumothorax, or hemothorax. Abdominal injuries include those of solid or hollow organs. Pelvic injuries may include fracture/dislocation, bladder rupture, and urethral injuries. Shoulder girdle or lower-extremity injuries are common, depending on the level of the impacting force.

REAR-IMPACT COLLISION

In the most common form of rear-impact collision, a stationary car is struck from the rear by another moving vehicle (see Figure 1-6). Also, a slower-moving car may be impacted from the rear by a faster-moving car. The sudden increase in acceleration produces posterior displacement of the occupants and possible hyperextension of the cervical spine if the headrest is not properly adjusted. There may also be rapid forward deceleration if the car suddenly strikes something in the front or if the driver applies the brakes suddenly. You should note deformity of the auto anterior and posterior as well as interior deformity and headrest position. The potential for C-spine injuries is great. Also be alert for associated deceleration injuries.

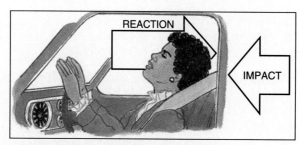

Figure 1-6 *Mechanism of neck injury in rear-impact collision.*

ROLLOVER COLLISION

During a vehicle rollover, the body may be impacted from any direction; thus the potential for injuries is great (see Figure 1-7). The chance for axial loading injuries of the spine is increased in this form of MVA. Rescuers must be alert for clues that imply that the car turned over (e.g., roof dents, scratches, debris, and deformity of roof posts). There are more lethal injuries in this form of accident because there is a greater likelihood of occupants being ejected. Occupants ejected from the car are 25 times as likely to be killed.

OCCUPANT RESTRAINT SYSTEMS

Restrained occupants are much more likely to survive because they are protected from much of the impact inside the auto and are restrained from being ejected from the auto. These occupants are, however, still susceptible to certain injuries. The lap belt is intended to go across the pelvis (iliac crests), not the abdomen. If the belt is in place and the victim is subjected to a frontal deceleration crash, his body tends to

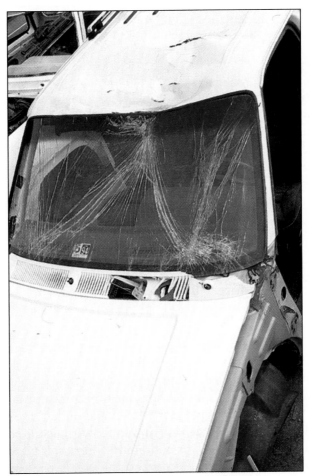

Figure 1-7 Rollover collision.
High potential for injury
Many mechanisms involved here
Victims frequently ejected if not restrained

fold together like a "clasp-knife" (see Figure 1-8). The head may be thrown forward into the steering wheel or dashboard. Facial, head, or neck injuries are common. Abdominal injuries occur if the lap belt is positioned improperly. The compression forces that are produced when a body is suddenly folded about the waist may injure the abdomen or the lumbar spine.

The three-point restraint or cross-chest lap belt (see Figure 1-9) secures the body much better than does a lap belt alone. The chest and pelvis are restrained, so life-threatening injuries are much less common. The head is not restrained, and therefore the neck is still subjected to stresses that may cause fractures, dislocations, or spinal cord injuries. Clavicular fractures (where the chest strap crosses) are common. Internal organ damage may still occur due to organ movement inside the body.

Like belt restraints, air bags (passive restraints) will reduce injuries in victims of MVCs in *most* but not all situations. Air bags are designed to inflate from the center of the steering wheel and the dashboard to protect the front-seat occupants in case of a frontal deceleration accident. If these function properly, they cushion

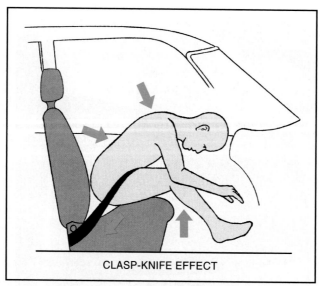

Figure 1-8 *Clasp-knife effect.*

the head and chest at the instant of impact. This is very effective in decreasing injury to the face, neck, and chest. You should still immobilize the neck until it has been adequately examined. Air bags deflate immediately, so they protect against only one impact. The driver whose car hits more than one object is unprotected after the initial collision. Air bags also do not prevent "down and under" movement, so drivers who are extended (tall drivers and drivers of small low-slung autos) may still impact with their legs and suffer leg, pelvis, or abdominal injuries. It is important for occupants to wear chest and lap belts even when the car is equipped with air bags. Research has recently shown that some drivers who appear uninjured after deceler-

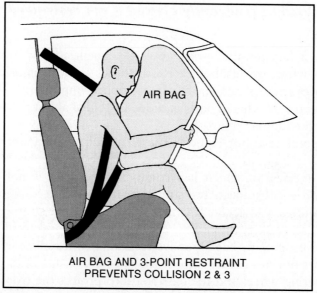

Figure 1-9 *Air bag and three-point restraint.*

ation accidents have been found to have serious internal injuries. A clue to which driver may have internal injuries is the condition of the steering wheel. A deformed steering wheel is just as important a clue in an auto equipped with an air bag as in those who are not. This clue may be missed because the deflated air bag covers the steering wheel. Thus a quick "lift and look" under the air bag should be a part of the routine examination of the steering wheel.

In summary, when at the scene of an MVC, you must note the type of collision and the clues that imply that high kinetic energy has been spent (e.g., deformities of the vehicle). Maintain a high index of suspicion for occult injuries and thus keep scene time to a minimum. These observations and clues are essential to quality patient care and must be relayed to medical direction and the receiving physician.

TRACTOR ACCIDENTS

Another large motorized vehicle with which you must be familiar is the tractor. The National Safety Council reports that one-third of all farm accident fatalities involve tractors. There are basically two types of tractors: the two-wheel drive and the four-wheel drive. In both the center of gravity is high, and thus the tractors are easily turned over (see Figure 1-10). The majority of fatal accidents are due to the tractor turning over and crushing the driver. Most overturns (85%) are to the side; these are less likely to pin the driver because he or she has a chance to jump or be thrown clear. Rear overturns, although less frequent, are more likely to entrap and crush the driver because there is almost no opportunity to jump free. The primary mechanism is the crush injury, and the severity depends on the part of the anatomy that is involved. Additional mechanisms are chemical burns from gasoline, diesel fuel, hydraulic fluid, or even battery acid. Thermal burns from hot engine parts or ignited fuel are also common.

Management consists of scene stabilization followed quickly by the primary survey and resuscitation. The following checklist is used in scene stabilization:

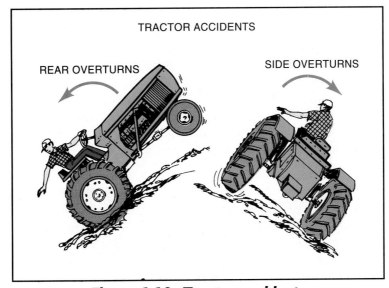

Figure 1-10 *Tractor accidents.*

1. Engine off
2. Rear wheels locked
3. Fuel situation and fire hazard addressed

While you are surveying the victim, other rescuers must stabilize the tractor. The center of gravity must be identified before any attempt is made to lift the tractor. The center of gravity of the two-wheel-drive tractor is located approximately 10 inches above and 24 inches in front of the rear axle. The center of gravity of a four-wheel-drive tractor is closer to the midline of the machine. Because tractors usually overturn on soft ground and their centers of gravity are tricky to determine, great care must be taken during lifting to avoid a second crush injury. Because of the weight of the tractor and the length of time (usually prolonged) pinned, anticipate serious injuries. Often, the patient will go into profound shock as the compressing weight of the tractor is removed—similar to what happens when anti-shock trousers are suddenly deflated. Rapid, safe management of tractor accidents requires special exercises in lifting heavy machinery as well as good trauma management.

SMALL-VEHICLE CRASHES

Other small vehicles that fall into the motion injury category include the motorcycle, all-terrain vehicle, and the snowmobile. The operators of these machines are not encased within them, and, of course, there are no restraining devices. When the operator is subjected to the classic head-on, lateral-impact, rear-end, or rollover collisions, his or her only form of protection is

1. Evasive maneuvering
2. Helmet usage
3. Protective clothing (e.g., leather clothes, helmet, boots)
4. Use of the vehicle to absorb kinetic energy (e.g., bike slide)

MOTORCYCLES: It is extremely important for motorcycle riders to wear helmets. Helmets help prevent head injury (which causes 75% of motorcycle deaths). However, helmets give no protection to the spine. The operator of a motorcycle involved in a crash is much like an ejected automobile occupant. Injuries depend on the part of the anatomy subjected to kinetic energy. Because of the lack of protective encasement, there is a higher frequency of head, neck, and extremity injuries. Important clues include deformity of the motorcycle, distance of skid, and deformity of stationary objects or cars. Again, a high degree of suspicion, appreciation of environmental clues (skid marks, vehicle deformity), identification of "load and go," and strict basic trauma life support (BTLS) protocols constitute the optimal standard of prehospital care.

ALL-TERRAIN VEHICLES: The ATV is one of the newer additions to the arsenal of trauma weapons. The ATV was designed as a vehicle to traverse rough terrain, used initially by ranchers, hunters, and farmers. Unfortunately, some people view the ATV as a fast toy. Careless misuse has resulted in an ever-increasing morbidity and mortality from accidents—sadly, frequently among the very young (see

Figure 1-11). The two basic designs are either three-wheeled or four-wheeled. The four-wheel design affords reasonable stability and handling, but the three-wheeled ATV has a high center of gravity and is very prone to rollover when turned sharply. The three most common mechanisms are

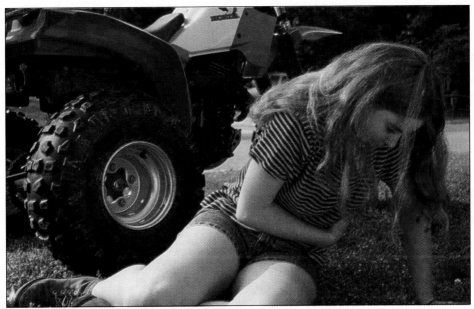

Figure 1-11 ATVs—not for children.

1. Vehicle rollover
2. Fall-off of rider or passenger
3. Forward deceleration of rider from vehicle impact with stationary object

The injuries produced depend upon the mechanism and the part of the anatomy that is impacted. The most frequent injuries are fractures, about half of which are above and half below the diaphragm. The major bony injuries involve the clavicles, sternum, and ribs. Be very suspicious for head or spinal injury.

SNOWMOBILES: Snowmobiles are used both as recreational and utility vehicles. The snowmobile has a low clearance and a low center of gravity. The injuries common to this vehicle are very similar to those that occur with the ATV. Turnovers are somewhat more common, and since the vehicle is usually heavier than the ATV, crush injuries are seen more frequently. Again, the injury pattern depends on the part of the anatomy that is directly involved. Be alert for possible co-existing hypothermia. A common injury with the snowmobile is the "hangman" or "clothes line" injury that results from running under wire fences. Be alert for occult cervical spine injuries and potential airway compromise.

PEDESTRIAN INJURIES: The pedestrian struck by a car almost always suffers severe internal injuries as well as fractures. This is true even if the vehicle is traveling at low speed. The mass of the auto is so large that high speed is not necessary to impart high-energy transfer. When high speed is involved the results are disastrous. There are two mechanisms of injury. The first is when the bumper of the auto strikes the body, and the second is when the body, accelerated by the transfer of forces strikes the ground or some other object. An adult usually has bilateral lower leg or knee fractures plus whatever secondary injuries occur when the body strikes the hood of the car and then later the ground. Children are shorter so the bumper is more likely to hit them in the pelvis or torso. They usually land on their heads in the secondary impact. When answering a call to an auto-pedestrian accident, be prepared for broken bones, internal injuries, and head injuries.

RAPID VERTICAL DECELERATION

The mechanism for falls is vertical deceleration. The types of injuries sustained depend upon three factors that you must identify and relay to medical direction. These factors are

1. Distance of fall

2. Anatomical area impacted

3. Surface struck

The primary groups involved in vertical falls are adults and children under the age of 5. In children, the falls most commonly involve males and occur mostly in the summer months in urban high-rise multiple-occupant dwellings. Predisposing factors include poor supervision, defective railings, and the curiosity associated with that age group. Head injuries are common in falls by children because the head is the heaviest part of the body and thus impacts first. Adult falls are generally occupational or due to the influence of alcohol or drugs. It is not uncommon for falls to occur during attempts to escape from fire or criminal activity. Generally, adults attempt to land on their feet; thus their falls are more controlled. In this landing form, the victim usually impacts initially on the feet and then falls backwards landing on the buttocks and outstretched hands. Classically, this "Lover's Leap" fall may result in the following potential injuries (see Figure 1-12.):

1. Fractures of the feet or legs

2. Hip injuries/pelvic injury

3. Axial loading to the lumbar and cervical spine

4. Vertical deceleration forces to the organs

5. Colles' fractures of the wrists

The greater the height, the greater the potential for injury. However, do not be deceived into believing that there is little risk for serious injury in a short-distance fall.

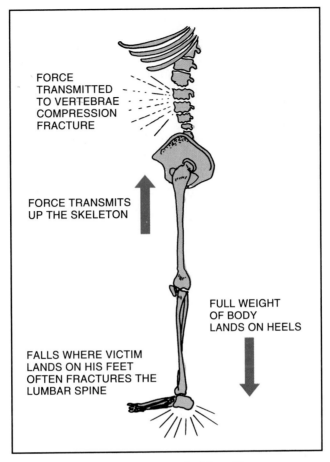

FORCE
TRANSMITTED
TO VERTEBRAE
COMPRESSION
FRACTURE

FORCE TRANSMITS
UP THE SKELETON

FULL WEIGHT
OF BODY
LANDS ON HEELS

FALLS WHERE VICTIM
LANDS ON HIS FEET
OFTEN FRACTURES THE
LUMBAR SPINE

Figure 1-12 *Axial loading.*

Surface density (concrete versus sawdust) and irregularity (gym floor versus staircase) also influence the potential for severity of injury. Relay information about distance fallen and surface struck to medical direction with other pertinent information.

PROJECTILE PENETRATION

Numerous objects are capable of producing penetration injuries. These range from the industrial saw blade that breaks off at an extremely high rpm rate to the foreign body hurled by a lawn mower. Most of such hurled objects are capable of penetrating the thorax or abdomen. However, the more common forms of penetrating wounds in the American society come from the knife and gun.

Knife wound severity depends on the anatomical area penetrated, blade length, and angle of penetration (see Figure 1-13). Remember, an upper abdominal stab wound may cause intrathoracic organ injury and stab wounds below the fourth intercostal space may have penetrated the abdomen. The golden rule with knife wounds that still have the blade inside is: Do not remove the knife.

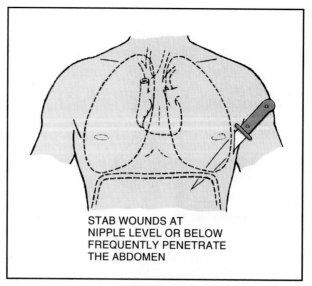

STAB WOUNDS AT
NIPPLE LEVEL OR BELOW
FREQUENTLY PENETRATE
THE ABDOMEN

Figure 1-13 *Stab wounds.*

Most penetration wounds inflicted by firearms are due to handguns, rifles, and shotguns. Important factors to obtain, if possible, is the type of weapon, caliber, and distance from which the weapon was fired.

USEFUL BALLISTIC INFORMATION

Caliber: the internal diameter of the barrel, and this corresponds to the ammunition used for the particular weapon.

Rifling: a series of spiral grooves in the interior surface of the barrel of some weapons. Rifling imparts a stabilizing spin to the missile.

Ammunition: case, primer, powder, and slug.

Bullet construction: usually solid lead alloy and may have a full or partial copper or steel jacket. The shape may be rounded, flat, conical, or pointed. The bullet nose may be soft or hollow (for expansion or fragmentation).

WOUND BALLISTICS

Because the kinetic energy (kinetic energy = 1/2 mass × velocity^2) produced by a projectile is mostly dependent upon velocity, weapons are classified as high or low velocity. Weapons with velocities less than 2,000 ft/sec are considered low velocity and include essentially all handguns and some rifles. Injuries from these weapons are much less destructive than from those that fire missiles that exceed that velocity. Low-velocity weapons are certainly capable of lethal injuries, depending on the body area struck. All wounds inflicted by high-velocity weapons carry the additional factor of hydrostatic pressure. This factor alone can increase the injury.

Factors that contribute to tissue damage include

1. *Missile size.* The larger the bullet, the more resistance and the larger the permanent tract.

2. *Missile deformity.* Hollow point and soft nose flatten out on impact, resulting in a larger surface area involved.

3. *Semijacket.* The jacket expands and adds to surface area.

4. *Tumbling.* Tumbling of the missile causes a wider path of destruction.

5. *Yaw.* The missile can oscillate vertically and horizontally about its axis, resulting in a larger surface area presenting to the tissue.

The wounds consist of three parts:

1. *Entry wound.*

2. *Exit wound.* Not all entry wounds will have exit wounds, and on occasion there may be multiple exits due to fragmentation of bone and missile; generally, the exit wound is larger and has ragged edges (see Figure 1-14).

3. *Internal wound.* Low-velocity projectiles inflict damage primarily by damaging tissue that the missile contacts; high-velocity projectiles inflict damage by tissue contact and transfer of kinetic energy to surrounding tissues (see Figure 1-15). Damage is related to

   a. Shock waves

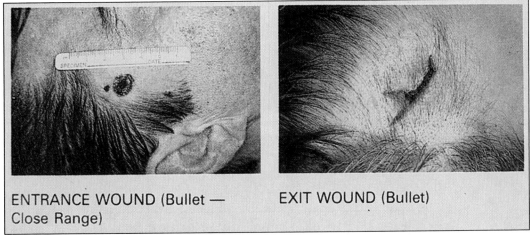

ENTRANCE WOUND (Bullet — Close Range)   EXIT WOUND (Bullet)

Figure 1-14 *Comparison of entrance and exit wounds.*

b. Temporary cavity, which is 30 to 40 times the bullet's diameter and creates immense tissue pressures

c. Pulsation of the temporary cavity, which creates pressure changes in the adjacent tissue.

Generally damage done is proportional to tissue density. Highly dense organs such as bone, muscle, and liver sustain more damage than less dense organs such as lungs. A key factor to remember is that once a bullet enters a body, its trajectory will not always be in a straight line. Any patient with a missile penetration of the head, thorax, or abdomen should be transported immediately. Personnel who have been shot while wearing a flak vest should be managed with caution; be alert for possible cardiac and other organ contusion.

In shotgun wounds, injury is determined by kinetic energy at impact that is influenced by

1. Powder

2. Size of pellets

3. Choke of muzzle

4. Distance to target

Velocity and kinetic energy dissipates rapidly as distance is traveled. At 40 yards the velocity is one-half the initial muzzle velocity.

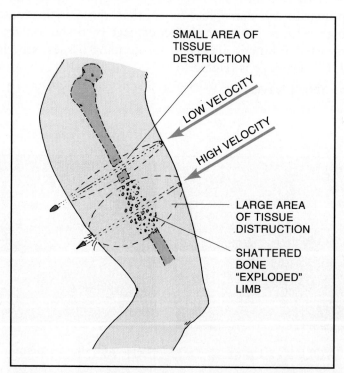

Figure 1-15 *High- versus low-velocity injury.*

BLAST INJURIES

Blast injuries in this country occur primarily in industrial settings such as grain elevator and gas fume explosions. However, as threat of terrorist activity can no longer be considered remote, blast injury management must be added to BTLS training and knowledge.

The mechanism of injury by blast/explosion is due to three factors:

1. Primary: initial air blast
2. Secondary: victim being struck by material propelled by the blast force
3. Tertiary: body being thrown and impacting on ground or other object

Injuries due to the primary air blast are almost exclusive to the air-containing organs. Auditory system usually involves ruptured tympanic membranes. Lung injuries may include pneumothorax, parenchymal hemorrhage, and especially, alveolar rupture. Alveolar rupture may cause air embolus that may be manifested by bizarre central nervous system symptoms. Gastrointestinal tract injuries may vary

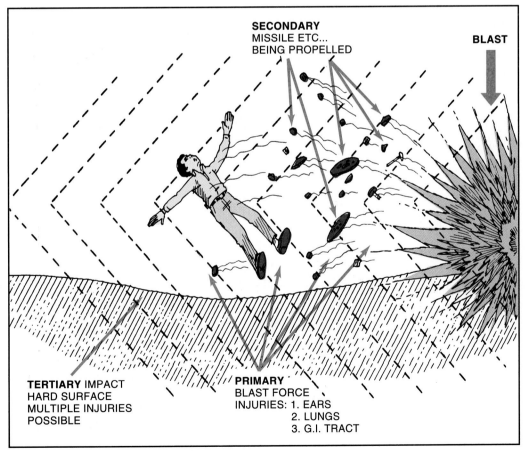

Figure 1-16 *Blast injury.*

from mild intestinal and stomach contusions to frank rupture (see Figure 1-16). Always suspect lung injuries in a blast victim.

Injuries sustained by the secondary factors are similar to those previously discussed, and tertiary injuries are much the same as to be expected from being ejected from an automobile.

SUMMARY

You must identify the mechanism of injury and consider it as part of the overall management of the trauma patient. What happened? What type of energy was applied? How much energy was transmitted? What part of the body was affected? If there is an MVC, you must consider the form of the crash as well as survey the vehicle's interior and exterior for damage. Tractor accidents require careful stabilization of the machine to prevent a second injury to the patient. Falls require identification of distance fallen, surface struck, and position of the patient upon impact. Stab wounds require a knowledge of the length of the instrument as well as the angle in which it entered the body. When evaluating a shooting victim you need to know the weapon, caliber, and distance from which fired. This information regarding the high-energy event (e.g., falls, vehicle damage) is also important to the emergency physician. Be sure to not only record your findings but also give a verbal report to the ED (Emergency Department) physician or trauma surgeon when you arrive. With this knowledge and a high index of suspicion, you can give your patient the greatest chance of survival.

BIBLIOGRAPHY

1. Greenberg, M. I. "Falls from Heights," *Journal of the American College of Emergency Physicians Emergency Procedures*, Vol. 7 (August 1978), pp. 300–301.

2. Huekle, D. F., and J. W. Melvin. "Anatomy, Injury, Frequency, Bio-mechanical Human Tolerance," Society of Automotive Engineers, Technical paper No. 80098, February 1980.

3. McSwain, N. E., Jr. "Kinematics of Penetrating Trauma," *Journal of Pre-Hospital Care*, Vol. 1 (October 1984), pp. 10–13.

4. McSwain, N. E., Jr., *Pre-Hospital Trauma Life Support*, 2nd ed., pp. 1–40. Akron, OH: Emergency Training, 1990.

5. National Highway Traffic Safety Administration. *Occupant Protection Facts.* Washington, D.C.: National Center for Statistics and Analysis, U.S. Department of Transportation, June 1989.

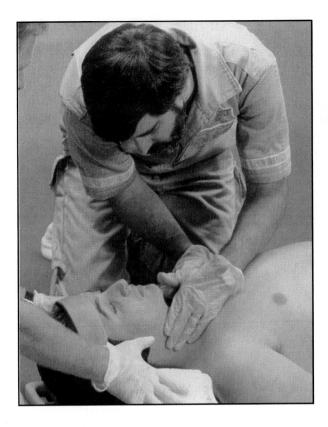

Assessment and Initial Management of the Trauma Patient

John E. Campbell, M.D., and Walt Alan Stoy, Ph.D., EMT-P

OBJECTIVES

At the conclusion of this chapter you should be able to:

1. State the purpose of each stage of an ambulance call.
2. Explain preliminary actions that should be performed prior to approaching a patient.
3. Recite the assessment priorities.
4. Describe when the primary trauma survey can be interrupted.
5. Describe when critical interventions should be made and where to make them.
6. Identify which patients have critical conditions and how they should be managed.
7. Recite the critical information needed for both primary and secondary trauma surveys.

It is heartbreaking to see a life lost, especially if that loss occurs due to treatment that is instituted too little or too late. For the severely injured patient, time is of the essence. The direct relationship between the timing of definitive (surgical) treatment and the survival of trauma patients was first described by Dr. R. Adams Cowley of the famous Shock-Trauma Unit in Baltimore, Maryland. He discovered that when seriously injured patients were able to gain access to the operating room within an hour of the time of injury, the highest survival rate was achieved (approximately 85%). He referred to this as the "golden hour."

You are trading minutes of the "golden hour" for every action done before the patient arrives in the operating room. This means that every action must have a life-saving purpose. Not only must you reduce evaluation and resuscitation to the most efficient and critical steps, but you must also develop the habit of assessing and treating every trauma patient in a planned logical and sequential manner. To accomplish these objectives, keep the following concepts in mind when approaching patients who are injured:

1. Trauma patients are not "treated" in the field. They are treated in the emergency department or operating room. Only critical interventions are made in the field.

2. Most preventable trauma fatalities are due to the patient not arriving in the operating room soon enough to be saved. Thus trauma care requires making the most efficient use of time and seeing that the patient is transported to the *appropriate* hospital as soon as possible.

As the first person to treat the patient, you are a critical member of the emergency medical service (EMS) system. The trauma victim's fate depends on the speed, judgment, and skill of your actions.

The "golden hour" begins when the victim is injured, *not* when EMS arrives at the scene. The minutes lost before EMS arrives are just as important as minutes lost because of disorganized actions at the scene. It is of utmost importance to manage every minute of the rescue process quickly and efficiently, beginning with the ambulance call. Yet, rapid management does not mean simply racing down the highway at breakneck speed, throwing the patient into the back of the ambulance, and racing to the nearest emergency department. You can best maximize the patient's chance of survival by properly performing specific duties during the six stages of an ambulance call (see Figure 2-1).

These six stages of an ambulance call are as follows:

1. PREDISPATCH: This is the first—and, unfortunately, the most ignored—stage of prehospital care. You can't provide life-saving care if you can't find the accident, if you don't know the shortest route, or if the ambulance or rescue vehicle is not ready to respond. Prior to responding to the field, you and your fellow providers must be well aware of your service area so that you can select the fastest, safest possible route to the scene. An alternate route should be known in case traffic conditions, weather, or other events make it unsuitable to travel the shortest route. Fast driving never makes up for lack of skills in map reading. Between runs you should be preparing the vehicle and essential equipment for the next call.

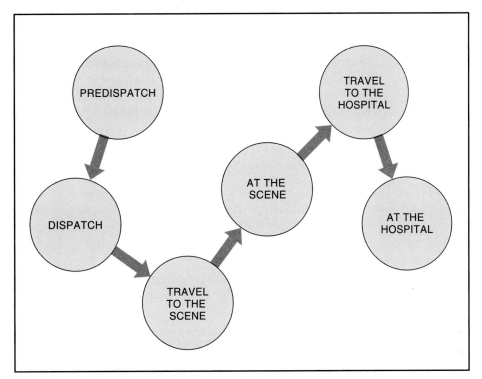

Figure 2-1 *Six stages of an ambulance call.*

2. DISPATCH: The rescue crew must have the proper information to rapidly respond to a call:

1. *The exact nature of the call:* Details as to what has happened. How many victims or potential victims? Are there dangers at the scene? Will special equipment be needed?

2. *The exact location of the call:* This cannot be overemphasized. If an exact address cannot be given, get directions that are as precise as possible.

3. *A call-back number:* This can be invaluable if you have trouble locating the scene of the accident. Units equipped with radio telephone switch station (RTSS) or cellular telephone can call directly to the scene while they are responding.

3. TRAVEL TO THE SCENE: A rapid yet careful response using good judgment concerning the fastest route should be the hallmark of the response to the scene. If needed, obtain further information from the dispatcher (or from a call-back to the scene) so while en route decisions about backup help and equipment can be made.

4. ACTIONS AT THE SCENE: Keeping scene safety in mind, quickly assess the overall situation upon arrival. Evaluate, resuscitate, and package the patient using the BTLS patient assessment priorities. The focus of the BTLS course is on this stage of the ambulance call.

5. TRAVEL TO THE HOSPITAL: Select the most suitable route and hospital according to your local protocols. The most experienced provider should remain at the patient's side and provide interventions and continuous monitoring. Notify Medical Direction if the patient's condition deteriorates during transport, and notify the receiving facility of the estimated time of arrival and any special needs. It is important to report to Medical Direction as early as possible. Frequently, critical members of the trauma team (surgeons, operating room crew, etc.) must be called to the hospital. Minutes lost waiting on the proper physician to arrive can be just as fatal as minutes lost waiting on the prehospital provider to arrive.

6. ACTIONS AT THE HOSPITAL: You should continue care until the emergency department staff assumes responsibility for the patient; *never leave a patient unattended.* Report pertinent information about the patient to the nurse or physician in charge. This should include a description of the scene, mechanisms of injuries, observed and suspected injuries, procedures performed, and changes in condition. Remain as long as needed. When no longer required for patient care, complete the written report (see Appendix C) and immediately prepare the vehicle for return to service.

TRAUMA ASSESSMENT

On-scene trauma assessment begins with certain actions before approaching the patient. Failure to perform preliminary actions may jeopardize your life as well as the patient.

PRELIMINARY ACTIONS AT THE SCENE

SCENE SURVEY

1. Assess the scene for hazards. Is the ambulance or rescue vehicle parked in the nearest safe place? Is it safe to approach the patient? If the scene is not safe, make it safe or do not enter! Does the patient require immediate movement because of hazards? Do not endanger yourself by acting rashly—think before you act! Is special equipment needed (turnout gear, breathing equipment) to approach the patient?

2. Note the number of patients.

   a. If there is more than one patient, call for more ambulances now. Usually one ambulance is needed for each seriously injured patient. If there are many patients, notify Medical Direction to initiate the disaster protocol. Remember, if there are multiple patients, change gloves between patients.

   b. Are all patients accounted for? If the patient(s) is unconscious, and there are no witnesses of the incident, look for clues (school books or diaper bag, passenger list in commercial vehicles) that other patients might be present. Carefully evaluate the scene for other patients. This is especially important at night or if there is poor visibility.

3. Note the mechanism of injury.

4. Does the patient require extrication? Is special extrication equipment needed?

ESSENTIAL EQUIPMENT: If possible, carry all essential medical equipment to the scene. This prevents loss of time returning to the vehicle. The following equipment is always needed for trauma patients:

1. Long backboard with attached head immobilization device

2. Cervical immobilization device

3. Oxygen and airway equipment (suction should be included with this)

4. Trauma box (bandage material, blood pressure cuff, stethoscope)

5. Personal protection equipment (glasses or face shield, rubber gloves—strongly consider use of gown and mask)

PATIENT ASSESSMENT AND MANAGEMENT PRIORITIES

Begin evaluation of the most seriously injured victim first—unless you have multiple casualties, in which case use multiple casualty incident (MCI) protocols. Be rapid but careful and gentle. Rough handling aggravates injuries. To make the most efficient use of time, prehospital patient assessment and management are divided into four steps, and each step contains certain priorities. These priorities are the foundation on which trauma care is built.

PRIMARY TRAUMA SURVEY: This is a rapid assessment to determine life-threatening conditions. The information gathered here is used to make decisions about critical interventions and time of transport. This assessment should be completed in 2 minutes or less and is so important that nothing is allowed to interrupt it except airway obstruction or cardiac arrest. Respiratory distress (other than airway obstruction) is not an indication to interrupt the primary survey because the cause of respiratory distress is frequently found during examination of the chest. Major bleeding should also be controlled at this time.

Assessment priorities you need to remember when conducting the primary survey are:

1. Total overview of the patient situation while approaching the patient

2. Evaluation of *airway*, C-spine control, and initial level of consciousness (LOC)

3. Evaluation of *breathing*

4. Evaluation of *circulation*

5. Brief examination of *abdomen, pelvis,* and *extremities*

CRITICAL INTERVENTIONS AND TRANSPORT DECISION: Upon completion of the primary survey, enough information is available to decide if a critical situation is present. *Patients with critical trauma situations are transported immediately.*

Most treatment will be done during transport. Certain interventions should be done on the scene (attempt removal of airway obstruction, stop major bleeding, seal sucking chest wounds, hyperventilate, etc.), but most treatment should wait until the patient is in the ambulance and transport has begun. *The minutes of the patient's "golden hour" must be used wisely—the critical patient often has none to spare!*

SECONDARY TRAUMA SURVEY: The secondary survey is a rapid, detailed evaluation to pick up all injuries, both obvious and potential. This assessment also establishes the baseline from which many treatment decisions will eventually be made. It is important to record the information discovered in this assessment. Critical patients should always have this assessment done during transport. If the primary survey has revealed no critical condition, this assessment may be performed on the scene. Even though the patient appears to be stable, the on-scene secondary survey should be kept to under 5 minutes, if possible.

    Assessment priorities for the secondary trauma survey are:

1. Vital signs
2. History of the patient and trauma event
3. Head-to-toes exam (including neurological)
4. Further bandaging and splinting
5. Continual monitoring

CRITICAL CARE AND REASSESSMENT: This includes the critical procedures performed on scene and during transport, the reassessment survey, and also communication with medical direction. The reassessment survey is an abbreviated exam to assess changes in the patient's condition.

    Assessment priorities for the reassessment survey are:

1. Level of consciousness
2. Airway exam
3. Breathing
4. Pulse, blood pressure, skin color/temperature
5. Abdomen exam
6. Focused assessment of injuries
7. Check of interventions

PATIENT ASSESSMENT USING THE PRIORITY PLAN

PRIMARY SURVEY

Once you determine that the patient may be safely approached, the assessment should proceed quickly (in fewer than 2 minutes) and smoothly. Remember, nothing interrupts the primary survey except treatment of airway obstruction or cardiac arrest. Unless delayed by extrication, total on-scene time should be under 10 minutes. For critical patients, the goal should be to have on-scene times of 5 minutes or less.

TOTAL OVERVIEW OF THE PATIENT SITUATION WHILE APPROACH-ING THE PATIENT: You should be evaluating your patient's situation even before you arrive at his side. Is the patient alert or in obvious distress? Does the patient have obvious major injuries? This initial appearance as you approach can give you a sense of the urgency of the situation, but no matter how gruesome the situation may appear; do not vary how you perform the primary survey. If you skip steps, you will miss injuries.

EVALUATE AIRWAY, C-SPINE CONTROL, INITIAL LEVEL OF CON-SCIOUSNESS: Assessment begins immediately, even if the patient is being extricated. Extrication should not interfere with patient care. The team leader should approach the patient from the front (face to face—so he does not turn his head to see you). A second rescuer immediately, gently, but firmly, stabilizes the neck in a neutral position. The team leader may need to initially stabilize the neck if there is not a second rescuer immediately available. The rescuer stabilizing the neck must not release the neck until he or she is relieved or a suitable stabilization device is applied. The team leader should say to the patient, "We are here to help you. What happened?" The patient's reply gives immediate information about both the airway and the level of consciousness. If the patient responds appropriately to questioning, you can assume that the airway is open and the level of consciousness is normal. If the patient cannot speak or is unconscious, further evaluation of the airway should follow. Look, listen, and feel for movement of air. Open the mouth and clear the airway if necessary. If the airway is obstructed, use an appropriate method to open it *before finishing the primary survey* (see Figure 2-2). Because of the ever-present danger of spinal injury, *never* extend the neck to open the airway of a trauma patient. Patients with airway difficulty or decreased level of consciousness (LOC) are in the "load-and-go" category. All patients with decreased LOC should be hyperventilated (24 per minute) if the patient will allow this to be done. The rescuer at the patient's head may use his knees to maintain immobilization of the patient's neck, freeing his hands to apply oxygen or use a bag-valve-mask to assist ventilation (see Figure 2-3). This is yet another reason that all equipment should be within immediate reach. When assisting or providing ventilation, be sure that the patient not only gets an adequate ventilatory rate, but also an adequate volume. *All* patients that have multisystem trauma should receive supplemental high-flow oxygen.

ASSESS BREATHING AND CIRCULATION: You can assess breathing and circulation at the same time. To do this, place your hand on the patient's neck to palpate the pulse while at the same time placing the other hand on the patient's chest to count respirations. You can gain much information when you perform this examination correctly. (Remember if the patient is not breathing, immediately deliver two full breaths and then check for a carotid pulse. If there is no pulse, begin cardiopulmonary resuscitation). After the neck has been immobilized and (if necessary) the airway opened with a modified jaw thrust, proceed with the evaluation of breathing and circulation in the following manner.

1. Place your ear over the patient's mouth so you can judge both the rate and quality of breathing. Is breathing too fast (more than 24 per minute) or too slow (fewer than 8 per minute)? Is the patient moving an adequate volume of air when breathing? Use the look, listen, and feel technique. Look at the movement of the chest

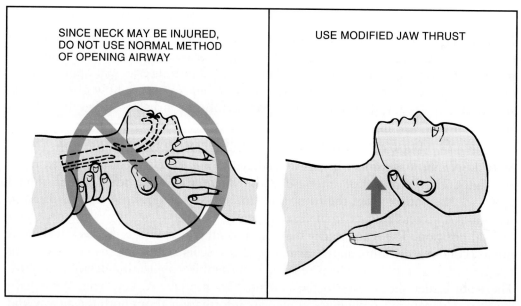

SINCE NECK MAY BE INJURED, DO NOT USE NORMAL METHOD OF OPENING AIRWAY

USE MODIFIED JAW THRUST

Figure 2-2 *Opening the airway using the modified jaw thrust. Maintain in-line stabilization while pushing up on the angles of the jaw with your thumbs.*

(or abdomen), listen to the sound of the air movement, and feel both the movement of air on your cheek and the movement of the chest wall with your hand. Any abnormality of breathing signals the need to search for the cause as well as administration of oxy-

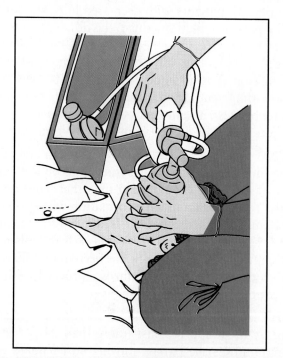

Figure 2-3 *Using your knees to maintain immobilization of the neck will free your hands to assist ventilation.*

NORMAL	ABNORMAL
ADULT	ADULT
12–20	<8 AND> 24
SMALL CHILD	SMALL CHILD
15–30	<10 AND> 35
INFANT	INFANT
25–50	<25 AND> 60

Table 2-1 *Normal and Abnormal Respiratory Rates*

gen and possibly breathing assistance (see Table 2-1). The rescuer at the head can apply the non-rebreather oxygen mask or bag-valve device (while stabilizing the neck with his knees) without interrupting your survey.

2. As soon as you have assessed the rate and quality of respiration, note the rate and quality of the carotid pulse and compare with your evaluation of the radial pulse (brachial in small child). Move next to evaluation of skin color/temperature. This information, combined with LOC, is the best early assessment of circulatory status and the presence of shock. The following generalizations about blood pressure have not been scientifically proven but from experience appear to be about right. If the pulse is present at the neck and the wrist, the blood pressure is greater than 80 mm Hg (it may be normal; judge by the strength of the pulse—it is not yet time to use the blood pressure cuff). If the pulse is present at the neck but not at the wrist, the blood pressure is between 60 and 80 mm Hg. This suggests late shock. Even if the pulse is present and strong at the neck and wrist, you may be able to diagnose early shock by other signs. Other signs of shock include rapid heart rate (more than 100 per minute), cold sweaty skin, pale appearance, confusion, weakness, or thirst. Remember, the patient with spinal shock may not be pale, cold, or sweaty and will not have a rapid pulse. The spinal shock patient will have a low blood pressure and paralysis.

3. Following assessment of the breathing and pulse, quickly assess (look and feel) the neck for injury (discoloration, swelling, or subcutaneous emphysema) to see if the neck veins are flat or distended and the trachea is in the midline. You may apply a rigid extrication collar at this time. *Note:* If the team leader elected to stabilize the neck, this duty should be transferred to another rescuer at this time.

4. Now look, feel, and listen to the chest. If there is any difficulty with respiration, the chest must be bared for examination. Look for deformity, contusions, abrasions, penetrations, paradoxical movement, burns, lacerations, and swelling (DCAPP-BLS). Feel for tenderness, instability, and crepitation (TIC). Note if the ribs rise with respiration or if there is only diaphragmatic breathing. Now listen to see if breath sounds are present and equal bilaterally. Listen with the stethoscope over the lateral chest about the fourth interspace in the midaxillary

line on one side, then immediately compare with the other side. An alternative is to listen to the anterior chest about the second interspace on both sides. The important determination is whether breath sounds are present and equal on both sides. If breath sounds are not equal (decreased or absent on one side), you should percuss the chest to determine if a tension pneumothorax or a hemothorax is present. If abnormalities are found during the chest exam (open chest wound, flail chest, respiratory difficulty), make the appropriate intervention (seal open wound, hand stabilize flail, give oxygen, assist ventilation).

EXAMINE ABDOMEN, PELVIS, AND EXTREMITIES:

1. Rapidly expose and look at the abdomen (distension, contusions, abrasions, penetrations), and gently palpate all four quadrants of the abdomen for tenderness.

2. Quickly check the pelvis. Look for deformity, contusions, abrasions, penetrations, burns, lacerations, and swelling (DCAP-BLS). Feel for tenderness, instability, and crepitation by pressing down on the symphysis and squeezing in on the iliac crests.

3. Assess both legs and then both arms looking for DCAP-BLS. Feel for TIC and for pulse, motor function, and sensation (PMS).

4. Stop active bleeding. If you have a three-rescuer team, rescuer 3 should have already done this, or at least begun to do this. Most bleeding can be stopped by direct pressure; use gauze pads and bandage or elastic wraps. Air splints or the pneumatic antishock garment (PASG) may be used to tamponade bleeding. Tourniquets may be needed in rare situations. In the past it has been taught that blood-soaked dressings should only have more dressings placed on top of them, but in some cases this only allows more bleeding. If a dressing becomes blood soaked, remove the dressing and redress once to be sure direct pressure is being placed on the bleeding area. It is important to report such excessive bleeding to the receiving physician. Do not use clamps to stop bleeders; this may cause injuries to other structures (nerves are present alongside arteries).

At this point enough information has been obtained to determine critical trauma situations that should be treated by load and go.

CRITICAL INTERVENTIONS AND TRANSPORT DECISION

To decide whether the patient falls into the "load-and-go" category, you need to determine whether the patient has any of the following critical injuries or conditions.

1. Head injury with decreased level of consciousness

   2. Airway obstruction unrelieved by mechanical methods (e.g., suction, finger sweep, even Heimlich maneuver or abdominal thrusts in desperate cases)
   3. Conditions resulting in possible inadequate breathing
      a. Large open chest wound (sucking chest wound)
      b. Large flail chest
      c. Tension pneumothorax
      d. Major blunt chest injury
   4. Traumatic cardiopulmonary arrest
   5. Shock
      a. Hemorrhagic
      b. Spinal
      c. Myocardial contusion
      d. Pericardial tamponade

This listing can be simplified further into conditions based on signs and symptoms:

   1. Decreased level of consciousness
   2. Abnormal respiration
   3. Abnormal circulation (shock)
   4. Signs of conditions that rapidly lead to shock:
      a. Tender, distended abdomen
      b. Pelvic instability
      c. Bilateral femur fractures

If the patient has one of the critical conditions listed above immediately transfer him to a long backboard, checking the back as you perform the log-roll maneuver. Apply oxygen, load into an ambulance (if available), and transport rapidly to the nearest appropriate emergency facility. Life-saving procedures may be needed but should not hold up transport. There are a few brief procedures that are done while at the scene: manage airway, control major bleeding, seal sucking chest wound, hand stabilize flail, hyperventilate, and begin CPR. However, most procedures are reserved for transport. *Weigh every field procedure against the time it will take to perform it.* Remember, you are spending minutes of the patient's golden hour; be sure the procedure is worth the cost. Nonlife-saving procedures such as splinting and bandaging must not hold up transport. Be sure to call Medical Direction early so that the hospital is prepared for the patient's arrival. If the primary survey fails to identify a critical trauma situation, you should transfer the patient to the backboard (check the back) and proceed with the secondary survey. There are exceptions:

   1. Consider the mechanism of injury before deciding that the patient is stable.
   2. Patients who are not critical should have their fractures splinted before moving to the backboard.

SECONDARY SURVEY

The critical patient has this exam performed during transport to the hospital while the patient who appears stable should have this exam done at the scene. Even if the patient appears stable and you decide to perform this exam at the scene, keep the overall scene time under 10 minutes. "Stable" patients may become "unstable" quite rapidly.

1. Record vital signs—record pulse, respiration, and blood pressure (obtain accurate recordings—count for 30 seconds and double; use the BP cuff now).

2. Obtain a history of the injury (your partner may already have done this):

   a. Personal observation.

   b. Bystanders.

   c. Patient. Look for a medic alert tag in unconscious patients. Take a *SAMPLE* history from conscious patients:

      S—symptoms

      A—allergies

      M—medications

      P—past medical history (other illnesses)

      L—last oral intake (when was the last time there was any solid or liquid intake)

      E—events preceding the accident

3. Perform a head-to-toes exam in more detail. The exam should consist of inspection, auscultation, palpation, and sometimes percussion.

   a. Begin at the head examining for DCAP-BLS, raccoon eyes, Battle's sign, and drainage of blood or fluid from the ears or nose. Assess the airway again.

   b. Check the neck again. Look for DCAP-BLS, distended neck veins, or deviated trachea. Check the pulse again. If not already done, apply a cervical immobilization device at this time.

   c. Recheck the chest. Be sure that breath sounds are still present and equal on each side. Recheck seals over open wounds. Be sure flails are well stabilized (hand stabilization is adequate until you are in the ambulance).

   d. Perform an abdominal exam. Look for signs of blunt or penetrating trauma. Feel for tenderness. Do not waste time listening for bowel sounds. If the abdomen is painful to gentle pressure during examination, you can expect the patient to be bleeding internally. If the abdomen is both distended and painful, you can expect hemorrhagic shock very quickly.

    e. Assess pelvis and extremities. Check for DCAP-BLS and TIC. Be sure to check and record PMS on all fractures. Do this before and after straightening any fracture. Angulated fractures of the upper extremities are usually best splinted as found. Most fractures of the lower extremities are *gently* straightened by using traction splints or air splints. Critical patients have all splints applied during transport.

4. Do a brief neurological exam.

    a. Level of consciousness (AVPU):

       A—alert

       V—responds to verbal stimuli

       P—responds to pain

       U—unresponsive

    b. Motor: Can the patient move fingers and toes?

    c. Sensation: Can he feel you when you touch his fingers and toes? Does the unconscious patient respond when you pinch his fingers and toes?

    d. Pupils: Are they equal or unequal? Do they respond to light? The neurological exam is very simple, but is frequently forgotten. It gives important baseline information that is used in later treatment decisions. Always perform and record the neurological exam.

5. If necessary, finish bandaging and splinting.

6. Continually monitor and reevaluate the patient.

Transport immediately if the secondary survey reveals any of the critical trauma situations listed on pages 32 and 33.

CRITICAL CARE AND REASSESSMENT EXAM

Critical care refers to all the interventions and procedures performed in response to the assessments that you perform. This refers to procedures performed on-scene and during transport.

1. Manage airway. All critical trauma patients should receive oxygen. Consider whether any further airway interventions are necessary (assisted ventilation, suction, stabilization of flail chest, etc.).

2. Apply monitor(s). If you are equipped with an automated external defibrillator or pulse oximeter, you should delay application until the patient is in the ambulance.

3. Bandage and splint. Critical patients have most dressings and splints applied during transport to conserve the "golden hour." Exceptions are pressure dressings to control bleeding

and dressings to stabilize impaled objects. Critical patients are splinted with the long spineboard initially and, unless delayed on scene, have other splints applied during transport.

The reassessment exam should be performed every 5 minutes in critical patients and every 15 minutes in stable patients. The reassessment exam should also be performed *anytime* the patient's condition worsens. Accurately record what you see and what you do. Record changes in the patient's condition during transport. Record the time that interventions are performed. Extenuating circumstances or significant details should be recorded in the comments or remarks section of the written report (review documentation in Appendix C).

CONTACTING MEDICAL DIRECTION

When you have a critical patient, it is extremely important to contact medical direction as early as possible. It takes time to get the appropriate surgeon and the operating room team in place and the critical patient has no time to wait. Always notify the receiving facility of your estimated time of arrival (ETA), the condition of the patient, and any special needs on arrival (see Appendix B).

SUMMARY

Patient assessment is the key to trauma care. The interventions required are not difficult; it is the timing of them that is often critical. If you know what questions to ask and how to perform the exam, you will know when to perform the life-saving interventions. This chapter has described a rapid, orderly, and thorough examination of the trauma patient with priorities of examination and treatment always in mind. The continuous practice of approaching the patient in the way described here will allow you to concentrate on the patient rather than trying to figure out what to do next. Optimum speed is achieved by teamwork. Teamwork is achieved by practice. During the predispatch stage, you should plan regular exercises in patient evaluation to perfect each team member's role in the priority plan. The following pages contain a brief outline of the critical questions that you should ask in the primary, secondary, and reassessment surveys as well as an algorithm for the primary survey by a three-member team.

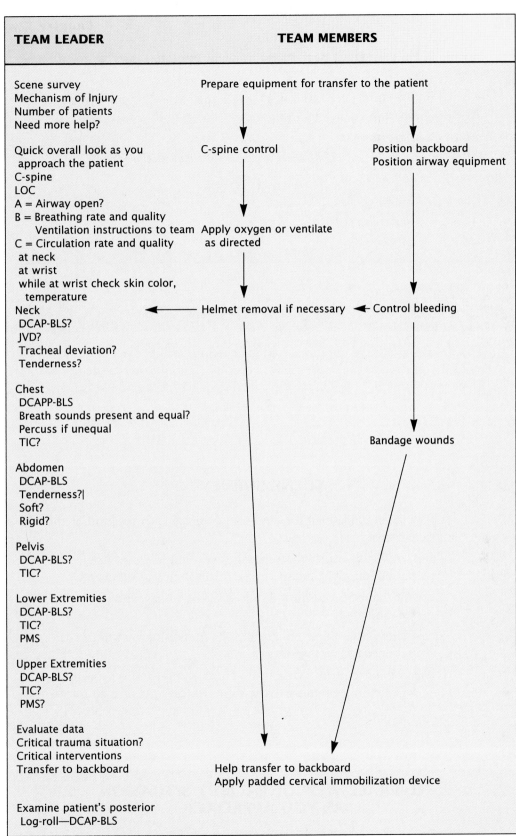

TEAM LEADER

Scene survey
Mechanism of Injury
Number of patients
Need more help?

Quick overall look as you
 approach the patient
C-spine
LOC
A = Airway open?
B = Breathing rate and quality
    Ventilation instructions to team
C = Circulation rate and quality
 at neck
 at wrist
 while at wrist check skin color,
  temperature
Neck
DCAP-BLS?
JVD?
Tracheal deviation?
Tenderness?

Chest
DCAPP-BLS
Breath sounds present and equal?
Percuss if unequal
TIC?

Abdomen
DCAP-BLS
Tenderness?|
Soft?
Rigid?

Pelvis
DCAP-BLS?
TIC?

Lower Extremities
DCAP-BLS?
TIC?
PMS

Upper Extremities
DCAP-BLS?
TIC?
PMS?

Evaluate data
Critical trauma situation?
Critical interventions
Transfer to backboard

Examine patient's posterior
Log-roll—DCAP-BLS

TEAM MEMBERS

Prepare equipment for transfer to the patient

C-spine control

Position backboard
Position airway equipment

Apply oxygen or ventilate
 as directed

Helmet removal if necessary ◄ Control bleeding

Bandage wounds

Help transfer to backboard
Apply padded cervical immobilization device

*The Basic Trauma Life Support Primary Trauma Survey Algorithm
for Three-Member Team*

Acronyms:

LOC—Level of consciousness

AVPU—Alert, responds to Verbal stimuli, responds to Painful stimuli, Unresponsive

JVD—Jugular venous distention

DCAPP—Deformities, contusions, abrasions, penetrations, paradoxical motion

DCAP—Deformities, contusions, abrasions, penetrations

BLS—Burns, lacerations, swelling

TIC—Tenderness, instability, crepitation

PMS—Pulses, motor, sensation

PRIMARY SURVEY

The following critical questions and instructions will get you the information you need to make the right decisions. Commit this to memory. Once you know it, you will have no problems with patient assessment.

SCENE SURVEY

Look, listen, and smell for anything dangerous to you and/or the victims.

Think of victims other than the ones you initially see. Ask patient and bystanders. Look for evidence of others.

Note mechanisms of injury. Look and ask patient and bystanders.

Decide now if you need more help. Base decision on number of patients and circumstances.

If the patient requires extrication, check motor and sensory of legs before beginning extrication (unless patient is in *immediate* danger and you must use rapid extrication protocol).

OVERALL VIEW OF PATIENT SITUATION AS YOU APPROACH

What is the patient's overall situation as you approach?

LEVEL OF CONSCIOUSNESS (AVPU)

Speak to the patient as you approach. Ask the patient not to move until you have completed your examination. Assure the patient that you are there to help him. His response gives you your first information as to LOC and airway. If the patient does not respond to your verbal stimuli, determine if he responds to pain or is unresponsive. Do this as you proceed through the primary survey. One of your teammates must stabilize the neck and be responsible for this and the airway until the patient is transferred to the backboard and the neck is stabilized with C-collar, body strapping, and head immobilizer.

AIRWAY

Is the airway open and clear?

BREATHING

Look, listen, and feel to determine if the patient is breathing and what is the rate and quality of the breathing. You do not stop to count at this time. Just get a "feel" for the rate and quality of the breathing.

VENTILATION INSTRUCTIONS

Now is the time to instruct your teammate (rescuer 2) how to assist the patient with respiration.

Have rescuer 2 stabilize the neck with his knees, freeing his hands to use suction, bag-valve mask, and so on.

Order oxygen for any patient with abnormal respiration, head injury, or shock.

Assist ventilation if the patient is hypoventilating.

Hyperventilate the patient with an altered level of consciousness.

CIRCULATION

Feel the rate and quality of the pulse at the neck and the wrist.
  Do not stop for an accurate count yet—just get a "feel" for
  rate and quality of the pulse.
Look and feel for the skin color, condition, and temperature.

NECK

Look for DCAP-BLS and feel for tenderness of the neck.
Look and feel of the neck veins. Note if flat or distended.
Look and feel of the trachea. Note if midline or deviated.

CHEST

Look for DCAPP-BLS and feel for TIC.
Listen to the chest high in the midaxillary line bilaterally.
Listen to see if the breath sounds are present and equal.
If breath sounds are not equal,
  Percuss the chest down the posterior axillary line *on the side
    with decreased breath sounds.*
  Listen for tympany (hyperresonance) or dullness.

ABDOMEN

Look at and feel the four quadrants of the abdomen.
Look for DCAP-BLS.
Feel for tenderness:
  Note if the abdomen is soft or hard (rigid).

PELVIS

Look for DCAP-BLS and feel for TIC.
Press down on symphysis and push in on the iliac crests.

LOWER EXTREMITIES

Look for DCAP-BLS.
Feel for TIC and PMS.

UPPER EXTREMITIES

Look for DCAP-BLS.
Feel for TIC and PMS.

BLEEDING

Look and feel for significant bleeding and obtain control.

You should note significant bleeding as you are going through the primary survey. Do not interrupt the survey to control yourself—instruct rescuer 3 to control with pressure dressings.

DECISION

Using the data that you have obtained up to this point, decide if this is a critical situation or is the patient stable.

If the patient is critical, move immediately to the backboard—do only *critical* interventions before transfer.

As a general rule, all interventions are done in the ambulance if it is immediately available.

If the patient appears stable, consider mechanisms of injury before deciding to do secondary survey on scene.

If the patient is stable, splint all fractures before moving to the backboard.

Even if the patient is stable, move to the backboard before beginning the secondary survey.

If you have to apply splints to a stable patient, one rescuer may obtain history and vital signs while the others are splinting.

EXAMINATION OF THE POSTERIOR

Do this during transfer to the backboard.
Look for DCAP-BLS.
Feel for TIC.

SECONDARY SURVEY

When performing the secondary survey, you must look, listen and feel from head to toes. Every patient gets a secondary survey: stable patients while at the scene, critical patients during transport. If other team members are available, the blood pressure and accurate pulse and respiratory rates may be taken by one of them prior to transport.
Obtain SAMPLE History now.

HEAD

Look and feel
For DCAP-BLS
For TIC
For Battle's sign
For blood or fluid in ears
For raccoon eyes
For blood or fluid from nose
For pupillary size, equality, reaction to light
For burns of face, nose hairs, mouth
For skin changes
For pallor
For cyanosis
For diaphoresis

REASSESS ABCS

AIRWAY

      Recheck patency.

      If burn victim, assess for signs of inhalation injury.

BREATHING

      Check rate (accurately and record).

      Check quality.

CIRCULATION

      Check pulse rate (accurately and record).

      Check pulse quality.

      Check blood pressure (done by partner if possible).

      Check skin color, condition, temperature.

NECK

(If collar has been applied, remove the front.) Look and feel for DCAP-BLS, tenderness, JVD (jugular venous distention), tracheal deviation.

CHEST

Look and feel for DCAPP-BLS and TIC.

      Listen for breath sounds in all lung fields.

If breath sounds unequal,

      Evaluate for tension pneumothorax and hemothorax.

ABDOMEN

Look for DCAP-BLS.

      Feel in all four quadrants for tenderness.

      Determine if the abdomen is soft or hard (rigid).

PELVIS

Look and feel for DCAP-BLS and TIC.

Gently compress over symphysis and push in laterally over iliac crests for TIC.

LOWER EXTREMITIES

Look and feel for DCAP-BLS and TIC.

Check PMS.

Check range of motion.

UPPER EXTREMITIES

Look and feel for DCAP-BLS and TIC.

Begin at the midline, checking clavicles, shoulders, arms, and hands.

Check PMS.

Check range of motion.

REASSESSMENT SURVEY

LEVEL OF CONSCIOUSNESS

Check LOC (AVPU).

Check pupillary size, equality, reaction to light.

REASSESS ABCS

Airway

    Recheck patency.

    If burn victim, reassess for signs of inhalation injury.

Breathing and circulation

    Recheck vital signs.

    Check quality of respiration.

    Neck

    If collar has been applied, remove the front.

    Look for JVD, tracheal deviation.

    Chest

    Listen for breath sounds in all lung fields.

    If breath sounds are unequal, evaluate for tension pneumothorax and hemothorax

    Check pulse rate (accurately and record).

    Check pulse quality.

    Check blood pressure.

    Check skin color, condition, temperature.

ABDOMEN

Feel in all four quadrants for tenderness.

Is the abdomen soft or hard (rigid)?

FOCUSED ASSESSMENT OF INJURIES

Check each of the identified injuries (lacerations for bleeding, PMS on all injured extremities, flails, pneumothorax, open chest wounds, etc.).

CHECK INTERVENTIONS

Check oxygen for rate.

Check seals on sucking chest wounds.

Check splints and dressings.

Check position of pregnant patients.

Check rate of hyperventilation of patients with decreased LOC.

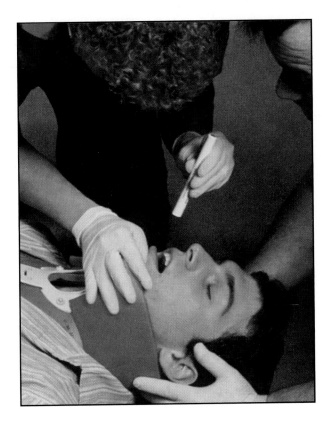

CHAPTER

Patient Assessment Skills

Donna Hastings, EMT-P

PRIMARY SURVEY

OBJECTIVES

At the conclusion of this skill station you should be able to:

1. Correctly perform the primary survey within 2 minutes.
2. Identify which patients require "load and go."
3. Describe when to perform critical interventions.

PROCEDURE

Short written scenarios will be used along with a model (to act as the patient). You will divide into teams to practice performing the primary survey, critical interventions, and transfer decisions. Each member of the team must practice being team leader at least once and preferably twice. The "Critical Information" represents the answers you should be seeking at each step of the survey.

CRITICAL INFORMATION—PRIMARY SURVEY

The following is a repeat of the information presented at the end of Chapter 2. These statements are so important that they are repeated in the first person as questions, just as you should ask them to yourself as you perform patient assessment. This is the least amount of information that you need as you perform each step of the primary survey. It may be helpful to copy these statements and questions and carry them with you when you are practicing patient assessment.

Scene Survey

Do I see, hear, or smell anything dangerous?

Are there any other victims? Ask patient and bystanders. Look for evidence of others.

I am surveying for mechanisms of injury. Look and ask patient and bystanders.

Do we need more help? This decision should be based on number of patients and circumstances.

Level of Consciousness (AVPU)

Say, "Please do not move until we have checked you for injuries."

Say, "We are here to help you. Can you tell us what happened?"

Airway

Is the airway open and clear?

Breathing

Is the patient breathing?

What is the rate and quality of respiration?

Ventilation Instructions

Order oxygen for any patient with abnormal respiration, head injury, or shock.

Assist ventilation if the patient is hypoventilating.

Hyperventilate the patient with an altered level of consciousness.

Circulation

What is the rate and quality of the pulse at the neck and the wrist?

What is the skin color, condition, and temperature?

Neck

Do I see or feel any DCAP-BLS or tenderness of the neck?

Do the neck veins look and feel flat or distended?

Does the trachea look and feel midline or deviated?

Chest

I am looking and feeling of the chest.

Is there DCAPP-BLS or TIC?

I am listening to the chest high in the midaxillary line bilaterally.

> Are the breath sounds present and equal?

If breath sounds are not equal,

> I am percussing the chest down the posterior axillary line on the side with decreased breath sounds.

> Is there tympany (hyperresonance) or dullness present?

Abdomen

I am looking at and feeling the abdomen.

> Is there any DCAP-BLS?

> I am feeling the four quadrants of the abdomen.

> Is the abdomen soft or hard (rigid)?

> Is there tenderness?

Pelvis

I am looking at and feeling (pressing down on symphysis and pushing in on the iliac crests) the pelvis.

> Is there DCAP-BLS or TIC?

Lower Extremities

I am looking at and feeling the legs.

> Is there DCAP-BLS or TIC?

> Is PMS (pulses, motor, sensation) normal?

Upper Extremities

I am looking at and feeling the arms.

> Is there DCAP-BLS or TIC?

> Is PMS normal?

Bleeding

> Do I see or feel any significant bleeding?

Decision

> Is this a critical situation?

> Are there interventions that I must make now?

Exam of the Posterior

This is done during transfer to the backboard.

> Is there any DCAP-BLS or TIC to the posterior?

SECONDARY SURVEY AND REASSESSMENT SURVEY

OBJECTIVES

At the conclusion of this skill station, you should be able to:

1. Correctly perform the secondary survey.
2. Identify which patients require "load and go."
3. Describe when to perform critical interventions.
4. Demonstrate proper communications with medical control.
5. Correctly perform the reassessment survey.

PROCEDURE

Short written scenarios will be used along with a model (to act as the patient). You will divide into teams to practice performing the secondary survey, making critical decisions and interventions, and performing the reassessment survey. Each member of the team must practice being team leader at least once and preferably twice. The "critical information" represents the answers you should be seeking at each step of the survey.

CRITICAL INFORMATION—SECONDARY SURVEY

This is a repeat of the information presented at the end of Chapter 2. These questions are so important that they are repeated in the first person, just as you should ask them as you perform patient assessment. This is the least amount of information that you need as you perform each step of the secondary survey and reassessment survey. It may be helpful to copy these questions and carry them with you when you are practicing patient assessment. Obtain SAMPLE History now.

Head

I am looking at and feeling the scalp and face.

> Is there DCAP-BLS or TIC?
>
> Are Battle's sign or raccoon eyes present?
>
> Is there blood or fluid draining from the ears or nose?
>
> What is pupillary size? Are they equal? Do they react to light?
>
> Is there pallor, cyanosis, or diaphoresis?

Airway

> Is the airway open and clear?
>
> If there are burns of the face, are there signs of burns in the mouth or nose?

Breathing

What is the rate and quality of respiration?

Circulation

What is the rate and quality of the pulse?

What is the blood pressure?

What is the skin color, condition, temperature?

Neck

I am looking at and feeling the neck.

Is there DCAP-BLS or tenderness of the neck?

Are the neck veins flat or distended?

Is the trachea midline or deviated?

Chest

I am looking at and feeling the chest.

Is there DCAPP-BLS or TIC?

I am listening to the chest.

Are the breath sounds present and equal?

If breath sounds are unequal,

I am percussing the chest. Is it hyperresonant or dull?

Abdomen

I am looking at and feeling the abdomen.

Is there DCAP-BLS?

Is there any tenderness?

Is the abdomen soft or hard (rigid)?

Pelvis

I am looking at and feeling the pelvis.

Is there DCAP-BLS or TIC?

Lower Extremities

I am looking at and feeling the legs.

Is there DCAP-BLS or TIC?

Is there normal PMS?

Is range of motion normal?

Upper Extremities

I am looking at and feeling the arms.

> Is there DCAP-BLS or TIC?
> Is there normal PMS?
> Is range of motion normal?

CRITICAL INFORMATION—REASSESSMENT SURVEY

Level of Consciousness

> What is the LOC?
> What is pupillary size? Are they equal? Do they react to light?

Reassess ABCs

Airway

> Is the airway open and clear?
> If there are burns of the face: Are there signs of burns in the
> mouth or nose?

Breathing and Circulation

> What is the rate and quality of respiration?
> What is the rate and quality of the pulse?
> What is the blood pressure?
> What is the skin color, condition, temperature?

Neck

> Is the trachea midline or deviated?
> Are the neck veins flat or distended?
> Is there increased swelling of the neck?

Chest

> Are the breath sounds present and equal?

If breath sounds are unequal,

> I am percussing the chest. Is it hyperresonant or dull?

Abdomen

Is the abdomen tender or distended?

Is the abdomen soft or hard (rigid)?

FOCUSED ASSESSMENT OF INJURIES

I am checking the injuries (mention each one). Has there been any change?

CHECK INTERVENTIONS

Ask the appropriate question for your patient.

Is the oxygen rate correct?

Is the open chest wound still sealed?

Are any of the dressings blood soaked?

Are the splints in good position?

Is the pregnant patient tilted to the left?

Is the patient being hyperventilated for decreased LOC?

ASSESSMENT AND MANAGEMENT OF THE TRAUMA PATIENT

OBJECTIVE

At the conclusion of this skill station you should be able to demonstrate the proper organized sequence of rapid assessment and management of the multiple-trauma patient.

PROCEDURE

Short written trauma scenarios will be used along with a model (to act as the patient). You will be divided into teams to practice the management of simulated trauma situations using the principles and techniques taught in the course. You will be evaluated in the same manner on the second day of the course. You will be expected to use all the principles and techniques taught in this course while managing these simulated patients. To familiarize yourself with the evaluation procedure, you will be given a copy of a scenario and a grade sheet. Review Chapter 2 and the primary and secondary surveys in this chapter.

GROUND RULES FOR TEACHING AND EVALUATION

1. You will be allowed to stay together in three-member groups (different-sized groups are optional) throughout the practice and evaluation stations.

2. You will have three practice scenarios. This allows each member of the team to be team leader once.

3. You will be evaluated as team leader once.

4. You will assist as a member of the rescue team during two scenarios in which another member of your team is being evaluated as team leader. You may assist but all assessments must be done by the team leader. This gives you a total of six scenarios from which to learn: three practice, one evaluation, and two assists while others are evaluated.

5. Wait outside the door until the instructor comes out and gives you your scenario.

6. You will be allowed to look over your equipment before you start your exam.

7. Be sure to ask about scene safety if not already given in the scenario.

8. Be sure to apply your personal protective gear.

9. If you have a live model for a patient, you must talk to that person just as you would a real patient. It is best to explain what you are doing as you examine the patient. Be confident and reassuring.

10. You must ask your instructor for things you cannot find out from your patient. Examples: Blood pressure, pulse, breath sounds.

11. Wounds and fractures must be dressed or splinted just as if they are real. Procedures must be done correctly (blood pressure, log-rolling, strapping, splinting, etc.).

12. If you need a piece of equipment that is not available, ask your instructors. They may allow you to simulate the equipment.

13. During practice and evaluation, you may be allowed to go (or may be directed) to any station but you cannot go to the same station twice.

14. You will be graded on
    a. Assessment of the scene
    b. Assessment of the patient
    c. Management of the patient
    d. Efficient use of time
    e. Leadership
    f. Judgment

g. Problem-solving ability

h. Patient interaction

15. When you finish your testing scenario, there is to be no discussion of the case. If you have any questions, they will be answered after the faculty meeting at the end of the course.

PATIENT ASSESSMENT PEARLS

1. Do not approach the patient until you have done a scene survey.

2. Do not interrupt the primary survey except for

   a. Airway obstruction or near obstruction

   b. Cardiac or respiratory arrest

3. Give ventilation instructions as soon as you assess the airway and breathing.

4. Hyperventilate (about 24 breaths per minute) all patients with decreased level of consciousness.

5. Assist ventilations for anyone who is hypoventilating (8 or fewer per minute).

6. Give oxygen to all multiple-trauma patients. If in doubt, give oxygen.

7. Transfer the patient to the backboard as soon as the primary survey is completed.

8. When primary survey is completed, decide if the patient is critical or stable. Critical trauma situations are characterized by

   a. Decreased level of consciousness

   b. Difficulty with breathing

   c. Shock

   d. Tender abdomen

   e. Unstable pelvis

   f. Bilateral femur fractures

9. If the primary survey reveals that the patient has a critical trauma situation, load the patient in the ambulance and transport.

10. If absolutely necessary, certain interventions may have to be done before transport. Remember that you are trading minutes of the patient's golden hour for those procedures. Use good judgment.

11. Critical patients get a secondary survey enroute to the hospital.

12. Stable patients get a secondary survey at the scene (on the backboard).

13. Transport immediately if your secondary survey reveals any of the critical trauma situations.

14. Critical patients should not have traction splints applied at the scene (it takes too long).

15. Call medical direction early if you have a critical patient (other physicians may have to be called from home to treat the patient).

16. Anytime the patient's condition worsens, perform the reassessment survey.

17. Anytime you make an intervention, repeat the reassessment survey.

18. Unconscious patients cannot protect their airways.

19. Transport pregnant patients with the backboard tilted slightly to the left. Do not let them roll over onto the floor.

20. Remain calm and think. Your knowledge, training, and concern are the most important tools you carry.

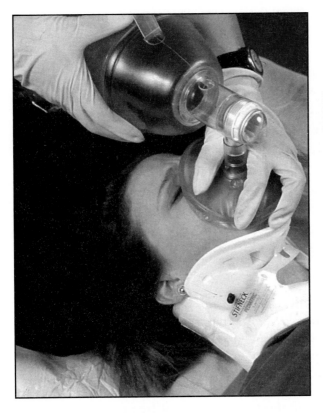

Initial Airway Management

John E. Campbell, M.D., F.A.C.E.P.

OBJECTIVES

At the conclusion of this chapter you should be able to:

1. Describe the anatomy and physiology of the respiratory system.
2. Define the following terms:
   a. Hyperventilation
   b. Hypoventilation
   c. Tidal volume
   d. Minute volume
   e. Delivered volume
   f. Compliance
3. Describe Sellick's maneuver and explain when it should and should not be used.
4. Describe the essential contents of an airway kit.
5. Explain the importance of observation as it relates to airway control.
6. Describe the recovery position and its indications.
7. Describe methods to deliver supplemental oxygen to the trauma patient.

Continued on next page

8. Briefly describe the indications and contraindications and the advantages and disadvantages of the following airway adjuncts:

a. Nasopharyngeal airways

b. Oropharyngeal airways

c. Bag-valve masks

d. Demand valves (that meet American Heart Association standards)

e. Blind-insertion airway devices (BIADs)

Of all the tasks expected of field teams caring for the trauma patient, none is more important than that of airway control. Maintaining an open airway and adequate ventilation in the trauma patient can be a challenge in any setting, but it can be almost impossible in the adverse environment of the field, with its poor lighting, the chaos that often surrounds an accident, the position of the patient, and perhaps hostile onlookers.

Airway control is a task that you must master, since it frequently cannot wait until you get to the hospital. Patients who are hypoxic, or underventilated, or both, are in need of immediate help—help that only you can give them in the initial stages of their care. It falls to you, then, to be fully versed in the basic structure and function of the airway, in how to achieve and maintain a patent airway, and in how to oxygenate and ventilate a patient.

Because of the unpredictable nature of the field environment, you will be called on to manage patient's airways in almost every conceivable situation; in wrecked cars, dangling above rivers, in the middle of a shopping center, at the side of a busy highway. You therefore need *options* and alternatives from which to choose. What will work for one patient may not work for another.

Whatever the methods required, you must always start with the basics. It is of little value—and in some cases downright dangerous—to apply "advanced" techniques of airway control before beginning basic maneuvers. The discussion of airway control in the trauma patient will be rooted in several fundamental truths: air should go in and out, oxygen is good, and blue is bad. Everything else follows from this.

ANATOMY

The airway begins at the tip of the nose and the lips and ends at the *alveolarcapillary membrane,* through which gas exchange takes place between the air sacs of the lung (the *alveoli)* and the lung's capillary network. The airway consists of chambers and pipes that conduct air and its 21% oxygen content to the alveoli during inspiration and carry away the waste *carbon dioxide* that diffuses from the blood into the alveoli.

The beginning of the respiratory tract, the *nasal cavity* and *oropharynx,* perform important functions (see Figure 4-1). Lined with moist *mucous membranes,* these areas serve to warm and filter inhaled gases. They are highly vascular and contain protective lymphoid tissue. Bypassing this portion of the respiratory tract through the use of an airway device will reduce the natural protection for the vulnerable lung, and you will have to assume some of those tasks. That is why suctioning of the airway, as well as the warming and humidification of gases, becomes of such importance in patients who have airway devices inserted.

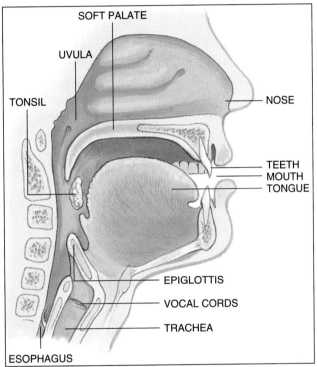

Figure 4-1 *Anatomy of the upper airway. Note that the tongue, hyoid bone, and epiglottis are attached to the mandible by a series of ligaments. Lifting forward on the jaw will therefore displace all these structures.*

The lining of the respiratory tract is delicate and highly vascular. It deserves every bit of respect you can give it, and that means preventing undue trauma, using liberally lubricated tubes, and avoiding unnecessary poking about. The *nasal cavity* is divided by a very vascular midline *septum* and on the lateral walls of the nose are "shelves" called the *turbinates.*

The teeth are the first obstruction we meet in the oral part of the airway. They may be more obstructive in some patients than in others. In any case, the same general principle always applies: Patients should have the same number of teeth at the end of an airway procedure as they had at the beginning.

The tongue is a large chunk of muscle and represents the next potential obstruction. These muscles are attached to the jaw anteriorly and, through a series of muscles and ligaments, to the *hyoid bone,* a "wishbonelike" structure just under the chin from which the cartilage skeleton (the *larynx)* of the upper airway is suspended. The *epiglottis* is also connected to the hyoid, and elevating the hyoid will lift upward on the epiglottis and open the airway further.

The epiglottis is one of the main anatomic landmarks in the airway. You must be familiar with it and be able to identify it by sight as well as by touch. It looks like a floppy piece of cartilage covered by mucosa—which is exactly what it is—and it feels like the tragus, the cartilage at the opening of the ear canal. Its function is unclear; it may be a "leftover" (i.e., vestigial) piece of anatomy. But it is important to you when you must assume control of the airway. The epiglottis is attached to the hyoid and thence to the mandible by a series of ligaments and muscles. In the unconscious patient, the tongue can produce some airway obstruction by falling back against the soft palate and even the posterior pharyngeal wall. However, it is the epiglottis that will produce complete airway obstruction in the supine unconscious patient whose jaw is relaxed and whose head and neck are in the neutral position. In such patients it will fall down against the glottic opening and prevent ventilation.

It is essential to understand this crucial fact in the management of the airway. To ensure a patent airway in an unconscious supine patient, the hyoid must be displaced anteriorly by lifting forward on the jaw ("chin lift," "jaw thrust"), or by pulling on the tongue. This will lift the tongue out of the way, and keep the epiglottis elevated away from the posterior pharyngeal wall and glottic opening (see Figure 4-2).

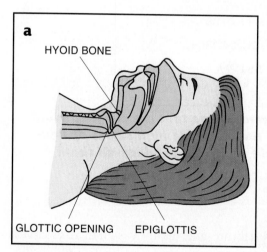
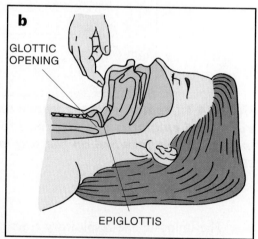

Figure 4-2 (a) *The epiglottis is attached to the hyoid and then to the mandible. When the mandible is relaxed and falls back, the tongue falls upward against the soft palate and the posterior pharyngeal wall, while the epiglottis falls over the glottic opening.* **(b)** *Extension of the head and lifting the chin will pull the tongue and the epiglottis upward and forward, exposing the glottic opening and ensuring a patent airway. In the trauma patient, only the jaw, or chin and jaw, should be displaced forward while the head and neck should be kept in alignment.*

The *vocal cords* are protected by the *thyroid cartilage,* a boxlike structure shaped like a "C," with the open part of the "C" representing its posterior wall, which is covered with muscle. When the cords vibrate, sound is produced. In some patients, the cords can close entirely in *laryngospasm,* producing complete airway obstruction. The thyroid cartilage can easily be seen in most people on the anterior surface of the neck as the laryngeal prominence.

Inferior to the thyroid cartilage is another part of the larynx, the *cricoid,* a cartilage shaped like a signet ring with the ring in front and the signet behind. It can be palpated as a small bump on the anterior surface of the neck inferior to the laryngeal prominence. Just behind the posterior wall of the cricoid cartilage lies the esophagus. Pressure on the cricoid at the front of the neck will close off the esophagus to pressures as high as 100 cm H_2O. Use this maneuver *(Sellick's maneuver)* to reduce the risk of gastric regurgitation and to prevent insufflation of air into the stomach during positive pressure ventilation by mouth-to-mouth, bag-valve mask, or demand valve (see Figures 4-3, 4-4a, and 4-4b). Do not use Sellick's maneuver if there is any danger of cervical spine injury. Applying pressure to the neck might cause too much movement in an unstable cervical spine.

The *tracheal rings,* C-shaped cartilaginous supports for the trachea, continue beyond the cricoid cartilage, and the trachea soon divides into the *left* and *right mainstem bronchi.* The open part of the C-shaped rings lies posterior against the esophagus. An impacted swallowed foreign body that remains in the esophagus, or a misplaced esophageal airway can create tracheal obstruction by pressing against the soft posterior tracheal wall and narrowing the lumen. The point at which the trachea divides is called the *carina.* It is important to note that the right mainstem

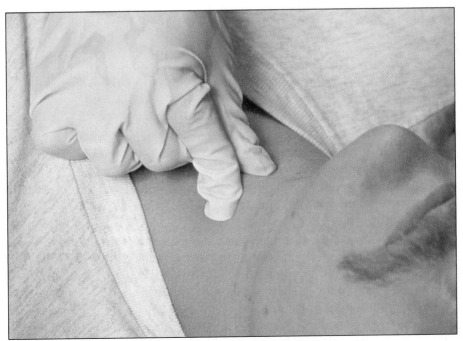

Figure 4-3 *Sellick's maneuver.*

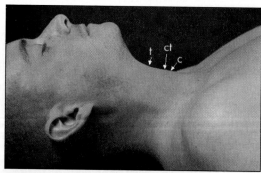

Figure 4-4a *External view of the anterior neck, showing the surface landmarks for the thyroid cartilage (laryngeal) prominence, cricothyroid membrane, and cricoid cartilage.*

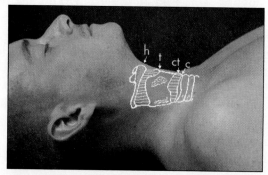

Figure 4-4b *Cut-away view showing the important landmarks of the larynx and upper airway: hyoid, thyroid cartilage, cricothyroid membrane, and cricoid cartilage.*

bronchus takes off at an angle that is slightly more in line with the trachea (see Figure 4-5). As a result, tubes or other foreign bodies that are poked or that trickle down the airway usually end up in the right mainstem bronchus.

To help protect the airway from becoming blocked and to reduce the risk of aspiration, the body has developed brisk reflexes that will attempt to expel any offending foreign material from the oropharynx, glottic opening, or the trachea. These areas are well supplied by sensitive nerves that can activate the swallowing, gag, and cough reflex. Activation of swallowing, gagging, or coughing by stimulation of the upper airway can cause significant cardiovascular stimulation as well as elevation in intracranial pressure.

The *lungs* are the organs through which this gas exchange takes place. They are contained within a "cage" formed by the ribs, and usually fill up the *pleural space*—the *potential space* between the internal chest wall and the lung surface. The lungs have only one opening to the outside, the *glottic opening*, the space between the vocal cords. Expansion of the chest wall (the cage) and movement of the diaphragm downward cause the lungs to expand (since the pleural space is airtight), and air rushes in through the *glottis*, the only opening to the outside. The air travels down the smaller and smaller tubes to the *alveoli*, where gas exchange takes place.

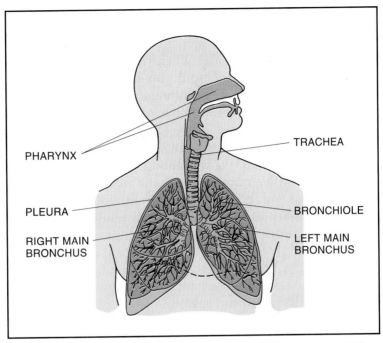

Figure 4-5 *Note that the right mainstem bronchus curves off at the carina at an angle slightly more in line with the trachea.*

VENTILATION

The movement of air or gases in and out of the lungs is called *ventilation*. At rest, adults normally take in about 450 to 500 cc with each breath. This is called the *tidal volume* and is measured by a respirometer. Multiplying that value by the number of breaths per minute (the respiratory rate) gives the *minute volume*, the amount of air breathed in and out each minute. This is an important value, and is normally 6 to 8 liters per minute (L/min). Anything greater than this resting value could be termed *hyperventilation*, and values lower than this, *hypoventilation*.

POSITIVE PRESSURE VENTILATION

Normal breathing takes place because the negative pressure inside the (potential) pleural space "draws" air in through the upper airway from the outside. In any patient who is unable to do this, or whose airway needs protecting, you may need to "pump" air or oxygen in through the glottic opening. This is called *intermittent positive pressure ventilation*. Positive pressure ventilation in trauma patients can take various forms, from mouth to mouth to bag-valve mask (or airway device). Pumping air into the oropharynx is no guarantee that it will go through the glottic opening and into the lungs. The oropharynx also leads to the esophagus, and pressure in the oropharynx of greater than 25 cm H_2O will open the esophagus and lead to air being pumped into the stomach (gastric insufflation). Bag-valve masks can produce pressures greater than this, and some older demand valves can produce pressures as high as 60 cm H_2O. This is why, if there is no danger of cervical spine injury, *Sellick's maneuver* (posterior pressure on the cricoid cartilage) is so very important as a basic airway procedure. When you need to ventilate a patient using intermittent positive pressure ventilation, you should know approximately how much volume you are delivering with each breath you give *(delivered volume)*. You can estimate the minute volume by multiplying this volume by the ventilatory rate. A demand valve that delivers oxygen at the rate of 100 L/min will have a delivered volume of 1660 cc each second that the valve is activated. Delivering over a liter of volume at a pressure of 60 cm H_2O will almost guarantee gastric insufflation and all the complications resulting from it. Bag-mask breathing may be no better; pressures generated by squeezing the bag may equal or exceed 60 cm H_2O.

Delivered volumes are usually less with bag resuscitators than with demand valves. There are two reasons for this. The average resuscitator bag holds only 1800 cc of gas, and that is the absolute limit to the volume that could be delivered if you were able to squeeze the bag completely. Using one hand, an average adult can squeeze approximately 1200 cc. The other reason for greater delivered volumes with demand valves is that a demand valve allows the rescuer to hold a mask on the face with both hands, thus decreasing mask leak. Keep in mind that these volumes, delivered from the ventilating port of these devices, equal the volumes delivered to the patient only if an endotracheal tube is in place. In other words, they do not take into account mask leak. When performing positive pressure ventilation with a mask, keep the following essentials in mind:

1. Supplemental oxygen must be provided for the patient during positive pressure ventilation.

2. Suction must be immediately available.

3. Ventilation must be done carefully to avoid gastric distension and to reduce the risk of regurgitation and possible aspiration. If there is no danger of spinal injury, you can help prevent these complications by using Sellick's maneuver.

4. Careful attention must be paid estimating the minute volume being delivered to the patient in trauma patients. A minute volume of at least 12 to 15 L should be provided. If an adult's hand will squeeze approximately 700 cc from a bag, "bagging" the patient every 3 or 4 seconds (15 to 20 times per minute would provide a minute volume of from 10.5 to 14 L. This should be enough to provide for the patients increased ventilatory needs. In the case of bag-mask breathing, up to 40% mask leak can be expected. Balloon mask designs can reduce this, and a two-person technique, in which one rescuer holds the mask in place with both hands while a second squeezes the bag, may better ensure adequate delivered volumes. During the stress of an emergency situation you will tend to ventilate patients at an increased rate but delivered volumes are often deficient. Pay attention

to delivered volumes as well, since rate alone cannot compensate for grossly inadequate ventilatory volumes.

COMPLIANCE

When air, or air containing oxygen, is delivered by positive pressure into the lungs of a patient, the "give" or elasticity of the lungs and chest wall will very much influence how easily it will be for the patient to breathe. If you are performing mask ventilation, a normal elasticity of the lungs and chest wall will allow air to enter the glottic opening and little gastric distension should result. However, if the elasticity is poor, ventilation will be harder to achieve. The ability of the lungs and chest wall to expand and therefore ventilate a patient is known as *compliance*. It is better to speak of "good compliance" or "bad compliance" rather than "high " or "low" compliance, since the latter terms can be somewhat confusing.

Compliance is an important concept, since it governs whether or not you can adequately ventilate a patient. Compliance can become bad (i.e., low) in some disease states of the lung or in patients who have an injury to the chest wall. In cardiac arrest, compliance will also become bad, due to poor circulation to the muscles. This makes ventilating the patient all the more difficult. A detectable worsening of compliance may be an early sign of tension pneumothorax.

AIRWAY EQUIPMENT

The most important rule to follow in regard to airway equipment is that it should be in working order and immediately available. It will do the patient no good if you have to run to get the suction apparatus. In other words, "be prepared." This is not difficult. Five basic pieces of equipment are necessary for the initial response to prehospital trauma calls:

1. Long backboard with attached head immobilization device
2. Cervical immobilization device
3. Airway kit
4. Trauma box (bandage material, BP cuff, stethoscope)
5. Personal protection equipment (glasses or face shield, rubber gloves)

The *airway kit* should be completely self-contained and should contain everything needed to secure an airway in any patient. Equipment now available is lightweight and portable. Oxygen cylinders are aluminum, and newer suction devices are less bulky and lighter. It is no longer acceptable to have suction units that are bulky and stored separate from a source of oxygen. Suction units should be contained in a kit with oxygen and other essential airway tools. A lightweight airway kit should consist of the following (see Figure 4-6):

1. Oxygen D cylinder, preferably aluminum
2. Portable, battery-powered or hand-powered suction unit

3. Oxygen cannulae and masks
4. Bag-valve-mask ventilating device
5. Pocket mask with supplemental oxygen intake

You should check all equipment each shift, and the kit should have a card attached to be initialed by the person checking it.

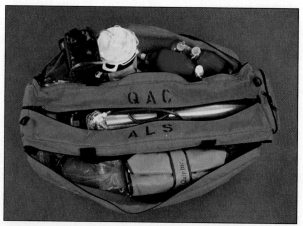

Figure 4-6 *An airway kit containing the essentials for airway management. Note that portable suction is included in this design. The total weight (with aluminum "D" oxygen cylinder) is approximately 10 kg (22 lb), about the same as a steel "E" oxygen cylinder.*

THE PATENT AIRWAY

One of the first maneuvers essential to caring for a patient is ensuring a *patent or open airway*. Without this, all other care is of little use. This must be done quickly, for patients can not tolerate hypoxia for more than a few minutes. The effect of hypoxia on an unconscious injured patient can be devastating, and if hypoxia is compounded by the absence of adequate perfusion, the patient is in even more difficult straits. Patients suffering from head trauma, not only may have hypoxic brain damage from airway compromise, but may also build up high levels of CO_2 that can increase blood flow to the injured brain causing swelling and increased intracranial pressure.

Ensuring an open airway in a patient can be a major challenge in the prehospital setting. Not only can trauma disrupt the anatomy of the face and airway, but resultant bleeding can lead to airflow obstruction as well as to obscuring airway landmarks. Add to this the risk of cervical spine injury, and the challenge is readily apparent. You must also remember that some airway maneuvers, including suction and insertion of naso and oropharyngeal airways, may stimulate a patient's protective reflexes and increase the likelihood of vomiting and aspiration, cardiovascular stimulation, and increased intracranial pressure. The first step in providing a patent

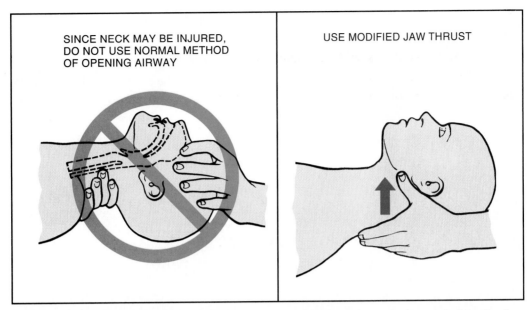

SINCE NECK MAY BE INJURED, DO NOT USE NORMAL METHOD OF OPENING AIRWAY

USE MODIFIED JAW THRUST

Figure 4-7a *Opening the airway using modified jaw thrust. Maintain in-line stabilization while pushing up on the angle of the jaw with your thumbs.*

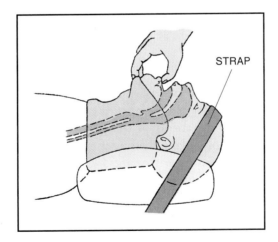

STRAP

Figure 4-7b *Jaw lift.*

airway in the unconscious patient is to ensure that the tongue and epiglottis are lifted forward and maintained in that position. This is done by either the modified jaw thrust (see Figure 4-7a) or the jaw lift (see Figure 4-7b). Either of these maneuvers will prevent the tongue from falling backward against the soft palate or posterior pharyngeal wall and will pull forward on the hyoid, lifting the epiglottis up out of the way. These are essential maneuvers for both basic and advanced airway procedures. Done properly, they will open the airway without the necessity of tilting the head backward or moving the neck.

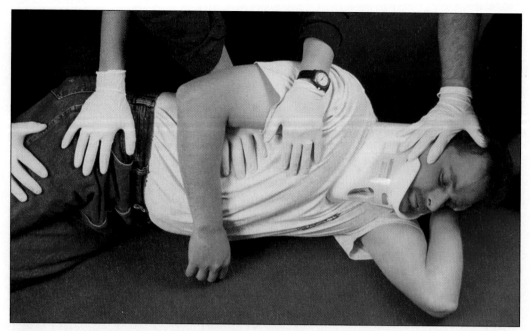

Figure 4-8 *The "recovery" position. When the patient is suspected of having sustained trauma, and when suction and immobilization devices are not yet available, use this position to prevent aspiration. You should have sufficient personnel available to move the patient carefully, with vertebral column kept in alignment.*

Recommending the maneuvers just mentioned assumes that the patient is supine and that there is an ability on the part of either the patient or the rescuer to clear the airway of blood or secretions. If the patient is unable to control the airway and suction is not available, place the patient carefully in the *recovery position* or left semiprone. This can be done with a rigid C-collar in place, with several rescuers to keep the vertebral column in alignment and prevent undue movement (Figure 4-8). In this position secretions can drain, the tongue and epiglottis are displaced forward, and the airway should remain patent. The risk of C-spine damage is less than the disaster that would occur should the patient vomit while supine. It is important to keep the head, neck, and vertebral column in alignment, but do not exert traction on head and neck.

In the rare instance where a patient has a foreign body obstruction of the airway and you are unable to remove it by suction or finger sweeps, you may be forced to do abdominal thrusts or the Heimlich maneuver. In this instance, the concern for cervical spine immobilization must come second to the fact that the patient will die within minutes if the airway is not cleared.

Constant vigilance and care are required for you to maintain a patent airway in your patient. There are several essentials for this task:

1. Continual observation of the patient.

2. An adequate suction device with large-bore tubing and attachment.

3. Airway adjuncts.

OBSERVATION

The patient who is injured is at risk of airway compromise even if completely conscious and awake. This is partially due to the fact that many patients have full stomachs, are anxious, and are prone to vomiting. You should have no difficulty understanding their plight when you consider that you bind them down on a hard surface with a rigid collar and fix their head and neck solidly to a board. Some patients will also be bleeding into their oropharynx and thus swallowing blood.

In view of these facts, you should constantly observe your patient for airway problems following injury. One team member must be responsible for both airway control and adequate ventilation for any patient who might be at risk of airway compromise.

The general appearance of the patient, the respiratory rate, and any complaints must be noted and attended to. In a spontaneous breathing patient, you must check frequently for the adequacy of tidal volume by feeling over mouth and nose and observing chest wall movements. Check the supplemental oxygen line periodically to ensure that oxygen is being delivered to the patient at a given flow rate or percentage. Clear blood and secretions. You must be alert for sounds that indicate trouble. Be alert for this danger sign: *noisy breathing is obstructed breathing.* Consider combative patients to be hypoxic until a systematic and rapid evaluation rules this out.

SUCTION

All patients who are injured and who have cervical immobilization in place should be considered at high risk for airway compromise. One of the greatest threats to the patent airway is that of vomiting and aspiration, particularly in patients who have recently eaten a large meal washed down with large quantities of alcohol. As a result, portable suction devices should be considered basic equipment for field trauma care and should have the following characteristics (see Figure 4-9):

1. They should be carried in a kit with an oxygen cylinder and other airway equipment; they should not be separated or stored remote from oxygen; otherwise, they represent an "extra" piece of equipment requiring extra hands.

2. They should be hand or battery powered rather than oxygen driven.

3. They should generate sufficient pressure and volume displacement that they can suction pieces of food, blood clots, and thick secretions from the oropharynx.

4. They should have tubing of sufficient diameter (0.8 to 1 cm) to handle whatever is suctioned from the patient.

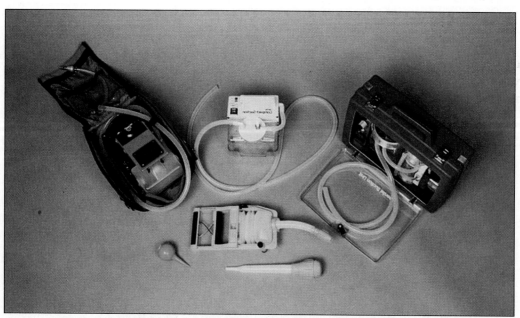

Figure 4-9 *Example of suction apparatus.*

Suction tips of more recent design are of large bore, particularly the new rigid "tonsil-tip" suckers that can handle most clots and bleeding. In some cases the suction tubing itself can be used to withdraw large amounts of blood or gastric contents. A 6-mm endotracheal tube can be used with a connector as a suction tip. The tube's side hole removes the necessity for a proximal control valve to interrupt suction.

AIRWAY ADJUNCTS

Equipment to aid in ensuring a patent airway will include various nasopharyngeal and oropharyngeal airways as well as blind-insertion airway devices (BIADs) such as esophageal gastric tube airway, pharyngotracheal lumen airway, and esophageal tracheal combitube. Insertion of these devices must be reserved for patients whose protective reflexes are sufficiently depressed to tolerate them. Care must be taken not to provoke vomiting or gagging, since both occurrences are bad for these patients. The nasopharyngeal airway will be better tolerated than the oropharyngeal. In fact, patients who are easily able to tolerate a proper-sized oropharyngeal airway should be considered candidates for insertion of a BIAD because their protective reflexes are so depressed that they cannot protect their trachea from aspiration.

Nasopharyngeal airways should be soft and of appropriate length. They are designed to prevent the tongue and epiglottis from falling against the posterior pharyngeal wall (see Chapter 5 for technique of insertion). With gentle insertion there should be few problems with this airway (see Figure 4-10). However, bleeding and trauma to the nasal mucosa are not infrequent. Mild hemorrhage from the nose after insertion of the airway is not an indication to remove it. In fact, it is probably better to keep the nasopharyngeal airway in place so as not to disturb the clot or reactivate the bleeding.

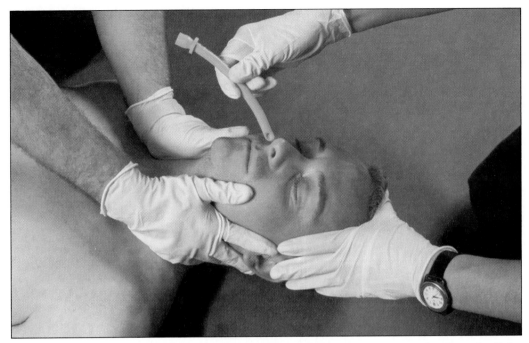

Figure 4-10 *The nasopharyngeal airway is inserted with the bevel slid along the septum or floor of the nasal cavity.*

Oropharyngeal airways are designed to keep the tongue off the posterior pharyngeal wall and thereby help maintain a patent airway (see Figure 4-11 and turn to Chapter 5 for techniques of insertion). Special oropharyngeal airways are available. One, the Williams airway intubator, has a large circular opening through which an endotracheal tube can be inserted or suctioning can be done. It is designed as an intubator guide. Other varieties of oropharyngeal airways include those with proximal ends that protrude from the lips and are designed to be used with balloon masks that seal the mouth and nose.

Esophageal Gastric Tube Airways (EGTA) are designed to be inserted into the esophagus at a level beyond the carina. A cuff is then inflated to reduce the likelihood of gastric distension or regurgitation during bag-valve mask or demand-valve mask ventilation (see Appendix A, "Optional Skills").

The *pharyngotracheal* (PTL) airway is a combination of the EOA and an endotracheal tube and represents an attempt to solve the problem of possible intratracheal placement of the EOA, as well as seeking to provide for tracheal ventilation should blind insertion result in intratracheal positioning. This is an airway device that incorporates two tubes and a balloon that can be inflated to fill the oropharynx (see Appendix A, "Optional Skills").

The esophageal tracheal combitube (Combitube®) is a double lumen tube like the PTL airway. It has both a distal balloon to seal the esophagus to help prevent regurgitation and a proximal balloon to seal the pharynx to help prevent air from escaping from the mouth and nose. The pharyngeal balloon can also help prevent blood and other foreign material from being aspirated (see Appendix A, "Optional Skills).

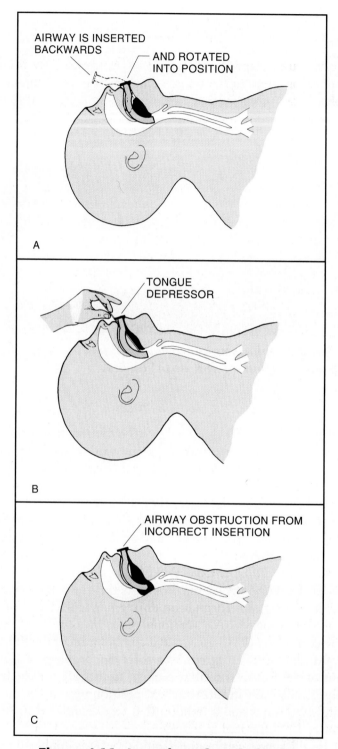

AIRWAY IS INSERTED
BACKWARDS
AND ROTATED
INTO POSITION

A

TONGUE
DEPRESSOR

B

AIRWAY OBSTRUCTION FROM
INCORRECT INSERTION

C

Figure 4-11 *Insertion of oral airway.*

OXYGENATION

Patients who are injured need supplemental oxygen, especially if they are unconscious. It is well recognized that patients suffering from head injury are frequently hypoxic. Supplemental oxygen can be supplied by simple face mask run at 10 to 12 L/min. This will provide the patient with about 40 to 50% oxygen. Non-rebreathing masks with a reservoir bag with oxygen flow rates into the bag of 12 to 15 L/min can provide 60 to 90% oxygen to the patient. Nasal cannulae are well tolerated by most patients, but provide only about 25 to 30% oxygen to the patient.

Supplemental oxygen must be used to ensure adequate oxygenation when you perform positive pressure ventilation. Oxygenation must be supplemented during mouth-to-mouth ventilation by running oxygen at 10 to 12 L/min through the oxygen nipple attached to most masks or by placing the oxygen tubing under the mask and running it at the same rate. Alternatively, you can increase the oxygen percentage delivered during mouth-to-mouth breathing by placing a nasal cannula on yourself. This increases the delivered oxygen percentage from 17% to about 30%.

Resuscitator bags require an oxygen flow rate of at least 15 L/min to increase the delivered oxygen from 21% (air) to 40 or 50%. The oxygen percentage delivered to the patient with 15 L/min running into the bag will depend on the rate of ventilation and the refilling time of the bag. Higher percentages will be delivered if the rate is slower and the bag is allowed to refill over 3 seconds. The importance of these factors will be reduced or eliminated if a large (2.5 L) bag reservoir is used or if a demand valve is connected to the reservoir port of the resuscitator bag. If the latter method is used, at no time should the demand valve be activated to fill the bag more quickly. This would produce continuous airway pressures that might be as high as 40 cm H_2O or more.

Oxygen-powered demand valves have the advantage of delivering 100% oxygen to the patient, but the older models do so at very high flow rates (100 L/min). Pressures in the oropharynx can be as high as 40 to 60 cm H_2O, and the use of these high-pressure devices can therefore result in gastric distention, with all its risks and potential for complications. Higher delivered volumes can be expected with these devices because it is possible to seal the mask on the face with both hands. However, with the demand valve it is not possible to feel compliance, and overdistension of the lungs may occur as well as further insufflation of oxygen into the stomach. Chest-wall movement, which is recommended as the endpoint of the inspiratory phase with demand valves, is neither an accurate nor an easily appreciated observation. Because of these disadvantages, high-pressure oxygen-powered resuscitator valves are not recommended for use in trauma patients. Newer demand valves that meet American Heart Association guidelines (oxygen flow rate of 40 L/min at a maximum pressure of 50 ± 5 cm H_2O) appear to provide equal oxygenation but less airway pressure (less gastric distention) than ventilation with a bag-valve device.

Bag-valve-mask devices, or resuscitator bags, are basically fixed-volume ventilators that deliver a volume of about 600 to 800 when squeezed with an adult hand. Several studies have shown that lower volumes are frequently delivered, and some experts recommend a two-person technique to overcome the problem of mask leak. The inflated or balloon face mask allows for a better seal on the face and thus less air leak when ventilating with a bag-valve device. Resuscitator bags offer the advantage of a better appreciation of the patient's compliance. Recent studies suggest that, with proper training, the new 40 L/min demand valves may be at least the equal of the resuscitator bags in this situation. You should follow your medical director's recommendations in instances such as this.

VENTILATION TECHNIQUES

MOUTH TO MOUTH

This is a most reliable and effective method of ventilation, with the advantage of requiring no equipment and a minimum of experience and training. In addition, delivered volumes are consistently adequate since mouth seal is effectively and easily maintained. In addition, compliance can be "felt" more accurately, and high oropharyngeal pressures are therefore less likely. The greatest disadvantage of mouth to mouth is the fact that it delivers only 17% oxygen. You can increase this by placing a nasal cannula on yourself and running it at 6 to 8 L/min, thereby increasing oxygen percentage to about 30%. Further disadvantages include the fact that many patients have copious secretions, bleeding, gastric regurgitation, or a combination of these. This makes this method of ventilation, however efficient, less attractive. The possibility of disease transmission has also become a concern.

MOUTH TO MASK

Most of the disadvantages of mouth-to mouth ventilation can be overcome by interposing a face mask between your mouth and that of the patient. Commercially designed pocket masks are particularly suited for the initial ventilation of many types of patients, and some have a side port for supplemental oxygen. Pocket ventilating masks have consistently been shown to deliver larger volumes than bag-mask devices and do so with a greater percentage of oxygen than mouth-to-mouth ventilation.

Mouth-to-mask ventilation has significant advantages over other methods, and should be more widely used (see Chapter 5).

DEMAND VALVE

In the past the high-pressure demand valves were considered too dangerous to use in multiple-trauma patients. Experience with the newer demand valves that meet American Heart Association guidelines (oxygen flow rate of 40 L/min at a maximum pressure of 50 ± 5 cm H_2O), suggests that these may now be the equal of bag-valve devices for ventilation (Figure 4-12). Because it is more difficult to feel lung

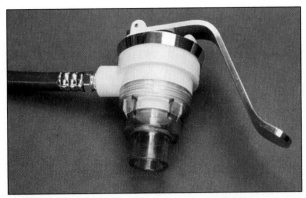

Figure 4-12 *The demand valve. This valve delivers a set flow of 40 L/min at maximum pressure of 50 ± 5 cm H₂O. Do not use unless it meets American Heart Association standards and is allowed by your medical director.*

compliance when ventilating with the newer demand valves, there is still some controversy about their use. Follow your medical director's advice on the use of demand valves.

BAG-VALVE MASK

This descendant of the anesthetic bag is a fixed-volume ventilator with an average delivered volume of about 700 cc. With a two-handed squeeze, over 1 L can be delivered to the patient. Allowing the bag to refill slowly (over 2 to 3 seconds) will substantially increase the percentage of oxygen when no reservoir, or a corrugated tube reservoir is used. The use of a 2.5 L bag reservoir, or the demand-valve reservoir system, removes the influence of rate or refilling time on the percentage of oxygen delivered to the patient.

The most important problem associated with the bag-mask devices is that of volumes delivered. Mask leak is a serious problem, decreasing the volume delivered to the oropharynx by sometimes 40% or more. In addition, masks of conventional design have significant dead space beneath them, thus increasing the challenge to you to provide an adequate volume to the patient. A newer design of a balloon mask which eliminates dead space beneath the mask and provides an improved seal over the nose and mouth has been shown in mannequin studies to decrease mask leak and improve ventilation. It is recommended particularly for trauma patients (see Figure 4-13).

A better seal can sometimes be obtained, and larger volumes delivered, with either a balloon or a conventional mask by the use of an extension tubing attached to the ventilating port of the bag-valve device. This permits the mask to be better seated on the face without a "levering" effect from the rigid ventilating port connector that tends to unseat the mask. With the extension in place, the bag can be more easily compressed, even against the knee or thigh, thus increasing the delivered volume and overcoming any mask leak (see Figure 4-14).

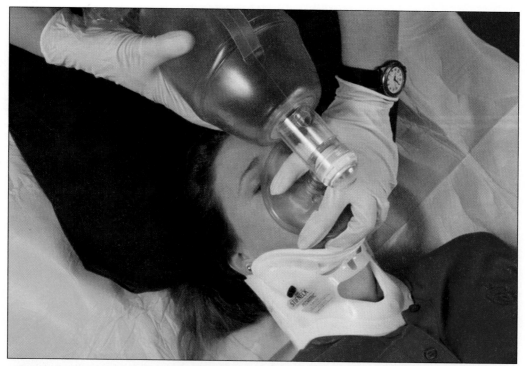

Figure 4-13 *The inflated or balloon mask has been shown to reduce mask leak and provide greater volumes during ventilation with bag-mask devices.*

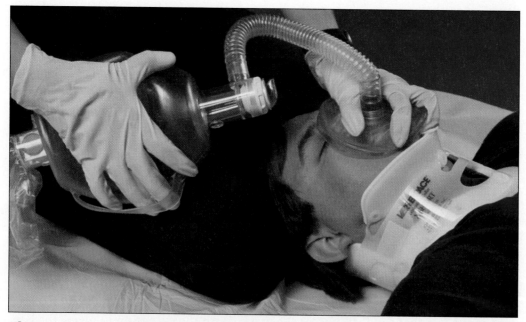

Figure 4-14 *A ventilating port extension attached to a ventilating bag permits a better mask seal and therefore greater delivered volumes. When the bag is compressed against the thigh, as shown here, delivered volumes may be increased further.*

SUMMARY

The trauma patients provide the greatest challenge in airway management. To be successful you must have a clear understanding of the anatomy of the airway as well as be proficient in techniques to open and maintain your patient's airway. You must have the correct equipment organized in a kit that is immediately available when you begin assessment of the trauma patient. To provide adequate ventilation for your patient, you must understand the concepts of tidal volume, minute volume, and lung compliance. Finally, you must become familiar with the various options for control of the airway and develop expertise in performing them.

BIBLIOGRAPHY

1. American Heart Association Committee on Emergency Cardiac Care. "Guidelines for Cardiopulmonary Resuscitation and Emergency Cardiac Care." *Journal of the American Medical Association,* Vol. 268 (1992), p. 2200.

2. Boidin, M. P. "Airway Patency in the Unconscious Patient." *British Journal of Anaesthesiology,* Vol. 57 (1985), pp. 306–310.

3. Jesudian, M. C. S., R. R. Harrison, R. L. Keenan, and others. "Bag-Valve-Mask Ventilation: Two Rescuers Are Better than One: Preliminary Report." *Critical Care Medicine,* Vol. 14 (1985), pp. 403–406.

4. Mosesso V. N., K. Kukitsch, and others. "Comparison of Delivered Volumes and Airway Pressures when Ventilation Through an Endotracheal Tube with Bag-Valve Versus Demand-Valve." *Prehospital and Disaster Medicine,* Vol. 9, no. 1 (1994), pp. 24–28.

5. Salem M. R., A. Y. Wong, M. Mani, and others. "Efficacy of Cricoid Pressure in Preventing Gastric Inflation During Bag-Mask Ventilation in Pediatric Patients." *Anesthesiology,* Vol. 40 (1974), pp. 96–98.

6. Stewart R. D., R. M. Kaplan, B. Pennock, and others. "Influence of Mask Design on Bag-Mask Ventilation." *Annals of Emergency Medicine,* Vol. 14 (1985), pp. 403–406.

7. White, S. J., R. M. Kaplan, and R. D. Stewart. "Manual Detection of Decreased Lung Compliance as a Sign of Tension Pneumothorax (abstr.)." *Annals of Emergency Medicine,* Vol. 16 (1987), p. 518.

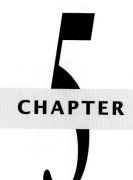

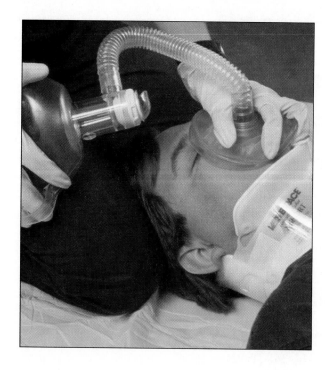

CHAPTER 5

Airway Management Skills

Donna Hastings, EMT-P

OBJECTIVES

Upon completion of this chapter you should be able to:

1. Suction the airway.
2. Insert a nasopharyngeal and oropharyngeal airway.
3. Use the pocket mask.
4. Use the bag-valve mask.

BASIC AIRWAY MANAGEMENT

PROCEDURES

SUCTIONING THE AIRWAY

Use of the hand-powered suction device may also be taught at this time.

1. Attach the suction tubing to the portable suction machine.
2. Turn the device on and test it.
3. Insert the suction tube through the nose or mouth without activating the suction.
4. Activate the suction and withdraw the suction tube.
5. Repeat the procedure as necessary.

INSERTING PHARYNGEAL AIRWAYS

Nasopharyngeal Airway

1. Choose the appropriate size. It should be the largest that will fit easily through the external nares.
2. Lubricate the tube.
3. Insert it straight back through the right nostril with the beveled edge of the airway toward the septum.
4. To insert in the left nostril, turn the airway upside down so that the bevel is toward the septum; then insert straight back through the nostril until you reach the posterior pharynx. At this point, turn the airway over 180 degrees and insert it down the pharynx until it lies behind the tongue.

Oropharyngeal Airway

1. Choose the appropriate size.
2. Open the airway:
   a. Scissor maneuver
   b. Jaw lift
   c. Tongue blade
3. Insert the airway gently without pushing the tongue back into the pharynx.
   a. Insert the airway upside down and rotate into place. This method should not be used for children.
   b. Insert the airway under direct vision using a tongue blade.

USING A POCKET MASK WITH SUPPLEMENTAL OXYGEN

1. Have your partner stabilize the neck in a neutral position (or apply a stabilization device).

2. Connect the oxygen tubing to the oxygen cylinder and the mask.

3. Open the oxygen cylinder and set the flow rate at 12 L/min.

4. Open the airway.

5. Insert the oral airway.

6. Place the mask on the face and establish a good seal.

7. Ventilate mouth-to-mask with enough volume (about 800–1000 cc) to cause the green light to come on in the recording mannequin.

USING THE BAG-VALVE MASK

1. Stabilize the neck with a suitable device.

2. Connect the oxygen tubing to the bag-valve system and oxygen cylinder.

3. Attach the oxygen reservoir to the bag-valve mask.

4. Open the oxygen cylinder and set the flow rate at 12 L/min.

5. Select the proper size mask and attach it to the bag-valve device.

6. Open the airway.

7. Insert the oral airway (do not insert if the patient has a gag reflex).

8. Place the mask on the face and have your partner establish and maintain a good seal.

9. Using both hands ventilate with about 800–1000 cc.

10. If you are forced to ventilate without a partner, use one hand to maintain a face seal and the other hand to squeeze the bag. This decreases the volume of ventilation because less volume is produced by only one hand squeezing the bag.

11. All trauma patients who have a decreased level of consciousness should be hyperventilated with 100% oxygen at a rate of one ventilation about every 2 seconds (24–30 breaths per minute). Using procedure steps 1–9, practice hyperventilation until you feel comfortable with the rhythm of ventilating at the rate of 24–30 breaths per minute.

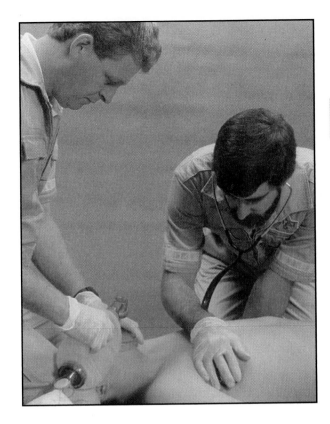

Thoracic Trauma

Andrew B. Peitzman, M.D., F.A.C.S.,
and Paul Paris, M.D., F.A.C.E.P.

OBJECTIVES

Upon completion of this chapter you should be able to:

1. Identify the major symptoms of thoracic trauma.

2. Describe the signs of thoracic trauma.

3. State the immediate life threatening thoracic injuries.

4. Explain the pathophysiology and management of an open pneumothorax.

5. Describe the clinical signs of a tension pneumothorax in conjunction with appropriate management.

6. Explain the hypovolemic and respiratory compromise pathophysiology and management in massive hemothorax.

7. Define flail chest in relation to associated physical findings and management.

8. Identify the triad of physical findings in the diagnosis of cardiac tamponade.

9. Explain the cardiac involvement and management associated with blunt injury to the chest.

10. Summarize other injuries and their appropriate management.

Twenty-five percent of trauma deaths are due entirely to thoracic injuries, and half of trauma victims with multiple injuries have an associated chest injury. Two-thirds of these patients with fatal thoracic trauma are alive when they reach the emergency department and only 15% require surgery. Thus, these are salvageable trauma victims. The goal of this chapter is to enable you to recognize signs and symptoms of major thoracic injury and provide appropriate care. Major thoracic injury may result from motor vehicle accidents, falls, gunshot wounds, crush injuries, stab wounds, or other mechanisms.

ANATOMY

The thorax is a bony cavity that is formed by 12 pairs of ribs that join posteriorly with the thoracic spine and anteriorly with the sternum. The intercostal neurovascular bundle runs along the inferior surface of each rib (see Figure 6-1).

The inner side of the thoracic cavity and the lung itself are lined with a thin layer of tissue, the pleura. The space between the two pleural layers is normally only a potential space. However, this space may be occupied by air, forming a pneumothorax, or blood, forming a hemothorax. This potential space can hold 3 liters of fluid in an adult.

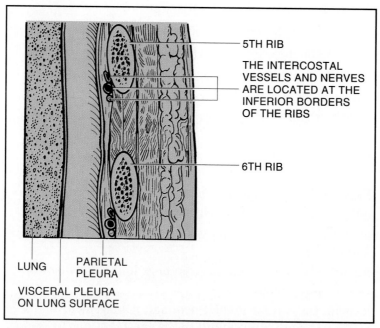

Figure 6-1 *Rib with intercostal vessels and nerve.*

As shown in Figure 6-2, one lung occupies each thoracic cavity. Between the two chest cavities is the mediastinum, which contains the heart, aorta, superior and inferior vena cava, trachea, major bronchi, and esophagus. The spinal cord is protected by the vertebral column. The diaphragm separates the thoracic organs from the abdominal cavity. The upper abdominal organs, including the spleen, liver, kidneys, pancreas, and stomach, are protected by the lower rib cage (see Figure 6-3). Any patient with a penetrating thoracic wound at the level of the nipples (fourth intercostal space) or lower should be assumed to have an abdominal injury as well as thoracic injury. Similarly, blunt deceleration injuries such as steering wheel injuries often injure both thoracic and abdominal structures.

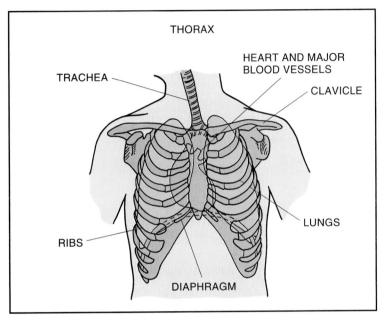

Figure 6-2 *Thorax.*

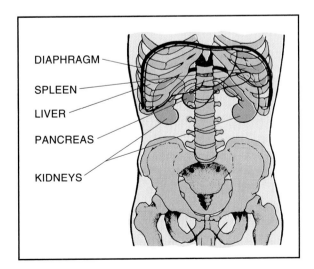

Figure 6-3 *Intrathoracic abdomen.*

PATHOPHYSIOLOGY

When evaluating a victim with probable thoracic trauma, always follow the BTLS assessment priorities (Chapter 2) to avoid missing life-threatening injuries. During the initial survey, search for the most dangerous injuries first to give your patient the best chance for survival. As with any trauma victim, the mechanism of injury is very important in caring for the thoracic trauma victim. Thoracic injuries may be the result of blunt trauma or penetrating objects. With blunt trauma, the force is distributed over a large area and visceral injuries occur from deceleration, sheering forces, compression, or bursting. Penetrating injuries, usually gunshot wounds or stab wounds, distribute the forces of injury over a smaller area. However, the trajectory of a bullet is often unpredictable, and all thoracic structures are at risk.

ASSESSMENT

The major symptoms of chest injury include shortness of breath, chest pain, and respiratory distress. The signs indicative of chest injury include shock, hemoptysis, cyanosis, chest wall contusion, flail chest, open wounds, distended neck veins, tracheal deviation, or subcutaneous emphysema. Check the lung fields for presence and equality of breath sounds, and life-threatening thoracic injuries should be identified immediately.

Major thoracic injuries to identify may be remembered as the "deadly dozen." The immediately life-threatening injuries include

1. Airway obstruction
2. Open pneumothorax
3. Tension pneumothorax
4. Massive hemothorax
5. Flail chest
6. Cardiac tamponade

Potentially life-threatening injuries include

7. Traumatic aortic rupture
8. Bronchial disruption
9. Myocardial contusion
10. Diaphragmatic tear
11. Esophageal injury
12. Pulmonary contusion

AIRWAY OBSTRUCTION

Airway management remains a major challenge in the care of any multiple-trauma victim. This has been discussed in Chapter 4. Always assume there is an associated cervical spine injury when securing the airway.

OPEN PNEUMOTHORAX

This is caused by a penetrating thoracic injury and may present as a sucking chest wound. The signs and symptoms are usually proportional to the size of the chest wall defect (see Figure 6-4).

Normal respiration involves a negative pressure being generated inside the chest by diaphragmatic contraction. As air is drawn through the upper airway, the lungs expand. With a large open wound of the chest, the path of least resistance for airflow is through the chest wall defect. This air will only enter the pleural space. It will not enter the lung and therefore will not contribute to oxygenation of the blood. Ventilation is impaired and hypoxia results.

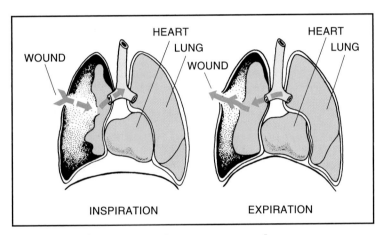

Figure 6-4 *Open pneumothorax.*

Management of Open Pneumothorax

1. Ensure an airway.
2. Promptly close the chest wall defect by any available means. You may accomplish this with a defibrillation pad, vaseline gauze, rubber glove, or plastic dressing. The risk of placing an occlusive dressing is that the patient may then develop a tension pneumothorax. To circumvent this problem, tape the occlusive dressing on three sides to produce a flutter valve: air can escape from the chest but will not enter. See Figure 6-5. A chest tube will be needed ultimately, followed by operative closure of the chest wall defect.
3. Administer oxygen.
4. Insert a large-bore I.V.
5. Monitor the heart if you carry monitoring equipment.
6. Transport rapidly to the appropriate hospital.

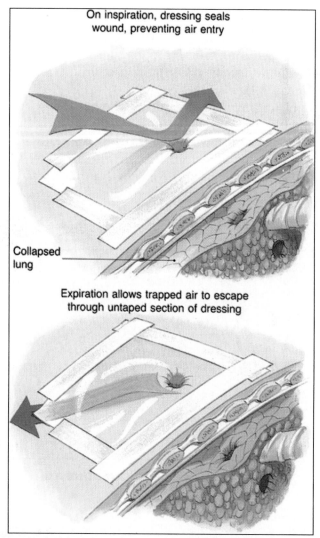

On inspiration, dressing seals
wound, preventing air entry

Collapsed
lung

Expiration allows trapped air to escape
through untaped section of dressing

Figure 6-5 *Treatment of sucking chest wound.*

TENSION PNEUMOTHORAX

This injury can occur, when a one-way valve is created, from either blunt or penetrating trauma. Air can enter but not leave the pleural space (see Figure 6-6). This causes collapse of the affected lung and will then push the mediastinum in the opposite direction with resultant kinking of the superior and inferior vena cava with loss of venous return to the heart. Shift of the trachea and mediastinum away from the side of the tension pneumothorax will also compromise ventilation of the other lung, although this is a late phenomenon.

Clinical signs of a tension pneumothorax include dyspnea, anxiety, tachypnea, diminished breath sounds and hyperresonance to percussion on the affected side, hypotension, and distended neck veins. Tracheal deviation is a late finding and its absence does not rule out the presence of a tension pneumothorax. The develop-

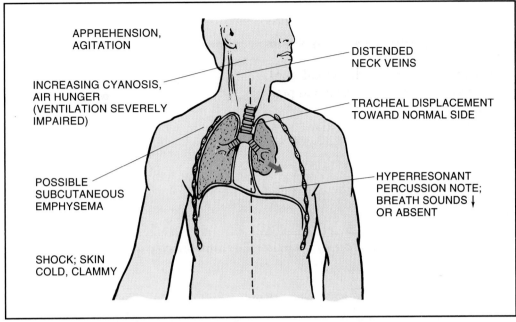

APPREHENSION, AGITATION

DISTENDED NECK VEINS

INCREASING CYANOSIS, AIR HUNGER (VENTILATION SEVERELY IMPAIRED)

TRACHEAL DISPLACEMENT TOWARD NORMAL SIDE

POSSIBLE SUBCUTANEOUS EMPHYSEMA

HYPERRESONANT PERCUSSION NOTE; BREATH SOUNDS ↓ OR ABSENT

SHOCK; SKIN COLD, CLAMMY

Figure 6-6 *Physical findings of tension pneumothorax.*

ment of decreased lung compliance (difficulty in squeezing the bag-valve device) should always alert you to the possibility of a tension pneumothorax.

Management of a Tension Pneumothorax

1. Establish an open airway.
2. Administer high-concentration oxygen.
3. Rapidly transport to the appropriate hospital so that chest decompression can be performed.
4. Notify Medical Direction.

MASSIVE HEMOTHORAX

Blood in the pleural space is a hemothorax (see Figure 6-7). A *massive hemothorax* occurs as a result of at least 1500 cc blood loss into the thoracic cavity. Each thoracic cavity may contain up to 3000 cc of blood. Massive hemothorax is more often due to penetrating than blunt trauma, but either injury may disrupt a major pulmonary or systemic vessel. As blood accumulates within the pleural space, the lung on the affected side is compressed. If enough blood accumulates (rare), the mediastinum will be shifted away from the hemothorax. The inferior and superior vena cava and the contralateral lung are compressed. Thus the ongoing blood loss is complicated by hypoxemia.

	TENSION PNEUMOTHORAX	HEMOTHORAX
PRIMARY PRESENTING SYMPTOM	DIFFICULTY BREATHING, THEN SHOCK	SHOCK, THEN DIFFICULTY BREATHING
NECK VEINS	USUALLY DISTENDED	USUALLY FLAT
BREATH SOUNDS	DECREASED OR ABSENT ON SIDE OF INJURY	DECREASED OR ABSENT ON SIDE OF INJURY
PERCUSSION OF CHEST	HYPERRESONANT	DULL
TRACHEAL DEVIATION AWAY FROM THE SIDE OF THE INJURY	MAY BE PRESENT AS A LATE SIGN	USUALLY NOT PRESENT

Table 6-1 *Comparison of Tension Pneumothorax and Hemothorax*

Signs and symptoms of massive hemothorax are produced by both hypovolemia and respiratory compromise. The patient may be hypotensive from blood loss and compression of the heart or great veins. Anxiety and confusion are produced by hypovolemia and hypoxemia. Clinical signs of hypovolemic shock may be apparent. The neck veins are usually flat secondary to profound hypovolemia, but may *rarely* be distended due to mediastinal compression. Other signs of hemothorax include decreased breath sounds and dullness to percussion on the affected side. See Figure 6-7 for comparison of tension pneumothorax and massive hemothorax.

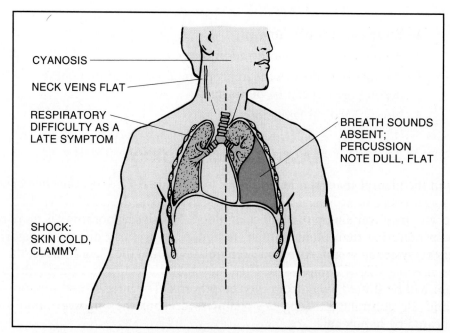

Figure 6-7 *Physical findings of massive hemothorax.*

Management of Massive Hemothorax

    1. Secure an airway.

    2. Apply high-flow oxygen.

    3. Rapidly transport to the appropriate hospital.

    4. Notify Medical Direction.

FLAIL CHEST

This occurs when three or more adjacent ribs are fractured in at least two places. The result is a segment of the chest wall that is not in continuity with the thorax. A lateral flail chest or anterior flail chest (sternal separation) may result. With posterior rib fractures, the heavy musculature usually prevents the occurrence of a flail segment. The flail segment moves with paradoxical motion relative to the rest of the chest wall (see Figures 6-8 and 6-9). The force necessary to produce this injury also bruises the underlying lung tissue and this pulmonary contusion will also contribute to the hypoxia. The patient is at risk for the development of a hemothorax or pneumothorax. With a large flail segment, the patient may be in marked respiratory distress. Palpation of the chest wall may reveal crepitus in addition to the abnormal respiratory motion.

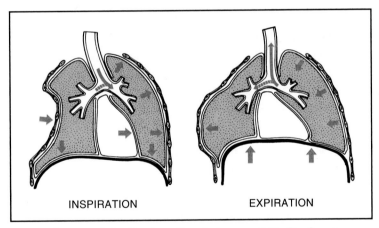

INSPIRATION   EXPIRATION

Figure 6-8 *Pathophysiology of flail chest.*

Management of Flail Chest

    1. Ensure an airway.

    2. Administer oxygen.

    3. Assist ventilation if required. Remember that pneumothorax is commonly associated with a flail chest.

    4. Rapidly transport to the appropriate hospital.

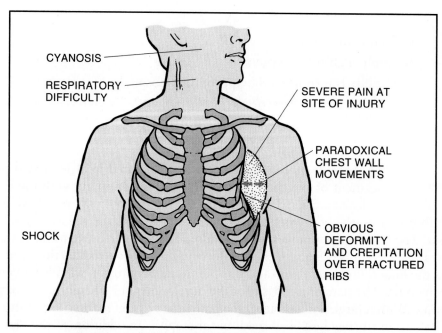

Figure 6-9 *Physical findings of flail chest.*

5. Stabilize the flail segment with manual pressure then bulky dressings taped to the chest wall. This is usually not necessary until the patient is stabilized on a backboard. Trying to maintain manual pressure on a flail segment while performing log-rolling may be dangerous to maintaining a stable spine (see Figure 6-10).

6. Notify Medical Direction.

7. Monitor the heart if you carry monitoring equipment. Associated myocardial trauma is frequent.

CARDIAC TAMPONADE

This injury is usually due to penetrating injury. The pericardial sac is an inelastic membrane that surrounds the heart. If blood collects rapidly between the heart and pericardium from a cardiac injury, the ventricles of the heart will be compressed. A small amount of pericardial blood may compromise cardiac filling. As the compression of the ventricles increases, the heart is less able to refill and cardiac output falls.

Diagnosis of cardiac tamponade classically relies upon the triad of hypotension, distended neck veins and muffled heart sounds. Muffled heart sounds may be very difficult to appreciate in the prehospital setting. The patient may have paradoxical pulse. If the patient loses his peripheral pulse during inspiration, this is suggestive of a paradoxical pulse and the presence of cardiac tamponade. The major

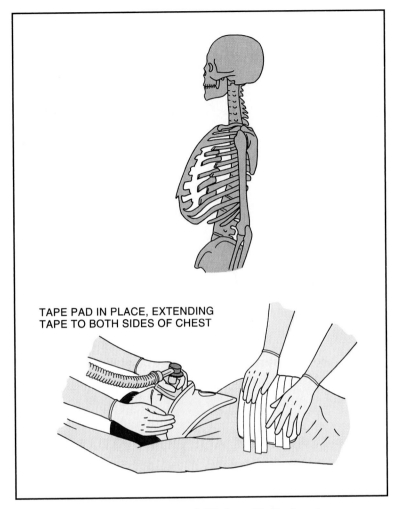

TAPE PAD IN PLACE, EXTENDING
TAPE TO BOTH SIDES OF CHEST

Figure 6-10 *Stabilizing flail chest.*

differential diagnosis in the field is tension pneumothorax. With cardiac tamponade, the patient will be in shock with a midline trachea and equal breath sounds (see
Figure 6-11).

Management of Cardiac Tamponade

1. Ensure an airway and administer oxygen.
2. This lesion is rapidly fatal and cannot be readily treated in
   the field. Load the patient and proceed rapidly to the
   appropriate hospital.
3. Notify Medical Direction.
4. Monitor the heart if you carry monitoring equipment.

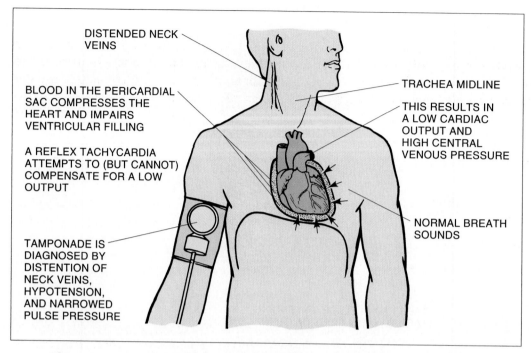

DISTENDED NECK VEINS

BLOOD IN THE PERICARDIAL SAC COMPRESSES THE HEART AND IMPAIRS VENTRICULAR FILLING

A REFLEX TACHYCARDIA ATTEMPTS TO (BUT CANNOT) COMPENSATE FOR A LOW OUTPUT

TAMPONADE IS DIAGNOSED BY DISTENTION OF NECK VEINS, HYPOTENSION, AND NARROWED PULSE PRESSURE

TRACHEA MIDLINE

THIS RESULTS IN A LOW CARDIAC OUTPUT AND HIGH CENTRAL VENOUS PRESSURE

NORMAL BREATH SOUNDS

Figure 6-11 *Pathophysiology and physical findings of cardiac tamponade.*

TRAUMATIC AORTIC RUPTURE

This is the most common cause of death in motor vehicle accidents or falls from heights. Ninety percent of these patients die immediately. For the survivors, salvage is feasible with prompt diagnosis and surgery. Traumatic thoracic aortic tears usually are due to deceleration injury with heart and aortic arch moving suddenly anteriorly, transecting the aorta where it is fixed at the ligamentum arteriosum. Of the 10% who do not exsanguinate promptly, the aortic tear will be contained temporarily by surrounding tissues and the adventitia. However, this is temporary and will usually rupture unless surgically repaired.

The diagnosis of a contained thoracic aortic laceration is impossible in the field and may be missed even in the hospital. The history from the scene is critically important since many of these patients have no obvious signs of chest trauma. Information regarding damage to the car or steering wheel with a deceleration injury or the height from which the patient fell are vital. Infrequently, the patient may present with upper extremity hypertension and diminished lower extremity pulses.

Management of Potential Aortic Tears

1. Ensure an airway.
2. Administer oxygen.
3. Rapidly transport to the appropriate hospital.
4. Notify Medical Direction.

TRACHEAL OR BRONCHIAL TREE INJURY

These injuries may be the result of penetrating or blunt trauma. Penetrating upper airway injuries often have associated major vascular injuries and extensive tissue destruction. Blunt trauma may present with subtle findings. Blunt injury usually ruptures the trachea or mainstem bronchus near the carina. Presenting signs of blunt or penetrating injury include subcutaneous emphysema of the chest, face, or neck or an associated pneumothorax or hemothorax.

Management of the Airway with Tracheal Injuries

This may be quite difficult, and emergency surgical intervention may be needed to obtain an airway. Thus, prompt transport to the hospital is important. Observing the patient for signs of a pneumothorax or hemothorax is also necessary.

MYOCARDIAL CONTUSION

This is a potentially lethal lesion resulting from blunt chest injury. Blunt injury to the anterior chest is transmitted via the sternum to the heart that lies immediately posterior to it (see Figure 6-12). Cardiac injuries from this mechanism may include valvular rupture, pericardial tamponade, or cardiac rupture, but myocardial contusion most commonly occurs. This bruising of the heart is basically the same injury as an acute myocardial infarction and also presents with chest pain, dysrhythmia, or cardiogenic shock (rare). In the field, cardiogenic shock cannot be distinguished from cardiac tamponade. The chest pain may be difficult to differentiate from the associated musculoskeletal discomfort that the patient also suffers as a result of the injury. All patients with blunt anterior chest trauma should be presumed to have a myocardial contusion.

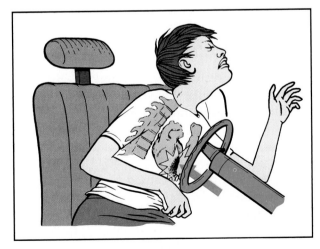

Figure 6-12 *Pathophysiology of myocardial contusion.*

Management of Myocardial Contusion

1. Administer oxygen.
2. Rapid transport to appropriate trauma center.
3. Monitor the heart if you carry monitoring equipment.

DIAPHRAGMATIC TEARS

Tears in the diaphragm may result from a severe blow to the abdomen. A sudden increase in intra-abdominal pressure, such as a seat belt injury or kick to the abdomen, may tear the diaphragm and allow herniation of the abdominal organs into the thoracic cavity. This occurs more commonly on the left than the right, since the liver protects the right hemidiaphragm. Blunt trauma produces large radial tears in the diaphragm. Penetrating trauma may also produce holes in the diaphragm, but these tend to be small.

Traumatic diaphragmatic hernia is difficult to diagnose even in the hospital. The herniation of abdominal contents into the thoracic cavity may cause marked respiratory distress. On examination, the breath sounds may be diminished and infrequently bowel sounds may be heard when the chest is auscultated. The abdomen may appear scaphoid if a large quantity of abdominal contents are in the chest.

Management of Diaphragmatic Rupture

1. Ensure an airway.
2. Administer oxygen.
3. Transport the patient to the hospital.
4. Notify Medical Direction.

ESOPHAGEAL INJURY

This injury is usually produced by penetrating trauma. Management of associated trauma including airway or vascular injuries is generally more pressing than the esophageal injury. However, esophageal injury is lethal if unrecognized in the hospital.

PULMONARY CONTUSION

This is a common chest injury resulting from blunt trauma. This bruising of the lung may produce marked hypoxemia. Management consists of assisted ventilation if indicated, oxygen administration, and transport.

OTHER CHEST INJURIES

Impalement injuries of the chest may be caused by any penetrating object, usually a knife. As in other areas of the body, the object should not be removed in the field. Stabilize the object, ensure an airway, and transport the patient.

Traumatic asphyxia is an important set of physical findings. The term is a misnomer since the condition is not caused by asphyxia. The syndrome results from a severe compression injury to the chest, such as a steering wheel injury, conveyor belt injury or compression of the chest under a heavy object. The sudden compression of the heart and mediastinum transmits this force to the capillaries of the neck and head. The victims appear similar to those of strangulation with cyanosis and swelling of the head and neck. The tongue and lips are swollen, and conjunctival hemorrhage is evident. The skin below the level of the crush injury to the chest will be pink unless there are other problems.

Traumatic asphyxia indicates that the patient has suffered a severe blunt thoracic injury and major thoracic injuries are likely to be present. Management includes (1) airway maintenance, (2) treating other injuries, and (3) rapid transport.

Similarly, *sternal fractures* indicate that the patient has suffered marked blunt trauma to the anterior chest. These patients should be presumed to have a myocardial contusion. Diagnosis can be made by palpation.

A *fracture of the scapula,* first or second rib requires a large force. The incidence of associated major thoracic vascular injury is high, and these patients should be given oxygen and promptly transported.

Simple pneumothorax may result from blunt or penetrating trauma. Fractured ribs are the usual cause in blunt trauma. This is caused by accumulation of air within the potential space between the visceral and parietal pleura. The lung may be totally or partially collapsed as the air continues to accrue in the thoracic cavity. In a healthy patient this should not acutely compromise ventilation, if a tension pneumothorax does not evolve. Patients with less respiratory reserve may not tolerate even a simple pneumothorax well.

Diagnosis of a pneumothorax is based on pleuritic chest pain, dyspnea, decreased breath sounds on the affected side and hypertympany to percussion. Close observation is required in anticipation of the patient developing a pneumothorax.

Simple rib fracture is the most frequent injury to the chest. If the patient does not have an associated pneumothorax or hemothorax, the major problem is pain. This pain will prohibit the patient from breathing adequately. On palpation, the area of rib fracture will be tender and may be unstable. Give oxygen and monitor for pneumothorax or hemothorax while encouraging the patient to breathe deeply.

SUMMARY

Chest injuries are common and often life-threatening in the multiple-trauma patient. If you follow the BTLS assessment priorities you will identify the injuries while performing the primary survey. The primary goals in treating the patient with chest trauma are (1) ensuring an airway while protecting the cervical spine, (2) administering high-flow oxygen, and (3) monitoring the vital signs. These are often "load-and-go" patients.

The thoracic injuries discussed are life threatening, but treatable by prompt intervention and transport to the appropriate hospital. It is mandatory that the injuries presented are recognized in the field and treated appropriately to salvage these patients.

BIBLIOGRAPHY

1. American College of Surgeons Committee on Trauma. *Advanced Trauma Life Support,* pp. 19–104. Chicago: American College of Surgeons, 1989.

2. Blair, E., C. Topuzulu, and R. S. Deane. "Major Chest Trauma." *Current Problems in Surgery* (May 1969), 2–69.

3. Jones, K. W. "Thoracic Trauma." *Surgical Clinics of North America* (1980), pp. 60–95.

4. Kirsh, M. M., D. M. Behrendt, M. B. Orringer, and others. "The Treatment of Acute Traumatic Rupture of the Aorta: A 10–Year Experience." *Annals of Surgery* (1976), pp. 184–308.

5. Richardson, J.D., L. Adams, and L. M. Flint. "Selective Management of Flail Chest and Pulmonary Contusion." *Annals of Surgery,* Vol. 196, no. 4 (1982), pp. 481–487.

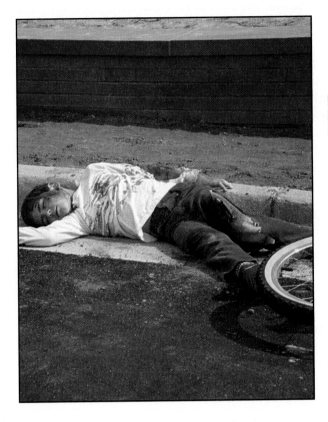

CHAPTER 7

Shock Evaluation and Management

Raymond L. Fowler, M.D., F.A.C.E.P, Paul E. Pepe, M.D., F.A.C.E.P., F.C.C.M., and Roger J. Lewis, M.D., Ph.D., F.A.C.E.P.

UPON COMPLETION OF THIS CHAPTER YOU SHOULD BE ABLE TO:

1. List the four components necessary for normal tissue perfusion.

2. Describe symptoms and signs of hemorrhagic shock.

3. Explain the pathophysiolgy of hemorrhagic shock and compare to the pathophysiology of "high-space" shock.

4. Describe the four common clinical shock syndromes.

5. Describe the management of

    a. External hemorrhage that can be controlled

    b. External hemorrhage that cannot be controlled

    c. Internal hemorrhage

    d. Nonhemorrhagic shock syndromes

6. Discuss the routine priorities in the prehospital management of shock.

7. Discuss the current indications and contraindications for the use of the antishock garment in the treatment of traumatic shock.

The management of shock has been the subject of intensive research during the past few years, and there have been many changes in the recommendations for prehospital treatment of the patient with hemorrhagic shock. While there have been some excellent studies on the treatment of hemorrhagic shock secondary to penetrating trauma, there has not been enough research on the treatment of hemorrhagic shock secondary to blunt trauma. This chapter represents the present knowledge about pathophysiology and treatment of traumatic shock.

BASIC PATHOPHYSIOLGY

The normal perfusion of body tissues requires four intact components:

1. An intact vascular system to deliver oxygenated blood throughout the body
2. Adequate air exchange in the lungs to allow oxygen to enter the blood
3. An adequate volume of fluid in the vascular system, including blood cells and plasma
4. A functioning pump: the heart

Maintenance of these components can be related to the basic tenets of emergency care:

1. Maintain the airway.
2. Control oxygenation and ventilation.
3. Control bleeding.
4. Maintain circulation.

All body tissues require oxygen. "Shock," as classically defined, is a condition that occurs when tissue perfusion with oxygen becomes inadequate. The loss of red blood cells in hemorrhaging patients results in less oxygen transport to the body tissues. The result is that the cells of the body become "shocked," and grave changes in body tissue begin to occur. Eventually, cell death follows.

Deprived of oxygen, cells begin to use "backup" processes that inefficiently utilize energy sources and produce toxic by-products. Although these "backup" (anaerobic) processes may postpone cellular death for a time, the oxygen lack is compounded by the toxic by-products that can poison certain cellular functions. Eventually, lactic acid spills over into the bloodstream and creates systemic acidosis that further disrupts cellular activity. With weakening respiratory muscle function, the patient may develop respiratory failure with worsening hypoxia.

In response to inadequate oxygen delivery, the body responds with increased sympathetic tone and release of circulating catecholamines (epinephrine and norepinephrine). These increase the heart rate, vasoconstrict peripheral blood vessels, and increase the respiratory rate.

Shock, therefore, is a cellular process with clinical manifestations. The patient with shock may be pale, diaphoretic, and tachycardic. At the cellular level, the patient's cells are starving for oxygen. "Shock," therefore, is a condition in which poor tissue perfusion may severely and possibly permanently damage the organs of the body. The clinical signs and symptoms of the patient in shock imply critical processes threatening every vulnerable cell in the patient's body, particularly those in vital organs.

ASSESSMENT: SIGNS AND SYMPTOMS OF SHOCK

When first considering the concept of shock, you must understand that "shock" is a condition that you can observe during assessment of the patient. The initial diagnosis of the shock state can be made from the physical assessment findings. Although shock states are often associated with systemic arterial hypotension (low blood pressure), a patient with a normal blood pressure may be in shock. Conversely, a patient with low blood pressure (e.g. 80 mm Hg systolic) may not be in shock. However, blood pressure should be monitored frequently as one tool to judge whether organ perfusion is adequate. Patients will vary as to the blood pressure needed to maintain *adequate* perfusion. The question of "how low can you go" and still maintain adequate perfusion has not been answered at this time. You must rely on medical direction for results of current research regarding shock. Assessment tools other than measuring the blood pressure must also be used to recognize the trauma patient in shock. The classic symptoms and signs associated with hemorrhage-associated shock include

1. Weakness: caused by tissue hypoxia and acidosis
2. Thirst: caused by hypovolemia (especially with relatively low fluid amounts in the blood vessels)
3. Pallor: caused by catecholamine-induced vasoconstriction and/or loss of red blood cells
4. Tachycardia: caused by catecholamines' effect on the heart
5. Tachypnea (elevated respiratory rate): caused in response to stress, catecholamines, acidosis, and hypoxia
6. Diaphoresis (sweating): caused by catecholamines' effect on sweat glands
7. Decreased urinary output: caused by hypovolemia, hypoxia, and circulating catecholamines (important to remember in interhospital transfers)
8. Diminished peripheral pulses: the "thready" pulse, caused by vasoconstriction, fast heart rate, and loss of blood volume
9. Hypotension: caused by hypovolemia, either absolute or relative (see later paragraphs for a discussion of "relative hypovolemia")
10. Altered sensorium (confusion, restlessness, combativeness, unconsciousness): caused by decreased cerebral perfusion, acidosis, and catecholamine stimulation

11. Cardiac arrest: caused by critical organ failure secondary to blood or fluid loss, hypoxia, and occasionally arrhythmia caused by catecholamine stimulation

To summarize, many of the symptoms of classic hemorrhage-associated shock are caused by the release of catecholamines. When the brain senses that there is not enough oxygen perfusion to the tissues, it sends messages down the spinal cord to the sympathetic nervous system and to the adrenal glands, which release circulating catecholamines (epinephrine and norepinephrine). The circulating catecholamines cause the tachycardia, anxiousness, diaphoresis, and vasoconstriction. The vasoconstriction shunts blood away from the skin to the vital organs, causing an initial rise in the blood pressure and causing the skin to be pale.

Decreased perfusion causes weakness and thirst initially and, later, a decreased level of consciousness (confusion, restlessness, or combativeness), worsening pallor, hypotension, and unconsciousness followed by cardiac arrest.

As shock continues, the prolonged tissue hypoxia leads to worsening acidosis. This acidosis can cause a loss of response to catecholamines, which may result in a drop in blood pressure. Eventually, the hypoxia and acidosis cause cardiac dysfunction and death.

Although the response to posttraumatic hemorrhage may vary from individual to individual, many patients will have the following classic patterns of "early" and "late" shock:

Early shock (loss of approximately 15 to 25% of the blood volume): enough to stimulate slight to moderate tachycardia, pallor, narrowed pulse pressure, thirst, weakness, and possibly delayed capillary refill

Late shock (loss of approximately 30 to 45% of the blood volume): enough to cause *hypotension* as well as the other symptoms of hypovolemic shock listed earlier

During the primary survey, "early" shock presents as a fast pulse with pallor and diaphoresis while "late" shock may present as weak pulse or loss of the peripheral pulse.

Prolonged capillary refill was previously thought to be useful for detecting early shock. Low blood volume and catecholamine-induced vasoconstriction cause decreased perfusion of the capillary bed in the skin. Capillary refill is tested by pressing on the palm of the hand or, in a child, squeezing the whole foot. The test is suspicious for shock if the blanched area remains pale for longer than 2 seconds. Scientific evaluation of this test has shown it to have a high correlation with late shock but of little value for detecting early shock. The test was associated with both frequent false positive as well as false negative results. Measurement of capillary refill is useful for small children in whom it is difficult to get an accurate blood pressure, but it is of little use for detecting early shock in adults.

THE "SHOCK SYNDROMES"

While the most common shock states seen in trauma patients are associated with hemorrhage and the accompanying hypovolemia, there are three other major causes of traumatic shock. These four shock states can be categorized according to their causes as follows:

1. *Low-volume shock* (absolute hypovolemia): caused by hemorrhage, or other major body fluid loss
2. *High-space shock* (relative hypovolemia): caused by spinal injury, syncope, severe head injury, vasomotor injury from hypoxia
3. *Mechanical (obstructive) shock:* caused by pericardial tamponade or tension pneumothorax
4. *Hypoxemic shock:* caused by respiratory failure from lung injury or airway obstruction/disruption

There are notable differences in the appearance of patients with these conditions, and it is critical that you be aware of the signs and symptoms that accompany each one.

LOW-VOLUME SHOCK (ABSOLUTE HYPOVOLEMIA)

Loss of blood from injury is called posttraumatic hemorrhage, and in addition to head injury, hemorrhagic shock is the number one cause of preventable death from injury. The amount of volume that the blood vessels *can* hold is many liters more than that which actually flows through the vasculature. The sympathetic nervous system keeps the vessels constricted, reducing their volume and maintaining blood pressure high enough to perfuse vital organs. If blood volume is lost, "sensors" in the major vessels signal the adrenal gland and the nerves of the sympathetic nervous system to secrete catecholamines, which cause vasoconstriction and thus further shrink the vascular space and maintain perfusion pressure to the brain and heart. If the blood loss is minor, the sympathetic system can shrink the space enough to maintain blood pressure. If the loss is severe, the vascular space cannot be shrunk down enough to maintain blood pressure, and hypotension occurs.

Normally, the blood vessels are elastic and are distended by the volume that is in them. This produces a radial artery pulse that is full and wide. Blood loss allows the artery to shrink in width, becoming more threadlike in size; hence the term "thready" pulse in shock.

HIGH-SPACE SHOCK (RELATIVE HYPOVOLEMIA)

As has been mentioned, the amount of volume that the blood vessels *can* hold is many liters more than the normal blood volume. Again, it is the "steady-state" action of the sympathetic nervous system that keeps the vascular bed mildly constricted to maintain perfusion to the heart and brain. Anything that disturbs the sympathetic nervous system resulting in the loss of this normal vasoconstriction can cause the vascular space to become much "too large" for the usual amount of blood. If the blood vessels dilate, the 5 liters or so of blood flowing through the normal adult's vascular space may not be sufficient to maintain blood pressure and vital tissue perfusion. Such a condition causing the vascular space to be too large for a normal amount of blood has been called "high-space shock" or "relative hypovolemia." Although several types of high-space shock exist (e.g., sepsis syndrome and drug overdoses), neurogenic shock, commonly called "spinal shock," will be addressed here. Patients with head injury and increased intracranial pressure usually develop *hypertension* to try to maintain cerebral perfusion (see Chapter 10), but as a *terminal event,* vasodilatation and hypotension develop.

Neurogenic shock occurs most typically after an injury to the spinal cord. Although circulating catecholamines (already present) may preserve the blood pressure for a short time, the disruption of the sympathetic nervous system outflow from the spinal cord results in loss of the normal vascular tone and an inability of the body to compensate for any accompanying hemorrhage. As opposed to other patients with hemorrhage-associated shock, these patients will have warm dry skin (due to vasomotor paralysis and vasodilatation) and no accompanying increases in heart rate or blood pressure (unless circulating catecholamines help to transiently mask the loss of sympathetic nervous system input). The patient may also have accompanying paralysis and/or sensory deficit corresponding to the spinal cord injury. You may also see a lack of chest wall movement and only simple diaphragmatic movements when the patient is asked to take a deep breath. The important point is that this form of shock does not have the typical picture of hemorrhagic shock, *even when associated with severe bleeding.* The neurological assessment is therefore very important, and you should not rely on typical "shock" symptoms and signs to suspect internal bleeding or accompanying hemorrhage-associated shock. Although low blood pressure and normal heart rate may be an indication, normal blood pressure and tachycardia can often be seen, especially early on in the course of patient care. Repeat assessments and clinical suspicion are important. A neurogenic shock patient may "look better" than his or her actual condition.

Certain overdoses (including drinking alcohol) can also result in vasodilation and relative hypovolemia. Very often injuries result after such intoxication, and their effect on typical clinical signs and symptoms (like spinal shock) should be considered. You may find that intoxication is an accompanying problem in many injury victims.

MECHANICAL OR OBSTRUCTIVE SHOCK

In the normal adult's resting state, the heart pumps *out* about 5 liters of blood per minute. This means, of course, that the heart also must take *in* about 5 liters of blood per minute. Therefore, any traumatic condition that slows or prevents the venous return of blood can cause shock by lowering cardiac output and thus oxygen delivery to the tissues. Likewise, anything that obstructs the flow of blood to or through the heart can cause shock. The following are some of the traumatic conditions that can cause mechanical shock:

Tension pneumothorax is so named because of the high air tension (pressure) that develops in the pleural space (between the lung and chest wall). This very high positive pressure is transmitted back to the right heart and prevents the venous return of blood. Shifting of mediastinal structures may also lower venous return. See Figure 7-1 and turn to Chapter 6 for a complete description of signs, symptoms, and treatment of tension pneumothorax.

Cardiac or pericardial tamponade occurs when blood fills the space around the heart, squeezing the heart and preventing the heart from filling or pumping well (see Figure 7-2). The net result is that the heart cannot fill properly and cardiac output falls. Pericardial tamponade may occur in more than 75% of cases of penetrat-

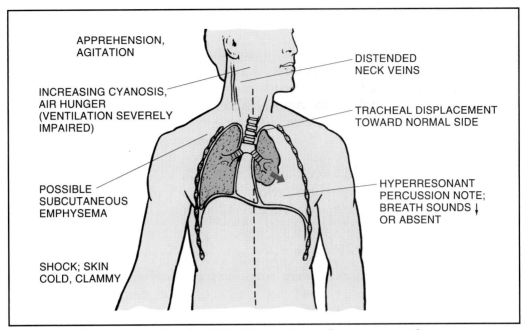

Figure 7-1 *Physical findings of tension pneumothorax.*

ing cardiac injury. *On-scene interventions should be avoided if the diagnosis is suspected because any time wasted on the scene could result in death of the patient.* Definitive surgical care in the nearest appropriate facility for pericardial decom-

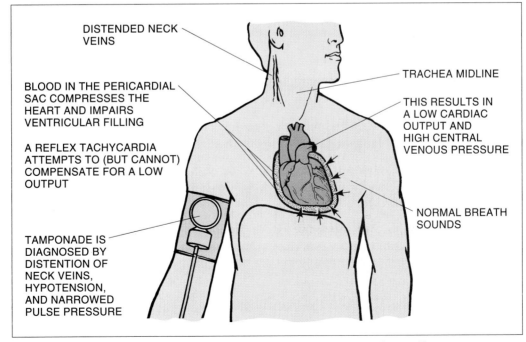

Figure 7-2 *Pathophysiology and physical findings of cardiac tamponade.*

pression may be the only life-saving measure available. See Chapter 6 for a more complete discussion.

Myocardial contusion can result in diminished cardiac output because the heart loses pumping ability due to direct injury. Myocardial contusion often can't be differentiated from cardiac tamponade in the field. Therefore, rapid transport, supportive care, and cardiac monitoring are the mainstays of therapy.

A word of caution is important here. Patients with shock from mechanical causes can be very near death. *Delay on the scene may prevent salvage of the patient.* Urban studies suggest that, in applicable cases, the time from development of a tamponade to circulatory arrest may be as little as 5–10 minutes. Survival following traumatic circulatory arrest, even in the best of trauma systems, is rarely achieved if surgery is not performed within 5–10 minutes.

HYPOXEMIC (RESPIRATORY) SHOCK

When massive aspiration, pulmonary contusion, pneumothorax, airway disruption/obstruction, or ventilatory insufficiency follow or accompany injury, the respiratory apparatus (lungs) may fail to deliver adequate oxygen levels to the blood. Therefore, even in the absence of excessive bleeding, mechanical obstruction to blood flow, or failure of the sympathetic nervous system, tissue oxygen perfusion may be critically impaired. While lung dysfunction is the most common cause of hypoxemia (e.g., blood or vomitus in the lungs), ventilatory insufficiency from flail chest wall segments, spinal cord injury, previous intoxication or a predisposing event (e.g., stroke), airway disruption (bronchial tear), pneumothorax, diaphragmatic tear, or other causes must also be considered. An open pneumothorax ("sucking chest wound") is a rare but highly reversible process that you should recognize and treat immediately. Patients with severe head injury may look as if they are breathing normally, but they may have hypoxemia because of inadequate respiratory patterns.

MANAGEMENT OF POSTTRAUMATIC SHOCK STATES

CONTROL BLEEDING: Red blood cells are necessary to carry oxygen. Control of bleeding must be obtained either by direct pressure or rapid transport to surgery.

GIVE OXYGEN: Cyanosis is an extremely late sign of hypoxemia, and may not occur at all if there has been extensive blood loss. *Give high-flow oxygen to all patients at risk for shock.*

TRANSPORT: Patients in shock are in the "load-and-go" category. Transport as soon as you finish the primary survey. Critical interventions can be done in the ambulance.

TREATMENT OF POSTTRAUMATIC HEMORRHAGE

Prehospital management of the patient in shock is controversial at this time. There is no question of the need for control of hemorrhage, supplemental oxygen, and early transport, but the indications for most other therapies is still being debated. Since the early days of modern shock treatment (about the middle of this century), intravenous crystalloid solutions (and sometimes colloid) have been tested and/or utilized to reverse the effects of hypovolemia. In addition, it has been previously proposed that intra-abdominal and pelvic bleeding may possibly be diminished by use of the pneumatic antishock garment, or military antishock trousers (PASG or MAST). Now, recent research suggests a modified approach. Patients may be thought of, roughly, in two categories: those with bleeding that you can control (e.g., extremity injury) and those with bleeding that you cannot control (e.g., internal injury). We will consider each type of bleeding and discuss current concepts of therapy of each type.

EXTERNAL HEMORRHAGE THAT CAN BE CONTROLLED: A patient with this type of injury is fairly easy to manage. Stop the bleeding by direct pressure. Only in the most extreme circumstances should a tourniquet be applied. A reasonable guide is that you should apply a tourniquet only to the extremity that you are prepared to sacrifice to save a life.

If the patient has clinical evidence of shock that persists after direct control of the bleeding, you should take the following steps:

1. Put the patient's body in a horizontal or slightly head-down position.
2. Administer high-flow oxygen.
3. Transport immediately and rapidly.
4. Apply the PASG, if local protocols recommend, until I.V. fluid therapy is available.
5. Monitor the heart and apply pulse oximetry if available.
6. Reassess frequently.

EXTERNAL HEMORRHAGE THAT CANNOT BE CONTROLLED: A patient with this type of injury must be rapidly transported to an appropriate facility where necessary procedures to gain surgical hemostasis can be performed. You must remember that elevating blood pressure can increase uncontrolled hemorrhage. To manage this patient, you should

1. Apply as much direct pressure as possible on the bleeding site (e.g., femoral artery, facial hemorrhage).
2. Put the patient's body in a horizontal or slightly head-down position.
3. Apply tourniquets to a bleeding extremity only as a desperate attempt to stop severe bleeding that cannot be otherwise controlled (discussed earlier).
4. Administer high-flow oxygen.
5. Transport immediately and rapidly.
6. Do not utilize the PASG in this setting.
7. Monitor the heart and apply pulse oximetry if available.
8. Reassess frequently.

Note: If assistance is not available, control of hemorrhage, even if minimal, should remain the priority. Other procedures become secondary if they interrupt attempts to maintain hemorrhage control.

INTERNAL HEMORRHAGE: The patient with uncontrolled internal hemorrhage is the classic critical trauma victim who will almost certainly die unless you rapidly transport to an appropriate facility where rapid operative hemostasis can be obtained. The results of the most current medical research regarding the management of patients with exsanguinating internal hemorrhage is that there exists *no substitute* for gaining surgical control of bleeding. Recent work regarding the use of the PASG and I.V. fluids in shock victims with presumed internal hemorrhage suggest the following:

1. Use of the PASG in the setting of uncontrolled internal exsanguination due to penetrating injury may increase mortality, especially in the setting of intrathoracic hemorrhage. The PASG raises blood pressure, and raising blood pressure in the setting of bleeding vessels within the thorax, abdomen, and pelvis probably increases internal bleeding, raising the chance of death due to exsanguination.

2. Any delay in providing rapid transport of such patients should not occur unless *absolutely* unavoidable, as in the case of a patient requiring prolonged extrication.

3. Moribund trauma patients (ones in very deep shock with blood pressures under 50 systolic) usually die, but the PASG may be indicated to maintain some degree of circulation. Treatment of this extreme amount of hemorrhage may override the concerns for increased hemorrhage secondary to the use of these interventions. However, this approach is still controversial. Local Medical Direction should guide such therapy.

The recommendations, therefore, for a patient with probable exsanguinating internal hemorrhage *secondary to penetrating injuries* are

1. Transport immediately and rapidly.
2. Put the patient's body in a horizontal or slightly head-down position.
3. Administer high-flow oxygen.
4. Do not utilize the PASG in this setting except as indicated by local Medical Direction.
5. Monitor the heart and apply pulse oximetry if available.
6. Reassess frequently.

Current published research has not yet adequately addressed the treatment of the patient with presumed internal hemorrhage in the setting of blunt injuries (motor vehicle mishaps, falls, etc.). This creates a dilemma because many patients with blunt injuries can lose a significant amount of blood and fluid from the intravascular space into the sites of large-bone fractures (hematoma and edema). This loss can be enough to cause shock, and yet the blood loss is usually self-limited. In theory, this situation should be treated with oxygen and rapid transport. These guidelines are subject to change pending ongoing research regarding treatment of shock. *Frequent patient assessments and local EMS Medical Direction should guide therapy.*

Note: It is a reasonable generalization that the patient who has "low-volume" shock syndrome *not due to hemorrhage* can generally be managed in the same manner as a patient with shock due to bleeding that can be controlled. An example of this type of patient would be one with shock due to severe diarrhea. Low-volume shock is the usual cause of death in these patients (acutely, such as in epidemic cholera). Since the loss of volume in this case is from the intestinal track and not from an injured vascular system, it is reasonable to treat such patients with PASG to restore vital signs toward normal.

TREATMENT OF NONHEMORRHAGIC SHOCK SYNDROMES (MECHANICAL AND HIGH SPACE)

Treatments for the other shock syndromes, namely, "mechanical" and "high-space" (relative) hypovolemia are somewhat different. All patients require high-flow oxygen, rapid transport, and shock positioning.

MECHANICAL SHOCK: The patient with mechanical shock must first be accurately assessed to determine the cause of the problem. The patient with *tension pneumothorax* needs prompt transport to appropriate hospital for decompression of the elevated pleural pressure.

The patient with suspected *pericardial tamponade* must be rapidly transported to an appropriate facility, because the time of onset of tamponade to the time of cardiac arrest can be a matter of minutes.

In two separate studies, one prospective and one retrospective, there was an increase in mortality of patients with tamponade when the PASG was applied in the prehospital setting. This may be due to the increase in field time taken to apply the PASG. By increasing peripheral resistance, the PASG also may decrease cardiac output, which may be another cause of increased mortality in such patients with an already low cardiac output. Therefore, the PASG is contraindicated in this setting.

Myocardial contusion rarely causes shock. Recent reports indicate that most contusions cause no clinical findings. However, severe contusion may cause acute heart failure, manifested by distended neck veins, tachycardia, or arrhythmias. These are the same signs seen with pericardial tamponade. These patients require rapid transport for proper care. Give high-flow oxygen and perform cardiac monitoring on the patient with suspected myocardial contusion.

HIGH-SPACE SHOCK: High-space shock, in theory, resembles controlled hemorrhage, in that there is relative hypovolemia with an "intact" vasculature (no leak). Therefore, initial management includes possible short-term use of the PASG. The patient's level of consciousness is a reasonable endpoint to follow. Be aware of possible internal injuries, and keep in mind that raising the blood pressure may increase internal bleeding in that situation.

CURRENT USES FOR THE PNEUMATIC ANTISHOCK GARMENT (PASG OR MAST)

The PASG is an inflatable compressive device that encircles the abdomen and legs. The PASG exerts its effect by compression of the arteries of the abdomen and legs, and this increases the peripheral vascular resistance (PVR). As PVR is a component of blood pressure (BP), BP typically rises with their application and inflation. However, as PVR rises, cardiac output (CO) may fall. Therefore, you must elevate PVR in settings of low BP with caution because of the possibility of lowering the cardiac output. Furthermore, if uncontrolled bleeding is occurring within the patient, raising the blood pressure may increase bleeding.

Until recently, it was commonplace to utilize the PASG for any patient with posttraumatic hypotension. Unfortunately, these well-intentioned recommendations came in the absence of real clinical proof for the effectiveness of PASG.

In the last few years, controlled clinical trials have been conducted to determine if PASG will improve vital signs, survival to hospital admission, and survival to discharge. The general consensus among informed medical personnel is that the PASG should probably not be applied in any clinical scenario in which bleeding cannot be controlled, such as in penetrating chest or abdominal trauma.

Do indications for PASG exist? In other words, is there an indication for elevating PVR in a patient? The patient with spinal shock has an inability to maintain vascular tone and could theoretically benefit from the use of PASG. Conceivably, a patient with anaphylaxis who has vasodilation due to histamine release might also benefit. However, there is no proof that the PASG helps in these clinical situations at this time.

It has been speculated that the PASG may be effective for the stabilization of pelvic and femur fractures. It is also possible that PASG *may* reduce pelvic hemorrhage in such situations. However, it must *still* be remembered that elevation of systolic pressure beyond 90 or 100 should be done only with caution in the setting of the patient with possible uncontrolled internal hemorrhage. Local Medical Direction should guide therapy.

SUMMARY

The patient with shock is often not diagnosed early enough. Shock may not be obvious until the patient is near death. The importance of careful assessment and reassessment cannot be overemphasized. You must understand the risk of any shock state to the patient. Further, you need to study and memorize the "shock syndromes," especially in regard to the rapid provision of the proper treatment for such conditions as internal hemorrhage, pericardial tamponade, and tension pneumothorax. Finally, you should be aware of the controversy regarding the use of I.V. fluid resuscitation and the PASG for cases of *uncontrolled* hemorrhage. Rely on your local Medical Direction to keep you current on the standard of care in these areas.

BIBLIOGRAPHY

1. Bickell, W. H., P. E. Pepe, M. L. Bailey, and others. "Randomized Trial of Pneumatic Anti-shock Garments in the Prehospital Management of Penetrating Abdominal Injury." *Annals of Emergency Medicine,* Vol. 16 (June 1987), pp. 653–658.

2. Bickell, W. H., M. J. Wall, P. E. Pepe, and others. "Immediate Versus Delayed Fluid Resuscitation for Hypotensive Patients with Penetrating Injuries." *The New England Journal of Medicine,* Vol. 331 (October 1994), pp. 1105–1109.

3. Kowalenko, T., S. Stern, S. Dronen, and X. Wang. "Improved Outcome with Hypotensive Resuscitation of Uncontrolled Hemorrhagic Shock in a Swine Mode." *Journal of Trauma,* Vol. 33 (1992), pp. 349–353.

4. Martin, R. R., W. H. Bickell, P. E. Pepe, and others. "Prospective Evaluation of Preoperative Fluid Resuscitation in Hypotensive Patients with Penetrating Truncal Injury: A Preliminary Report." *Journal of Trauma,* Vol. 33 (September 1992), pp. 354–362.

5. Mattox, K. L., W. H. Bickell, P. E. Pepe, and others. "Prospective Mast Study in 911 patients." *Journal of Trauma,* Vol. 29 (1989), pp. 1104–1112.

6. Pepe, P. E. "Anti-shock Garments: More Harm than Good." *Journal of Critical Illness,* Vol. 7 (1992), pp. 166–168.

7. Pepe, P. E., and M. K. Copass. "Prehospital Care." In American College of Surgeons Committee on Trauma, *Early Care of the Injured,* ed. E. E. Moore, pp. 34–55. Toronto: B. C. Decker, 1990.

8. Pepe, P. E., and R. F. Maio. "Evolving Challenges in Prehospital Trauma Services: Current Issues and Suggested Evaluation Tools." *Prehospital and Disaster Medicine,* Vol. 8 (1993), pp. S25–S34.

9. Pepe, P. E., K. L. Mattox, R. P. Fischer, and C. M. Matsumoto. "Geographical Patterns of Urban Trauma According to Mechanism and Severity of Injury." *Journal of Trauma,* Vol. 30 (September 1990), pp. 1125–1132.

10. Schriger, D. L., and L. J. Baraff. "Capillary Refill—Is It a Useful Predictor of Hypovolemic States?" *Annals of Emergency Medicine,* Vol. 20 (June 1991), pp. 601–605.

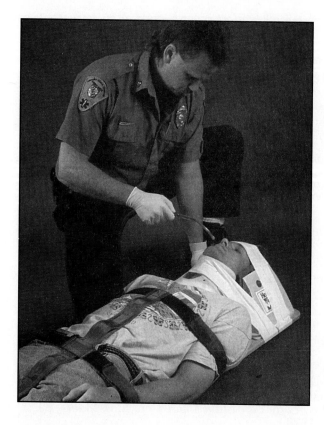

Spinal Trauma

James J. Augustine, M.D., F.A.C.E.P.

OBJECTIVES

Upon completion of this chapter you should be able to:

1. Explain the normal anatomy and physiology of the spinal column and spinal cord.

2. Describe three mechanisms of injury that require spinal column immobilization.

3. Using clinical observations, differentiate spinal shock from hemorrhagic shock.

4. Describe the process of spinal immobilization from extrication to transportation.

5. Explain how unusual circumstances affect spinal immobilization and give examples.

6. Explain the importance of maintaining the patient's airway while immobilized.

There are current estimates of a cost of about $1.5 million to support a spinal cord injury patient for a lifetime. The question is: Which one of the patients whom you treat, who has fallen, wrecked, been beaten, shot, or stabbed, will you need to be supporting for the rest of their life? The answer is: You don't know! Even after years of research, no formula or technique has been devised to predict which trauma patient has the unstable fracture or cord injury that will be aggravated by improper handling. The only safe course of action is constant suspicion of spinal injury combined with proper patient handling and packaging. In this chapter we review this process.

THE NORMAL SPINAL COLUMN AND CORD

SPINAL COLUMN

It is important to begin by differentiating the spinal column from the spinal cord. The spinal column is a bony tube composed of 33 vertebrae (see Figure 8-1). It supports the body in an upright position, allows us to make use of our extremities, and protects the delicate spinal cord. The column's 33 vertebrae are aligned in an S-shaped curve and are identified by their location: 7 cervical (the C-spine), 12 thoracic (the T-spine), and 5 lumbar (the L-spine) and the remainder fused together as the posterior portion of the pelvis (sacrum and coccyx). The vertebrae are then numbered in each section from the head down to the pelvis. The third cervical vertebrae from the head is designated C-3, the sixth called C-6, and so forth. The thoracic vertebrae are T1 through T12, and each attaches to 1 of the 12 pairs of ribs. The lumbar vertebrae are numbered L1 through L5, with L5 being the last vertebra

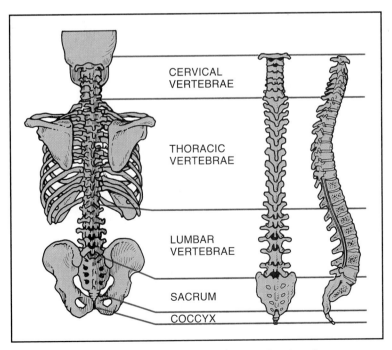

CERVICAL
VERTEBRAE

THORACIC
VERTEBRAE

LUMBAR
VERTEBRAE

SACRUM

COCCYX

Figure 8-1 *Anatomy of the spinal column*

above the pelvis. The vertebrae are each separated by a fibrous disc that acts as a shock absorber. The alignment is maintained by strong ligaments between the vertebrae, and by muscles that run along the length of the bony column from head to pelvis (the same muscles strained when lifting improperly). The S-curve is most prominent at the C5-6 and T12-L1 levels in adults, making these areas the most susceptible to injury.

SPINAL CORD

The spinal cord is an electrical conduit, an extension of the brainstem that continues down to the level of the first lumbar vertebra. The cord is 10–13 mm in diameter and is suspended in the middle of the spinal column (see Figures 8-2 and 8-4). The cord is soft and flexible, like a cotton rope, and is surrounded and bathed by cerebrospinal fluid along its entire length. The fluid and the flexibility

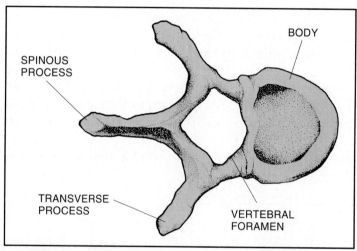

Figure 8-2 *Vertebra viewed from above. The spinal cord passes through the vertebral foramen.*

provide some protection from injury to the cord. The cord is composed of specific bundles of nerve tracts, much as a rope is composed of individual strands of fiber, which are arranged in a predictable manner. The spinal cord passes down the vertebral canal, and gives off pairs of nerve roots that exit at each vertebral level (see Figures 8-3 and 8-4). The roots lie next to the intervertebral discs and the lateral part of the vertebrae, making the nerve roots susceptible to injury with trauma to these areas (see Figure 8-4). The nerve roots carry sensory signals from the body to the spinal cord and then to the brain. The roots also carry signals from the brain to specific muscles causing them to move. These signals pass back and forth rapidly, and some are strong enough to cause actions on their own, called reflexes. This reflex system is demonstrated by a strong tap below the knee causing the lower leg to jerk. If you accidentally put your finger on a hot burner,

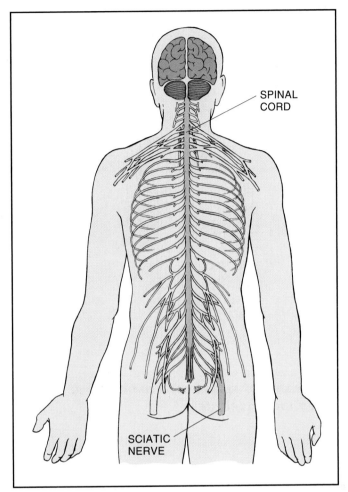

Figure 8-3 *Spinal cord. The spinal cord is a continuation of the central nervous system outside the skull.*

your reflex system causes your hand to move even before your brain receives the warning message. Strong signals can also overwhelm the spinal cord's ability to keep signals moving separately to the brain, which is why a trauma patient with a fractured hip may complain of knee pain, or a patient with a ruptured spleen may complain of shoulder pain.

The integrity of spinal cord function is tested by motor, sensory, and reflex functions. Sensory levels are the most accurate at predicting the level of spinal cord injury. Muscle strength is another function that is easy to assess in the conscious patient. Reflexes are helpful for distinguishing complete from partial spinal cord injuries, but are best left for hospital assessment. The spinal cord is also an integrating center for the autonomic nervous system, which assists in controlling heart rate, blood vessel tone, and blood flow to the skin. Injury to this component of the spinal cord results in "spinal shock," which will be discussed later.

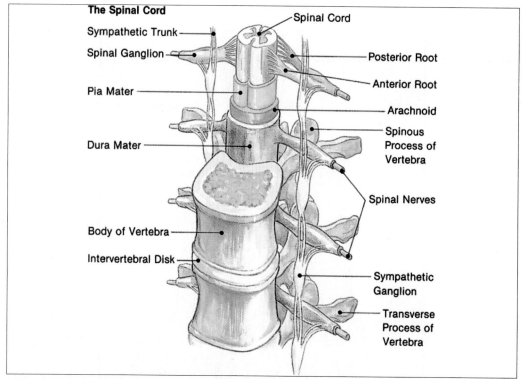

Figure 8-4 *Relationship of spinal cord to vertebra. Note how the nerve roots exit between the vertebrae.*

KINEMATICS OF BLUNT SPINAL INJURY

A normal healthy spinal column can be severely stressed and maintain its integrity without damage to the spinal cord. But certain mechanisms of trauma can overcome the protective defenses, injuring the spinal column and cord. The most common mechanisms are hyperextension, hyperflexion, compression, and rotation. Rarely, lateral stress or distraction will injure the cord. These mechanisms and their subsequent injuries are illustrated in Table 8-1.

SPINAL COLUMN INJURY

The head is a relatively large ball perched on top of the neck. Sudden movement of the head or trunk will produce flexion, extension, or lateral stresses that may damage the bony or connective tissue components of the spinal column. Injury to the spinal column presents in several ways. Pain is the most common symptom, but it may be completely absent or unnoticed by the patient. This is especially true if the patient has other painful injuries. Local muscle spasm may occur. Injury to individual nerve roots occurs and results in localized pain, paralysis, or sensory loss. Spinal cord injury is of greatest concern, but it is important to remember that only 14% of all *column* injuries have evidence of spinal *cord* dam-

DESCRIPTION	DIAGRAM	EXAMPLES
HYPEREXTENSION EXCESSIVE POSTERIOR MOVEMENT OF HEAD OR NECK		FACE INTO WINDSHIELD IN MVC ELDERLY PERSON FALLING TO THE FLOOR FOOTBALL TACKLER DIVE INTO SHALLOW WATER
HYPERFLEXION EXCESSIVE ANTERIOR MOVEMENT OF HEAD ONTO CHEST		RIDER THROWN OFF OF HORSE OR MOTORCYCLE DIVE INTO SHALLOW WATER
COMPRESSION WEIGHT OF HEAD OR PELVIS DRIVEN INTO STATIONARY NECK OR TORSO		DIVE INTO SHALLOW WATER FALL OF GREATER THAN 10–20 FEET ONTO HEAD OR LEGS
ROTATION EXCESSIVE ROTATION OF THE TORSO OR HEAD AND NECK, MOVING ONE SIDE OF THE SPINAL COLUMN AGAINST THE OTHER		ROLLOVER MVC MOTORCYCLE ACCIDENT
LATERAL STRESS DIRECT LATERAL FORCE ON SPINAL COLUMN, TYPICALLY SHEARING ONE LEVEL OF CORD FROM ANOTHER		"T-BONE" MVA FALL
DISTRACTION EXCESSIVE STRETCHING OF COLUMN AND CORD		HANGING CHILD INAPPROPRIATELY WEARING SHOULDER BELT AROUND NECK SNOWMOBILE OR MOTORCYCLE UNDER ROPE OR WIRE

Table 8-1 *Mechanisms of Spinal Injury*

age. In the cervical spine region it is much more common to have cord injury, with almost 40% of column injuries having cord damage. In contrast, 63% of spinal cord injuries have evidence of spinal column damage. This means that almost half of the patients with some degree of paralysis will have no obvious bone or ligament injury (even by X-ray) to the spinal column. The unconscious trauma patient carries a high risk (15–20%) of spinal column injury. The injuries are frequently in more than one place, and therefore the unconscious patient should be immediately and consistently immobilized. Those requiring immobilization include patients who had lap and shoulder belts in place, had air bags activated, and also those found walking at the scene.

SPINAL CORD INJURY

Spinal cord injury is devastating. It is most common in patients aged 16 to 35, typically those who are active and productive. Out of the thousands of cord injuries per year, 56% involve motor vehicle accidents (including pedestrians), 19% falls, 12% penetrating wounds, 7% recreational activities, and the remaining 6% from all other causes. Under age 16, falls are the most common cause of spinal injury. Under age 8, the relatively large size of the head makes the upper end of the cervical cord, an extremely devastating level, the most common site of injury.

Spinal cord injury results in a defect in the signal conducting function, presenting as a loss of motor function and reflexes, loss or change in sensation, and/or spinal shock. The delicate structure of the nerve tracts in the cord make it very sensitive to any form of trauma. What is termed *primary* damage occurs at the time of the trauma itself. Primary damage is from the cord being cut, torn, or crushed or its blood supply being cut off. This damage is usually irreversible despite the best trauma care. *Secondary* damage occurs from injury to blood vessels, swelling, compression of the cord from surrounding hemorrhage, hypotension, or generalized hypoxia. Emergency efforts are directed at preventing secondary damage through careful packaging of the patient and attention to the ABCs.

Injury to the cervical spinal cord can produce spinal shock. Spinal shock is the malfunction of the autonomic nervous system in regulating blood vessel tone and cardiac output. Classically, this means a patient is hypotensive, with normal skin color and temperature and an inappropriately slow heart rate. In the healthy patient, blood pressure is maintained by the controlled release of catecholamines (epinephrine and norepinephrine) from the adrenal glands. Catecholamines cause constriction of the blood vessels, increase the heart rate and strength of heart contraction, and stimulate sweat glands. Sensors in the aortic and carotid arteries monitor the blood pressure. The brain and spinal cord signal the adrenal glands to release catecholamines to keep the blood pressure in the normal range. In pure *hemorrhagic shock,* these sensors detect the hypovolemic state and compensate by constricting the blood vessels and speeding the heart rate. The high levels of catecholamines thus produced cause pale skin, tachycardia, and sweating. The mechanism of shock from spinal cord injury is just the opposite. There is no blood loss, but there is no signal going to the adrenals (the spinal cord cable is out) so no catecholamines are released. The blood vessels dilate and blood pools, and the blood pressure cannot be maintained. The brain cannot correct this because it cannot get the message to the adrenal glands. The patient with spinal shock cannot show the signs of pale skin, fast heart beat, and sweating because the cord injury prevents release of catecholamines. Since spinal shock is caused by blood vessel dilation, it frequently responds to anti-shock trousers that work by circumferential compression of the blood vessels in the lower part of the body. This use is discouraged unless you are *sure* that there is no internal bleeding (review Chapter 7). Intra-abdominal injury and bleeding can be difficult to determine because the spinal-shock patient usually has no sensation in the abdomen. The multiple-trauma patient may have both spinal shock and hemorrhagic shock. Spinal shock is a diagnosis of exclusion, after all other potential causes of shock have been ruled out. In the prehospital setting, spinal shock is treated the same as hemorrhagic shock.

PATIENT ASSESSMENT

All trauma patients are evaluated in the same manner using the assessment priority plan of which evaluation of spinal cord function is a part. Clues to spinal cord injury are given in Table 8-2. The neurological exam (except for level of consciousness) is performed in the secondary survey. This is frequently done after the victim is loaded into the ambulance. The exception to this is the patient that requires extrication. Before beginning extrication you should check sensory and motor function in the hands and feet, and document these findings later in the written report. Not only does this preextrication neurological exam alert you to any spinal injury, but it also provides documentation if there was loss of function before extrication was begun. It is a sad fact that there are a few reports of patients with spinal injuries

CLUES TO SPINAL CORD INJURY ON PATIENT ASSESSMENT
THE FOLLOWING ARE INDICATORS THAT THE SPINE MAY HAVE BEEN INJURED. THESE PATIENTS SHOULD BE IMMOBILIZED.

MECHANISM OF TRAUMA:
*BLUNT TRAUMA ABOVE THE CLAVICLES
*DIVING ACCIDENT
*MOTOR VEHICLE OR BICYCLE ACCIDENT
*FALL
*STABBING OR IMPALEMENT ANYWHERE NEAR THE SPINAL COLUMN
*SHOOTING OR BLAST INJURY TO THE TORSO
*ANY VIOLENT INJURY WITH FORCES THAT COULD ACT ON THE SPINAL COLUMN OR CORD

WHEN THE PATIENT COMPLAINS OF:
*NECK OR BACK PAIN
*NUMBNESS OR TINGLING
*LOSS OF MOVEMENT OR WEAKNESS

WHEN ON EXAM YOU FIND:
*PAIN ON MOVEMENT OR PALPATION OF THE SPINAL COLUMN
*OBVIOUS DEFORMITY OF BACK OR SPINAL COLUMN
*GUARDING AGAINST MOVEMENT OF BACK
*LOSS OF SENSATION
*WEAK OR FLACCID MUSCLES
*LOSS OF CONTROL OF BLADDER OR BOWELS
*ERECTION OF THE PENIS (PRIAPRISM)
*SPINAL SHOCK

Table 8-2 *Clues to Spinal Cord Injury on Patient Assessment*

who have claimed that the injuries were caused by their rescuers. Unfortunately, you will probably not have time to perform the preextrication neurological exam on the patient who requires rapid extrication.

The neurological exam has already been covered in Chapter 2 and will be further expanded in Chapter 10, but we will review the most important elements here: the exam of peripheral neurological function is kept brief and simple. If the conscious patient cán move his fingers and toes, the motor nerves are intact. Anything less than normal sensation (tingling or decreased sensation) is suspicious for cord injury. The unconscious patient may withdraw if you pinch his fingers and toes. If so, you have demonstrated intact motor and sensory nerves and thus an intact cord. Flaccid paralysis, even in the unconscious head injury patient, usually means cord injury. Document these important findings.

PATIENT MANAGEMENT

Based on the mechanism of injury, it is appropriate to place the head and neck in a neutral position as the rescuer first approaches the patient. The neck is then maintained in stabilization until the patient is securely strapped to the long backboard (see Figure 8-5). In general, any patient with an injury above the clavicles should be treated for potential cervical spine injury. Suspect thoracic and lumbar spine injuries from sudden deceleration accidents or direct torso injuries. Patients who have had seizures or who are "found down" should also be immobilized. Preparation for managing spinal column or cord injury can begin when dispatched to the scene of a motor vehicle accident, fall, explosion, head injury, or neck injury.

The most easily applied and readily available method of cervical immobilization is with your hands or knees. They should be placed to stabilize the neck in rela-

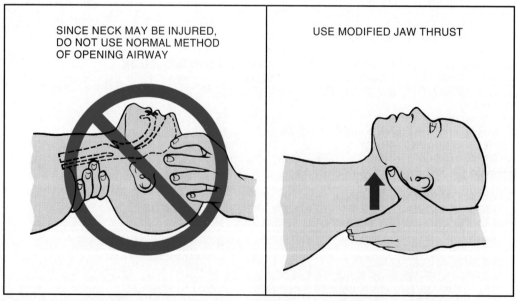

SINCE NECK MAY BE INJURED, DO NOT USE NORMAL METHOD OF OPENING AIRWAY

USE MODIFIED JAW THRUST

Figure 8-5 *Modified jaw thrust. By using this maneuver, you may maintain stabilization of the neck while opening the airway.*

tion to the long axis of the spinal column. **Pulling traction** is not a prehospital option, and the term "traction" is not an appropriate description for the immobilization of the spine. **Traction** will usually result in further instability of any spinal column injury. If an appropriately sized cervical immobilization collar is available, you can place it on the patient as airway assessment is being done. These one- or two-piece collars are not definitive devices for cervical spine control, but should be used only as a reminder that cervical immobilization is necessary, and to prevent gross neck movement. The rescuer's hands can be removed only when the head and spinal column has been definitively immobilized on a spinal board with an attached immobilization device. For the conscious patient, positioning the head and neck in the position of patient comfort is a good guideline. Patient management then proceeds with initial assessment and interventions.

In the critically unstable patient, rapid extrication from a vehicle or structure may be necessary. This form of extrication is used for patients whose primary assessment indicates a critical degree of ongoing danger. Indications for rapid emergency extrication are when

1. Scene survey identifies a condition that may immediately endanger the patient or rescuers:
   a. Fire or immediate danger of fire
   b. Danger of explosion
   c. Rapidly rising water
   d. Structure in danger of collapse
   e. Continuing toxic exposure
2. Primary survey of the patient identifies a condition that requires immediate intervention that cannot be done in the entrapped area:
   a. Airway obstruction that cannot be relieved by jaw thrust or finger sweep
   b. Cardiac or respiratory arrest
   c. Chest or airway injuries requiring ventilation or assisted ventilation
   d. Deep shock or bleeding that cannot be controlled

Rapid extrication requires multiple rescuers who remove the patient along the long axis of the body, using their hands to maintain cervical immobilization. (See Chapter 9.) When the rapid extrication technique is used, the written report should be reviewed by your medical director.

LOG-ROLL

This technique is used for moving a patient onto a backboard. It is commonly used because it is easy to perform with a minimum number of rescuers. As yet no movement technique has been devised that maintains complete spinal immobilization while moving a patient onto a backboard. Properly performed, the log-roll technique will minimize movement of the spinal column as well as any other technique.

The log-roll technique moves the spinal column as a single unit with the head and pelvis. It can be performed on victims lying prone or supine. Using three or more rescuers, controlled by the rescuer at the patient's head, the patient (with the arms by his or her side) is rolled onto the uninjured side, a board is slid underneath, and the patient is rolled face up onto the board. The log-roll technique is then completed when the patient's head, chest, and pelvis are secured to the board. The log-roll technique is useful for most trauma patients, but is contraindicated for those patients with a fractured pelvis who may aggravate the injury with their weight rolled onto the pelvis. Pelvic fracture patients should instead be lifted carefully onto a board using four or more rescuers. Log-roll must be modified for patients with painful arm, leg, and chest wounds who should be rolled onto their uninjured side.

In certain situations, once the patient is packaged onto the backboard, the board and patient may have to be rolled up on to his or her side (see Figure 8-6a to 8-6c). Women who are more than 20 weeks pregnant should always be transported with the backboard tilted 20–30 degrees to the patient's left side to keep the uterus off the inferior vena cava. Patients with airway problems, who are not intubated, are better transported on their side. This is especially critical when there is uncontrolled bleeding into the airway or if there is massive face or neck trauma. In these situations gravity assists with the drainage of fluids out of the airway and may prevent aspiration if the patient vomits. Because of the danger of vomiting, unconscious patients who are not intubated should be transported on their side.

Cervical spine immobilization is completed only when the head and body are secured to a long backboard. Inadequate strapping will torque the neck against the body if the patient moves, rolls, is dropped, or is rotated. Once the patient is secured to the board, a rescuer must be present and capable of rolling the board if the patient begins to vomit or loses his or her airway. Placing and strapping a patient on the board effectively paralyzes the patient's ability to protect the airway, and therefore the rescuer is responsible. This rule continues in effect in the emer-

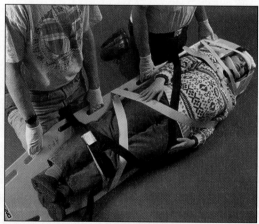

Figure 8-6a *Pregnant patient immobilized and board tilted to the left.*

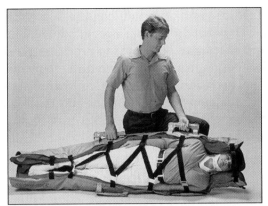

Figure 8-6b *Patient in vacuum backboard turned on side. Notice that the body is maintained in a straight line.*

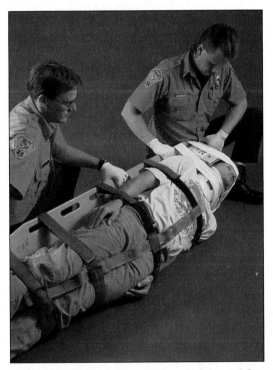

Figure 8-6c *Immobilized patient turned on side. This may be necessary for the patient who is vomiting. The patient must be secured well enough so that the spine remains straight.*

gency department, where an emergency staff person must assume responsibility for airway protection. Definitive immobilization occurs when the body is strapped securely to the board with cushions, blanket, or towel rolls maintaining the head, cervical spine, torso, and pelvis in line. Sandbags have been used for head immobilization and perform well when the patient is kept supine. However, if the board is tilted or the patient and board are rotated (as to prevent aspiration when the patient vomits), the weight of the sandbags may cause an extreme amount of head movement (see Figure 8-7). Therefore sandbags are an extremely poor option for prehospital immobilization. Lighterweight bulky objects, such as towel rolls, blanket rolls, or head cushions are a better tool for this job. When applied properly, these devices allow removal of the front portion of the cervical collar and observation of the neck, as in the patient with open neck wounds. Commercial cervical immobilization devices may be left in place on the spineboard.

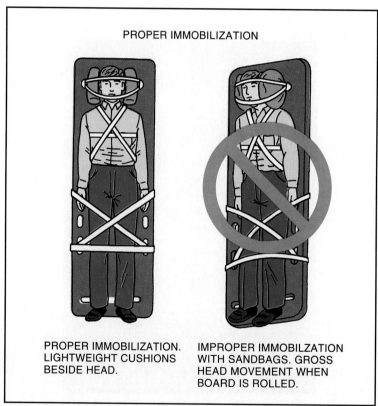

Figure 8-7 *Proper immobilization.*

Recent studies have suggested that a true neutral position on a long backboard for an adult is obtained with the use of 1 to 2 inches of occipital padding. This slightly elevates the head and tends to make the patient more comfortable. This is accomplished with the head pad on a cervical immobilization device or the padding that is used with many short board devices. Some padding is a necessity in elderly patients who have a natural flexed posture of their necks.

SPINAL IMMOBILIZATION DEVICES

There is a wide range of devices currently marketed to provide immobilization for injured patients (Figure 8-8). No device has yet been proven to excel over all others, and no device will ever be produced that can immobilize all patients. No device is better than the crew that is using it, so training with the available tools is the most critical factor in providing good patient care.

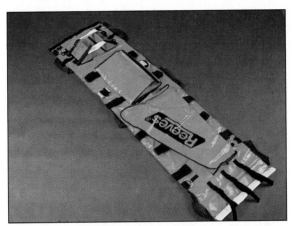

Figure 8-8a. *Reeves sleeve*

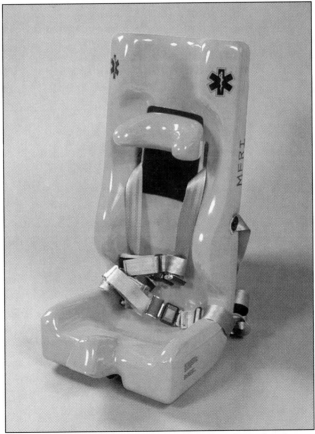

Figure 8-8b. *Pediatric immobilization device*

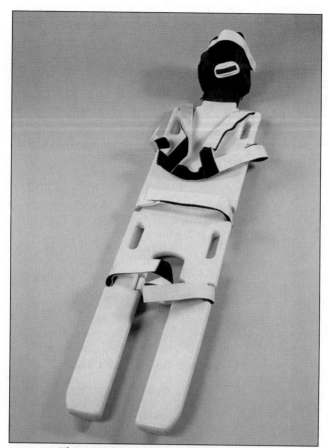

Figure 8-8c. *Miller body splint*

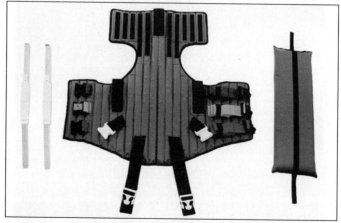

Figure 8-8d. *Kendrick immobilization device*

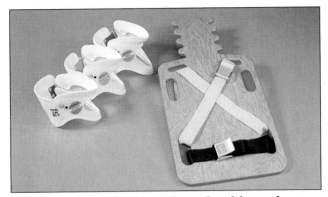

Figure 8-8e(1)   *Short backboard.*

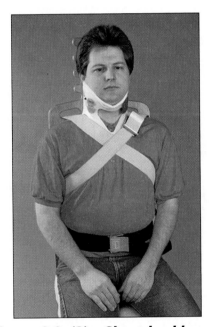

Figure 8-8e(2)   *Short backboard.*

SPECIAL SITUATIONS

Immobilization must occasionally be performed in special circumstances. These include

1. Patients in closed spaces
2. Patients in water
3. Patients in a prone or standing position
4. Pediatric patients
5. Elderly patients

6. Patients in protective helmets
7. Very large or obese patients
8. Patients with disfiguring or penetrating neck wounds

Closed-space rescues are performed in a manner appropriate for the clinical condition of the patient. The only general rules that can be applied to these rescues are to prevent gross cervical spine movement and to move patients in line with the long axis of the body (see Figure 8-9). Safety of the rescuer is of prime importance in all closed-space rescue. Asphyxia, poison gas, or cave-ins are dangers of closed-space rescue. Never enter a closed space until you are properly equipped (air pack, etc.) and you are sure of scene safety.

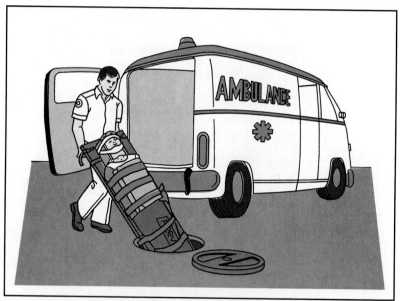

Figure 8-9 *Closed-space rescue. Special devices such as the Reeves sleeve are useful in this situation.*

You can perform water rescues by moving the patient in line, preventing gross cervical movement. When the rescuers are in a stable position for immobilizing the patient, the backboard is floated under the patient and the patient is then secured and removed from the water (see Figure 8-10).

Prone and standing patients are immobilized in a manner that minimizes spinal column movement, ending with the patient in the conventional supine position. Prone patients are log-rolled onto a long board with careful coordination of head and chest rescuers. Seated patients may be immobilized using short backboards or their commercial adaptations. Used appropriately, these provide initial stabilization of the cervical and thoracic spine, and then facilitate the movement of the patient onto a long backboard. Standing patients may be placed against the long board while upright and then while supporting the head and torso, gently lowered to the supine position and strapped in place. For immobilizing the pediatric patient, it is best to provide initial immobilization with the rescuer's hands, and then use cushions or towel rolls to help

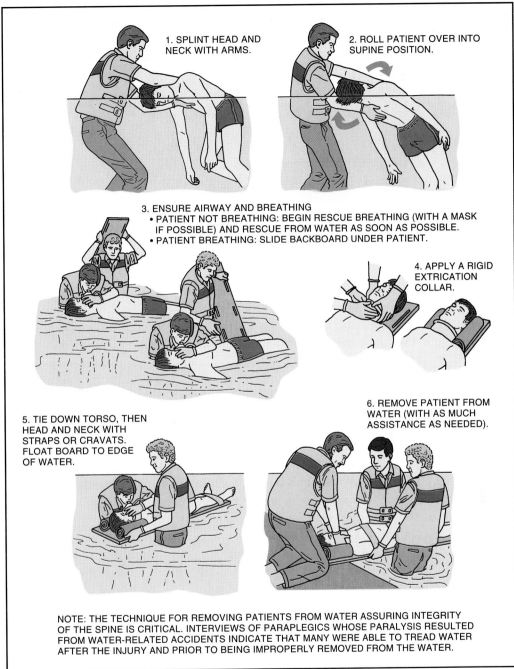

1. SPLINT HEAD AND NECK WITH ARMS.

2. ROLL PATIENT OVER INTO SUPINE POSITION.

3. ENSURE AIRWAY AND BREATHING
   • PATIENT NOT BREATHING: BEGIN RESCUE BREATHING (WITH A MASK IF POSSIBLE) AND RESCUE FROM WATER AS SOON AS POSSIBLE.
   • PATIENT BREATHING: SLIDE BACKBOARD UNDER PATIENT.

4. APPLY A RIGID EXTRICATION COLLAR.

5. TIE DOWN TORSO, THEN HEAD AND NECK WITH STRAPS OR CRAVATS. FLOAT BOARD TO EDGE OF WATER.

6. REMOVE PATIENT FROM WATER (WITH AS MUCH ASSISTANCE AS NEEDED).

NOTE: THE TECHNIQUE FOR REMOVING PATIENTS FROM WATER ASSURING INTEGRITY OF THE SPINE IS CRITICAL. INTERVIEWS OF PARAPLEGICS WHOSE PARALYSIS RESULTED FROM WATER-RELATED ACCIDENTS INDICATE THAT MANY WERE ABLE TO TREAD WATER AFTER THE INJURY AND PRIOR TO BEING IMPROPERLY REMOVED FROM THE WATER.

Figure 8-10 *Extricating suspected diving accident victim.*

secure on an appropriate board or device. Some pediatric trauma specialists suggest padding beneath the *back and shoulders* on the board in the child under the age of 3 (see Figure 8-11). These children normally have a relatively large head that flexes the neck when placed on a straight board. Padding under the back and shoulders will prevent this flexion and also make the child more comfortable.

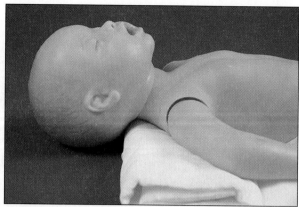

Figure 8-11 *Most children require padding under back and shoulders to keep the cervical spine in a neutral position.*

Children who have sustained trauma while immobilized in a child safety seat may be packaged in the safety seat for transport to the hospital. Using towel or blanket rolls, cloth tape, and a little reassurance, you can secure the child in the safety seat and then belt the seat into the ambulance. This technique minimizes movement of the child and provides a secure method for child transport in the ambulance. Some autos come with built-in child-restraint seats that cannot be removed. Children in such seats will have to be extricated onto a spine board or other pediatric immobilization device. For the child who is frightened and struggling there may be no good way to obtain immobilization.

Elderly patients require flexibility in packaging techniques. Many elderly patients have arthritic changes of the spine and very thin skin. Such patients will be very uncomfortable when placed on a backboard. Some arthritic spines are so rigid that the victim cannot be laid straight on the board, and some elderly victims have rigid flexion of the neck that will result in a large gap between the head and the board. The rescuer can make use of towels, blankets, and pillows to pad the elderly patient and prevent movement and discomfort on the backboard (see Figure 8-12). This is a situation where the vacuum backboard (which conforms to the shape of the patient) works very well.

Athletes and cyclists wearing helmets are another special set of patients. Large helmets used in these sports must be removed at some point to allow complete assessment and care. Helmets used in different sports present different management problems for rescuers. Football and ice hockey helmets are custom fitted to the individual. Unless special circumstances exist, such as respiratory distress coupled with inability to access the airway, the helmet should not be removed in the prehospital setting. Athletic helmet design will generally allow easy airway access once the face guard is removed. The face guard can easily be cut off using EMS-type scissors (see Figure 8-13). The athlete wearing shoulder pads has his or her neck in a neutral position when on the backboard with the helmet in place. If the helmet is removed, padding must be inserted under the head to keep the neck from extending (see Figure 8-14). After arrival at the emergency facility the cervical spine can be X-rayed with the helmet in place. Once the spine is evaluated, the helmet can be removed by stabilizing the head and neck, removing the cheek pads, releasing the

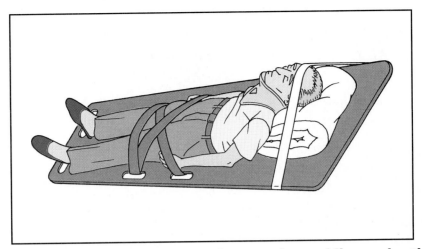

Figure 8-12 *Elderly patients often require padding under the shoulders and head to stabilize the spine.*

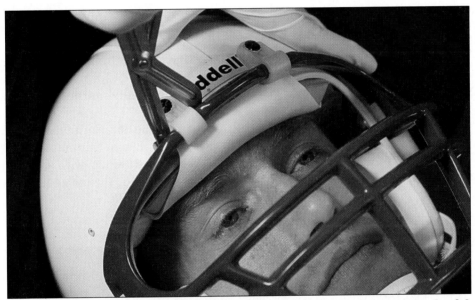

Figure 8-13 *The face guard of football helmets can be removed with rescue scissors or a screwdriver.*

air inflation system, and then sliding the helmet off in the usual manner.

In contrast, motorcycle helmets must often be removed in the prehospital setting. The removal technique is modified to accommodate the different design. Motorcycle helmets are often designed with a continuous solid face guard that limits airway access. These helmets are not custom designed, and frequently are poorly fitted to the victim. Their large size will usually produce significant neck flexion if left in place when the victim is placed on a backboard (see Figure 8-15). Motorcycle accidents are usually associated with much more violent forces than athletic injuries. The motorcycle helmet will make it difficult to stabilize the neck in a neutral position, may obstruct

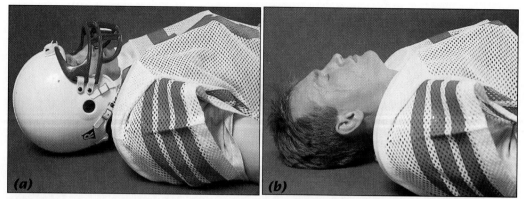

Figure 8-14 *(a) Patients with shoulder pads and helmets are usually best immobilized with the helmet in place. The spine is maintained in a neutral position with a minimum of movement. (b) Patients with shoulder pads must have padding under the head to maintain a neutral position if the helmet is removed.*

access to the airway, and may hide injuries to the head or neck; it should be removed in the prehospital setting using the techniques taught in Chapter 9.

Very large or obese patients may not fit appropriately in standard equipment. Rescuers must be flexible, even using sheets of plywood and head cushions or towel rolls to stabilize. In cold weather climates, patients in bulky warm clothing will need to be snugly secured to prevent excessive movement.

Patients with penetrating or disfiguring wounds of the neck or lower face must be continually observed. Cervical collars will prevent continued examination of the wound site, and they may compromise the airway in wounds with expanding hematomas or subcutaneous air. If the mandible is fractured, the collar may again

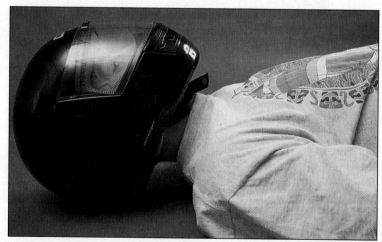

Figure 8-15 *Full-face helmets obstruct access to the patient's airway. Notice that the helmet flexes the neck in a patient who is not wearing shoulder pads.*

cause airway compromise. Therefore, in this class of patients, it may be wise to avoid collars, using manual stabilization and then head cushion devices or blanket rolls for cervical immobilization.

Trauma patients with paralysis or spinal shock have lost vascular control and thus cannot control blood flow to the skin. They may lose heat rapidly. Unless the weather is very warm, such patients should be covered to prevent hypothermia.

AIRWAY INTERVENTION

When the rescuer performs spinal immobilization in any manner, the patient loses some of his ability to maintain his own airway. As mentioned earlier, the rescuer must then assume this responsibility until the patient has a controlled airway or has the spinal column cleared in the emergency department and is released from the immobilizing equipment (see Figure 8-16). This is particularly critical in children, who have a greater potential for vomiting and aspiration following a traumatic injury.

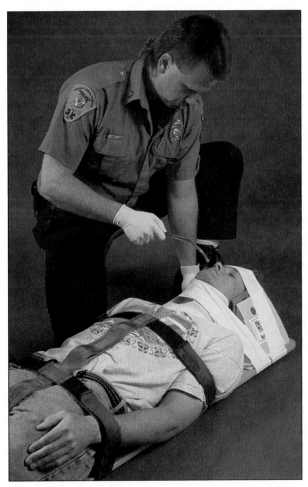

Figure 8-16 *You are responsible for the patient's airway once the patient is immobilized.*

Your priority plan should include airway control with *manual* immobilization, using the method that you are most skilled at performing. In weighing the risks and benefits of each airway procedure, recall that the risk of dying with an uncontrolled airway is greater than the risk of inducing spinal cord damage using a careful approach to airway control.

SUMMARY

Spinal cord injury is a devastating consequence of modern-day trauma. Unstable or incomplete damage to the spinal column or cord is not predictable, and therefore trauma victims who are unconscious or have any mechanism of injury affecting the head, neck, or trunk should have their spines immobilized. Special cases require special techniques. You should transport pregnant patients and patients with continued airway bleeding with the backboard turned to the side. You may have to use special padding to stabilize the spines of pediatric and elderly patients. Leave the helmet in place on patients wearing helmets and shoulder pads. Remove the helmet if the patient is wearing a helmet but no shoulder pads. Once you have immobilized the patient, you are responsible for controlling the airway and must be prepared at all times to intervene should the patient vomit or have evidence of airway compromise.

BIBLIOGRAPHY

1. Aprahamian, L. "Experimental Cervical Spine Injury Model: Evaluation of Airway Management and Splinting Techniques." *Annals of Emergency Medicine*, Vol. 13 (1994), p. 584.

2. Henry, G. L., and N. Little. *Neurologic Emergencies*. New York: McGraw-Hill, 1985.

3. Illinois State Medical Association, *Guidelines for Helmet Fitting and Removal in Athletes*. Chicago: The Association, 1990.

4. Jacobs, L. M. "Prospective Analysis of Acute Cervical Spine Injury." *Annals of Emergency Medicine*, Vol. 15 (1986), p. 44.

5. Johnson, R. M. "Clinical Orthoses, A Guide to Their Selection and Use." *Clinical Orthopedics*, Vol. 154 (1981), p. 34.

6. Podolsky, S. "Efficacy of Cervical Spine Immobilization Methods." *Journal of Trauma*, Vol. 23 (1983), p. 461.

7. Seaman, P. J. "Log-roll Technique." *Emergency*, Vol. 24 (1992), p. 18.

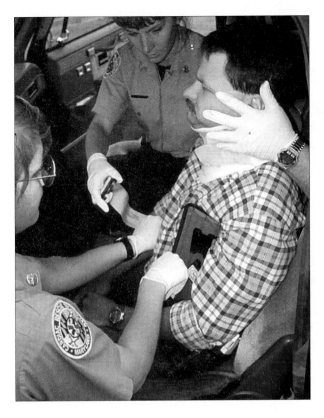

CHAPTER 9

Spine Management Skills

Donna Hastings, EMT-P

OBJECTIVES

Upon completion of this chapter you should be able to:

1. Explain when to use spinal immobilization.
2. Perform spinal immobilization with a short backboard.
3. Perform log-rolling of a victim onto a long backboard.
4. Properly secure a victim to a long backboard.
5. Immobilize a victim from a standing position.
6. Immobilize the head and neck when a neutral position cannot safely be attained.
7. Perform emergency rapid extrication.
8. Explain when helmets should and should not be removed from injured patients.
9. Properly remove a motorcycle helmet.
10. Demonstrate proper stabilization of the neck in patients who are wearing shoulder pads and helmets.

PATIENTS REQUIRING SPINAL IMMOBILIZATION

1. Any patient incurring trauma with obvious neurological deficit such as paralysis, weakness, or paresthesia (numbness or tingling)

2. Any patient incurring trauma who complains of pain in the head, neck, or back

3. Any patient incurring trauma who is unconscious

4. Any patient incurring trauma who may have injury to the spine but in whom evaluation is difficult due to altered mental status (e.g., drugs, alcohol)

5. Any unconscious patient who may have incurred trauma

6. Any patient incurring trauma with facial or head injuries

7. Any trauma patient subjected to deceleration forces

When in doubt, immobilize the patient.

Patients requiring immobilization must have it done before they are moved at all. In the case of an automobile accident, you must immobilize the patients before removing them from the wreckage. More movement is involved in extrication than at any other time, so you must immobilize the neck and spine before beginning extrication. *Remember:* Excessive traction can cause permanent paralysis. Your goal is to immobilize the spine and prevent further harm. Except in situations requiring rapid emergency extrication, always try to document sensation and motor function in the extremities before movement of the patient.

SPINAL IMMOBILIZATION USING THE SHORT BACKBOARD

The short backboard is used for patients who are in a position (such as an automobile) that does not allow for use of the long backboard. There are several different devices of this type: some devices have different strapping mechanisms from the one explained here. You must first practice with a piece of equipment before employing it in an emergency.

1. Remember that the priorities of evaluation and management are done before the immobilization devices go on.

2. One rescuer must, if possible, station himself behind the patient, place his hands on either side of the patient's head, and immobilize the neck in a neutral position. This step is part of the ABCs of evaluation. It is done at the same time that you begin evaluation of the airway.

3. When you have the patient stable enough to begin splinting, you must apply a semirigid extrication collar. If you have enough people, this can be done while someone else is doing the ABCs of evaluation and management.

4. Position the backboard behind the patient. The first rescuer continues to immobilize the neck while the short backboard is being maneuvered into place. The patient may have to be moved forward to get the backboard into place; great care must be taken that moves are coordinated so as to support the neck and back.

5. Secure the patient to the board: there are usually two straps for this. Bring each strap over a leg, down between both legs, back around the outside of the same leg, across the chest, and then attach them to the opposite upper straps that were brought across the shoulders.

6. Tighten the straps until the patient is held securely.

7. Secure the patient's head to the board by wide tape or elastic wraps around the forehead. Apply padding under the neck and head as needed to maintain a neutral position.

8. Transfer the patient to a long backboard. Turn the patient so that his back is to the opening through which he is to be removed. Someone must support his legs so that the upper legs remain at a 90-degree angle to the torso. Position the long backboard through the opening until it is under the patient. Lower the patient back onto the long backboard and slide the patient and the short backboard up into position on the long backboard. Loosen the straps on the short board and allow the patient's legs to extend out flat and then retighten the straps. Now secure him to the long backboard with straps, and secure his head with a padded immobilization device. When he is secured in this way, it is possible to turn the whole board up on its side if the patient has to vomit. The patient should remain securely immobilized.

These steps are illustrated in Figures 9-1 through 9-13.

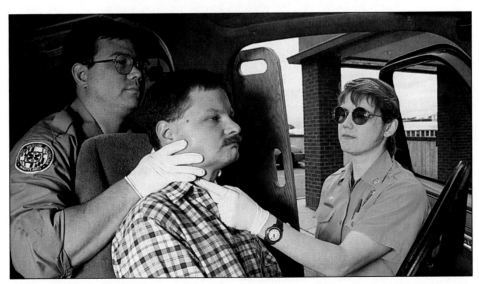

Figure 9-1 *Stabilize the neck and perform the primary survey.*

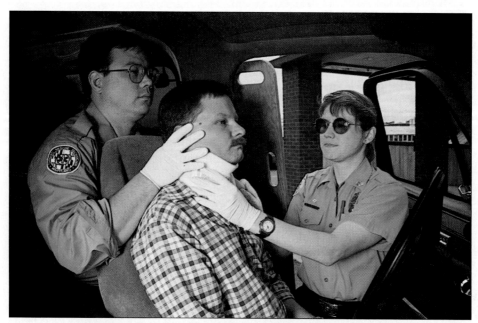

Figure 9-2 *Apply a semirigid extrication collar.*

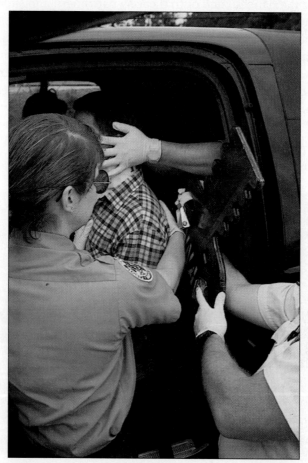

Figure 9-3 *Position the short backboard behind the patient. Coordinate all movement so that the spine is kept immobile.*

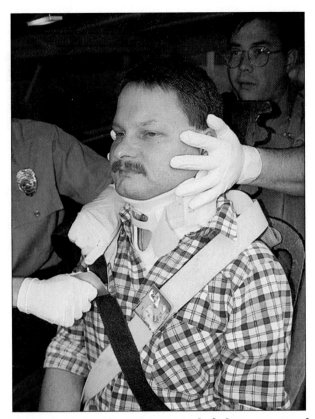

Figure 9-4 *Apply straps and tighten securely.*

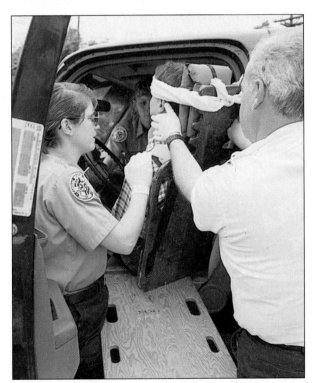

Figure 9-5 *Turn the patient carefully; then lower onto the long backboard.*

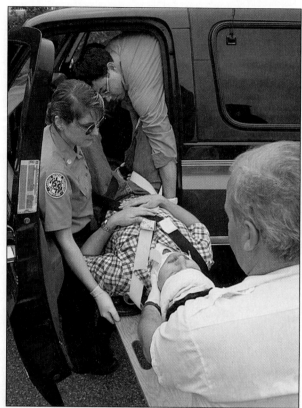

Figure 9-6 *Slide the patient and the short backboard up into position on the long backboard. Loosen the straps and allow the legs to extend out flat; then retighten the straps. Secure the patient and the short backboard to the long backboard. Apply padded immobilization device to secure the patient's head and neck.*

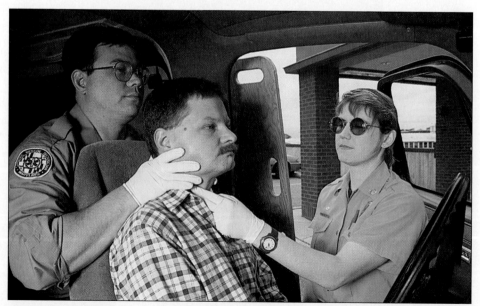

Figure 9-7 *Kendrick extrication device (KED). Stabilize the neck and perform the primary survey.*

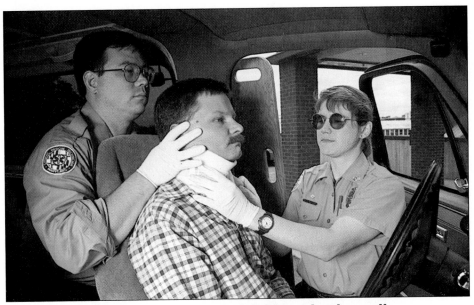

Figure 9-8 *Apply a semirigid extrication collar.*

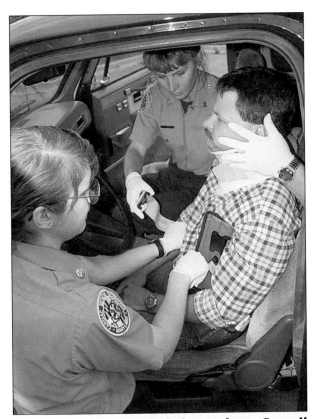

Figure 9-9 *Position the device behind the patient. Coordinate all movements so that the spine is kept immobile. Position the chest panels up well into the armpits.*

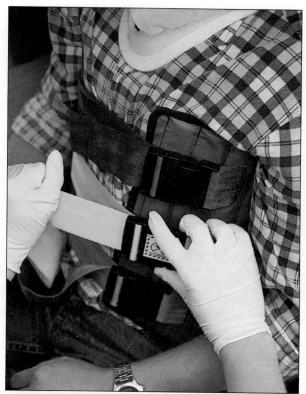

Figure 9-10 *Tighten the chest straps.*

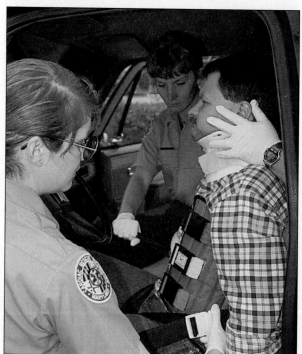

Figure 9-11 *Loop each leg strap around the ipsilateral (same side) leg and back to the buckle on the same side. Fasten snugly.*

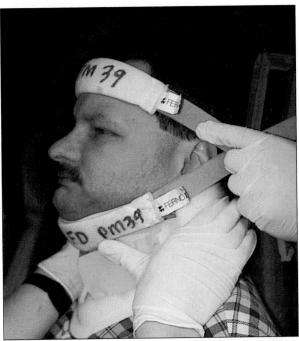

Figure 9-12 *Apply firm padding as needed between the head and the headpiece to keep the head in a neutral position. Bring the head flaps around to the side of the head and secure firmly with straps, tape, or elastic wrap.*

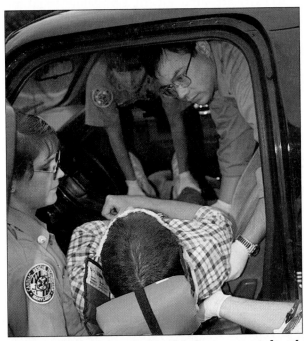

Figure 9-13 *Turn the patient and the device as a unit; then lower onto a long backboard. Slide the patient and the device up into position on the board. Loosen the leg straps and allow the legs to extend out flat; then retighten the straps. Secure the patient and the device to the backboard.*

1. When you are placing the straps around the legs on a male, do not catch the genitals in the straps.

2. Do not use the short board as a "handle" to move the patient. Move both patient and board as a unit.

3. When you are applying the horizontal strap (long backboard) around a woman, place the upper strap above her breasts and under her arms, not across the breasts.

4. When you are applying the lower horizontal strap on a pregnant woman, place it across the pelvis and not across the uterus.

5. Injuries may force you to modify how you attach the straps.

6. The patient must be secured well enough to have no motion of the spine if the board is turned on its side. Do not tighten straps so tight as to interfere with breathing.

RAPID EXTRICATION

Patients left inside vehicles after an accident are usually stabilized on a short backboard (or extrication device) and then transferred onto a long backboard. Although this is the best way to extricate anyone with a possible spinal injury, there are certain situations where a more rapid method must be used.

SITUATIONS REQUIRING EMERGENCY RAPID EXTRICATION

Your scene survey identifies a condition that may immediately endanger the victim or you.

EXAMPLES

1. Fire or immediate danger of fire
2. Danger of explosion
3. Rapidly rising water
4. Structure in danger of collapse
5. Continuing toxic exposure

Your primary survey of the patient identifies a condition that requires immediate intervention that cannot be done in the vehicle.

EXAMPLES

1. Airway obstruction that you cannot relieve by jaw thrust or finger sweep
2. Cardiac or respiratory arrest
3. Chest or airway injuries requiring ventilation or assisted ventilation
4. Deep shock or bleeding that you cannot control

This procedure is used only in a situation where the victim's life is in immediate danger. Whenever you use the procedure, it should be noted in the written report and you should be prepared to defend your actions at a review by your Medical Direction physician. This is an example of "desperate situations often demand desperate measures."

TECHNIQUE

1. One rescuer must, if possible, station himself behind the patient, place his hands on either side of the patient's head, and stabilize the neck in a neutral position. This step is part of the ABCs of evaluation. It is done at the same time that you begin evaluation of the airway.

2. Do a rapid survey; then quickly apply a cervical collar. You should have the collar with you when you begin.

3. If your scene survey or your primary survey of the patient reveals an immediate life-threatening situation, go to the emergency rapid extrication technique described shortly. This requires at least four and preferably five or six persons to perform well.

4. Immediately slide the long backboard onto the seat and, if possible, at least slightly under the patient's buttocks.

5. A second rescuer stands close beside the open door of the vehicle and takes over control of the cervical spine.

6. Rescuer 1 or another rescuer is positioned on the other side of the front seat ready to rotate the patient's legs around.

7. Another rescuer is also positioned at the open door by the patient. By holding the upper torso, he works together with the rescuer holding the legs to turn the patient carefully.

8. The patient is turned so that his back is toward the backboard. His legs are lifted and his back is lowered to the backboard. The neck and back are not allowed to bend during this maneuver.

9. Using teamwork, the patient is carefully slid to the full length of the backboard and his legs are carefully straightened.

10. The patient is then moved immediately away from the vehicle (to the ambulance if available) and resuscitation is begun. He is secured to the backboard as soon as possible.

These steps are illustrated in Figures 9-14 through 9-21.

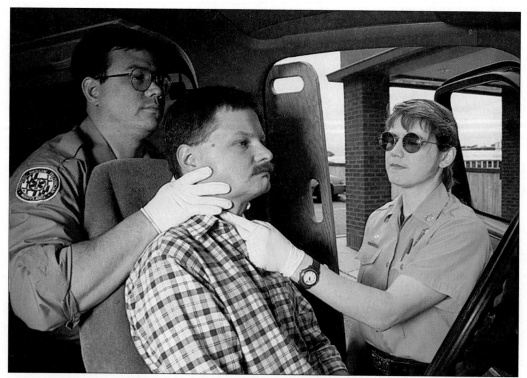

Figure 9-14 *Stabilize the neck and perform the primary survey.*

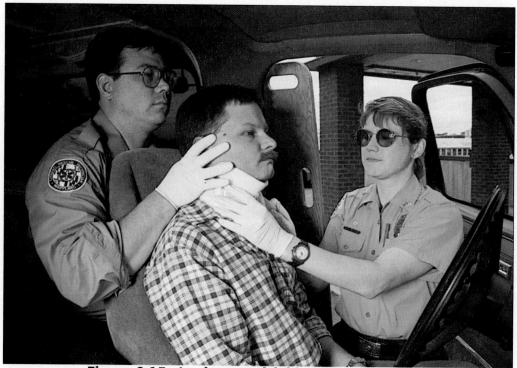

Figure 9-15 *Apply a semirigid extrication collar.*

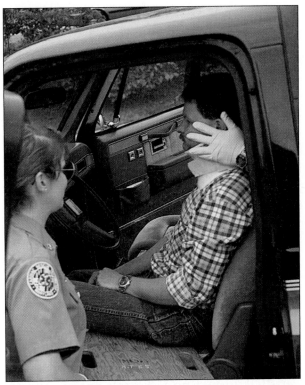

Figure 9-16 *Slide the long backboard onto the seat and slightly under the patient.*

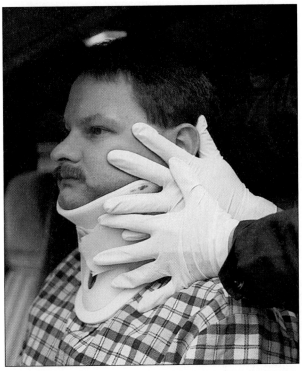

Figure 9-17 *A second rescuer stands close beside the open door of the vehicle and takes over control of the cervical spine.*

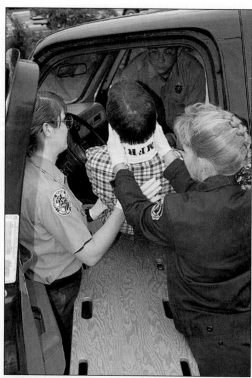

Figure 9-18 *Carefully supporting the neck, torso, and legs, the rescuers turn the patient.*

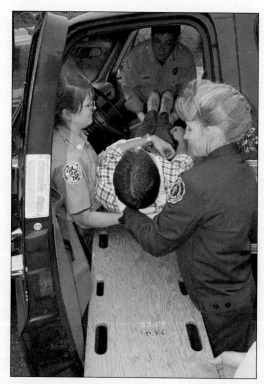

Figure 9-19 *The legs are lifted and the back is lowered to the backboard.*

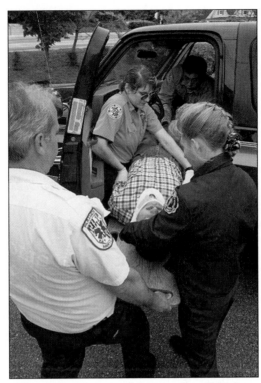

Figure 9-20 *Carefully slide the patient to the full length of the backboard.*

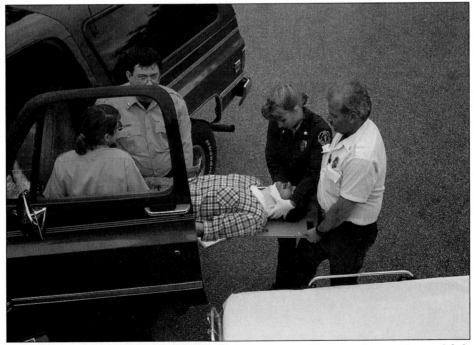

Figure 9-21 *The patient is immediately moved away from the vehicle and into the ambulance, if available. Secure the patient to the backboard as soon as possible.*

SPINAL IMMOBILIZATION USING THE LONG BACKBOARD

LOG-ROLLING THE SUPINE PATIENT

These steps are illustrated in Figures 9-22 through 9-29.

1. Rescuer 1 maintains the spine immobilized in a neutral position. Do not apply traction. A semirigid extrication collar is applied. Even with the collar in place, rescuer 1 maintains the head and neck in a neutral position until the log-rolling maneuver is completed.

2. The patient is placed with his legs extended in the normal manner and his arms (palms inward) extended by his sides. The patient will be rolled up on one arm with that arm providing proper spacing and acting as a splint for the body.

3. The long backboard is positioned next to the body. If one arm is injured, place the backboard on the injured side so that the patient will roll upon the uninjured arm.

4. Rescuers 2 and 3 kneel at the patient's side opposite the board.

5. Rescuer 2 is positioned at the midchest area and Rescuer 3 is by the upper legs.

6. With his knees, rescuer 2 holds the patient's near arm in place. He then reaches across the patient and grasps the shoulder and the hips, holding the patient's far arm in place. Usually, it is possible to grasp the patient's clothing to help with the roll.

7. With one hand, rescuer 3 reaches across the patient and grasps the hip. With his other hand, he holds the feet together at the lower legs.

8. When everyone is ready, rescuer 1 gives the order to roll the patient.

9. Rescuer 1 carefully keeps the head and neck in a neutral position (anterior-posterior as well as laterally) during the roll.

10. Rescuers 2 and 3 roll the victim up on his side toward them. The patient's arms are kept locked to his side to maintain a splinting effect. The head, shoulders, and pelvis are kept in line during the roll.

11. When the patient is upon his or her side, rescuer 2 (or rescuer 4, if available) quickly examines the back for injuries.

12. The backboard is now positioned next to the patient and held at a 30- to 45-degree angle by rescuer 4. If there are only three rescuers, the board is pulled into place by rescuer 2 or 3. The board is left flat in this case.

13. When everybody is ready, rescuer 1 gives the order to roll the patient onto the backboard. This is accomplished keeping head, shoulders, and pelvis in line.

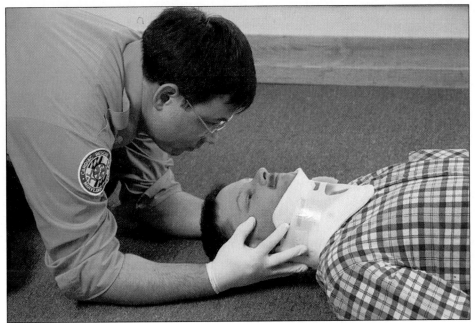

Figure 9-22 *Rescuer 1 maintains the neck immobilized in a neutral position.*

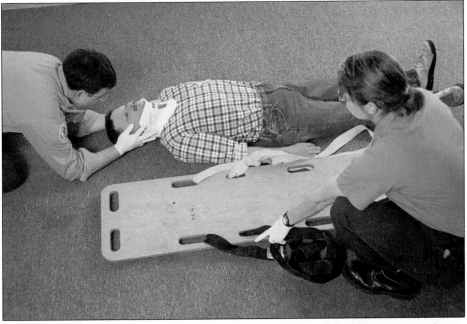

Figure 9-23 *The long backboard is positioned beside the patient.*

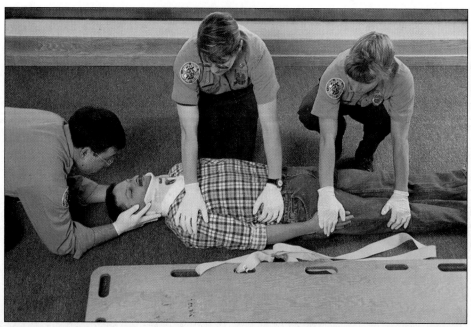

Figure 9-24 *Rescuer 2 and rescuer 3 assume their positions at the patient's side opposite the board.*

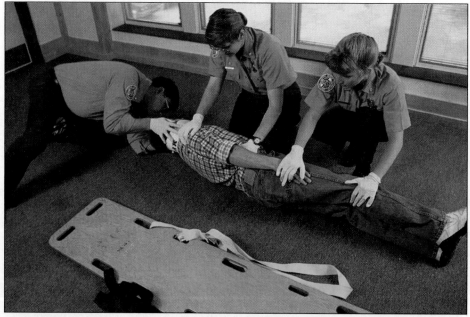

Figure 9-25 *The patient is carefully rolled upon his side.*

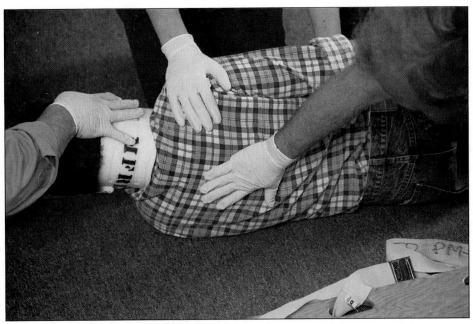

Figure 9-26 *Quickly examine the back for injuries.*

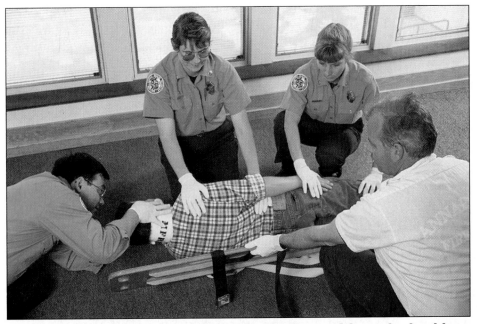

Figure 9-27 *If another person is available, he positions the backboard next to the patient at a 30- to 45-degree angle.*

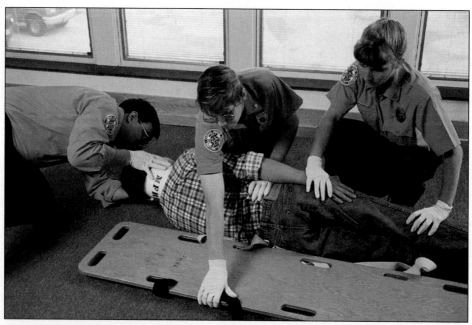

Figure 9-28 *If no other help is available rescuer 2 or 3 positions the backboard and leaves it flat.*

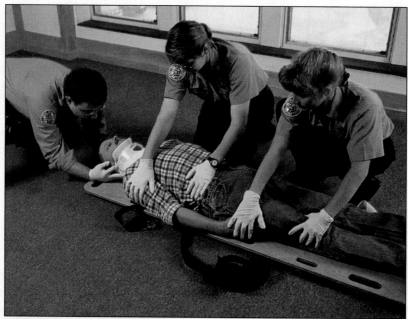

Figure 9-29 *At rescuer 1's order, the patient is rolled onto the backboard. All movements are coordinated so that the spine is kept straight at all times.*

LOG-ROLLING THE PRONE (FACE DOWN) PATIENT

The status of the airway is critical for decisions concerning the order of the log-rolling procedure. There are three clinical situations that dictate how you should proceed.

1. The patient who is not breathing or who is in severe respiratory difficulty must be log-rolled immediately to manage the airway. Unless the backboard is already positioned, you must log-roll the patient, manage the airway, then transfer the patient to the backboard (in a second log-rolling step) when ready to transport.

2. The patient with profuse bleeding of the mouth or nose must not be turned to the supine position. Profuse upper airway bleeding in a supine patient is a guarantee of aspiration. This patient will have to be carefully immobilized and transported prone or on his side, allowing gravity to help keep the airway clear.

3. The patient with an adequate airway and respiration should be log-rolled directly onto a backboard.

LOG-ROLLING THE SUPINE PATIENT WHO HAS AN ADEQUATE AIRWAY

See Figure 9-30.

1. Rescuer 1 immobilizes the neck in a neutral position. When placing the hands on the head and neck, the rescuer's thumbs always point toward the patient's face. This prevents having the rescuer's arms crossed when the patient is log-rolled. A semirigid extrication collar is applied.

2. A rapid survey is done (including the back) and the patient is placed with his legs extended in the normal manner and his arms (palms inward) extended by his sides. The patient will be rolled up on one arm, with that arm acting as a splint for the body.

3. The long backboard is positioned next to the body. The backboard is placed on the side of rescuer 1's lower hand (if rescuer 1's lower hand is on the patient's right side, the backboard is placed on the patient's right side). If the arm next to the backboard is injured, carefully raise the arm above the victim's head so he does not roll on the injured arm.

4. Rescuers 2 and 3 kneel at the patient's side opposite the board.

5. Rescuer 2 is positioned at the midchest area and rescuer 3 is by the upper legs.

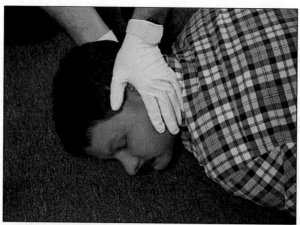

Figure 9-30 *When immobilizing the neck of the prone (or supine) patient, your thumbs always point toward the face (not the occiput). This prevents having your arms crossed when the patient is rolled over.*

6. Rescuer 2 grasps the shoulder and the hip. Usually, it is possible to grasp the victim's clothing to help with the roll.

7. Rescuer 3 grasps the hip (holding the near arm in place) and the lower legs (holding them together).

8. When everyone is ready, rescuer 1 gives the order to roll the patient.

9. Rescuer 1 carefully keeps the head and neck in a neutral position (anteroposterior as well as laterally) during the roll.

10. Rescuers 2 and 3 roll the patient up on his side away from them. The patient's arms are kept locked to his side to maintain a splinting effect. The head, shoulders, and pelvis are kept in line during the roll.

11. The backboard is now positioned next to the patient and held at a 30- to 45-degree angle by rescuer 4. If there are only three rescuers, the board is pulled into place by rescuer 2 or 3. The board is left flat in this case.

12. When everyone is ready, rescuer 1 gives the order to roll the patient onto the backboard. This is accomplished keeping the head, shoulders, and pelvis in line.

SECURING THE PATIENT TO THE BACKBOARD

There are several different methods of securing the victim using straps. Two examples of commercial devices for full body immobilization are the Reeves sleeve and the Miller body split. The Reeves sleeve is a heavy-duty sleeve that a standard backboard will slide into. Attached to this sleeve are:

1. A head immobilization device
2. Heavy vinyl-coated nylon panels that go over the chest and abdomen and are secured with seat-belt-type straps and quick-release connectors
3. Two full-length leg panels to secure the lower extremities
4. Straps to hold the arms in place
5. Six handles for carrying the patient
6. Metal rings (2500-lb strength) for lifting the victim by rope

When the patient is in this device, he remains immobilized when lifted horizontally, vertically, or even carried on his side (like a suitcase). This device is excellent for the confused, combative victim who must be restrained for his safety.

The Miller body split is a combination backboard, head immobilizer, and body immobilizer. Like the Reeves sleeve, it does an excellent job of full-body immobilization with a minimum of time and effort.

There are several different commercial strapping systems available. As with all equipment, you should become familiar with your strapping system before using it in an emergency situation.

APPLYING AND SECURING A LONG BACKBOARD TO A STANDING PATIENT

METHOD 1

1. One person stands behind the patient and immobilizes the head and neck in a neutral position. Apply a semirigid extrication collar and maintain immobilization in a neutral position.
2. A long backboard is placed on the ground behind the patient.
3. Other rescuers stabilize the shoulders and trunk and allow the victim to carefully sit down on the backboard.
4. The patient is carefully lowered back onto the backboard maintaining stabilization of the head, neck, and trunk.
5. The patient is centered on the backboard and secured.

METHOD 2

1. Rescuer 1 stands in front of the patient and immobilizes the head and neck in a neutral position. Apply a semirigid cervical collar. Rescuer 1 continues to maintain immobilization in a neutral position.
2. Rescuer 2 places a long backboard against the patient's back.
3. Rescuer 3 secures the patient to the board using nylon straps. These must cross over the shoulders and the pelvis and legs to prevent movement when the board is tilted down.

4. Place padding behind the patient's head to maintain a neutral position and apply and secure a blanket roll or commercial head immobilizer using elastic wraps or wide tape.

5. Carefully tilt the board back onto a stretcher and secure the legs.

IMMOBILIZING THE HEAD AND NECK WHEN A NEUTRAL POSITION CANNOT SAFELY BE ATTAINED

If the head or neck is held in an angulated position and the patient complains of pain on any attempt to straighten it, you should immobilize it in the position found. The same is true of the unconscious patient whose neck is held to one side and does not easily straighten with gentle traction. You cannot use a cervical collar or commercial head immobilizer in this situation. You must use pads or a blanket roll and careful taping to immobilize the head and neck in the position found.

HELMET MANAGEMENT

IMPORTANT POINTS ABOUT HELMET REMOVAL

1. Patients wearing both helmets and shoulder pads can usually have their spines maintained in a more neutral position by leaving the helmet in place and padding and taping the helmet to the backboard.

2. Face masks on helmets can be removed with EMS-type scissors.

3. Patients wearing helmets but no shoulder pads can usually have their spines maintained in a more neutral position by removing the helmet.

4. Full-face motorcycle-type helmets must be removed to evaluate and manage the airway.

REMOVING A MOTORCYCLE HELMET FROM A PATIENT WITH A POSSIBLE CERVICAL SPINE INJURY

See Figures 9-31 and 9-32.

1. Position yourself above or behind the victim, place your hands on each side of the helmet, and immobilize the head and neck by holding the helmet and the patient's neck.

2. Your partner positions himself to the side of the patient and removes the chin strap. Chin straps can usually be removed easily without cutting them.

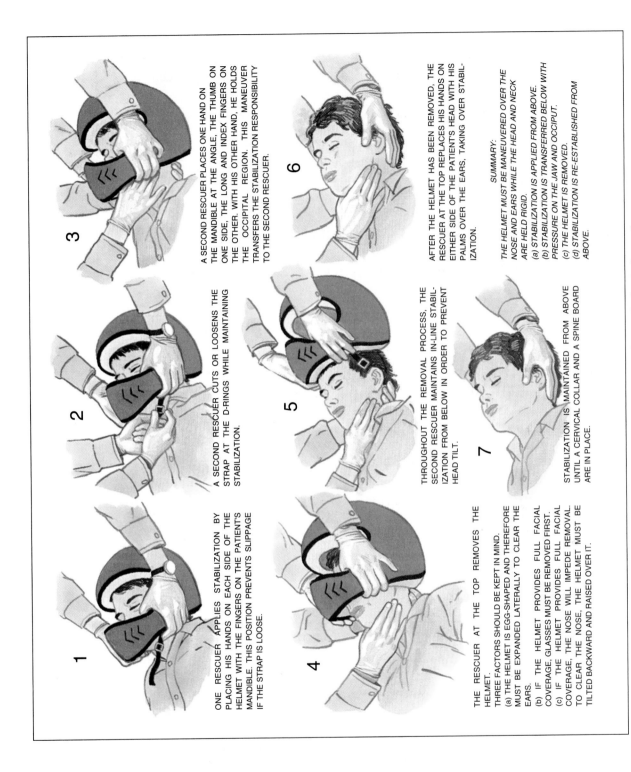

1 ONE RESCUER APPLIES STABILIZATION BY PLACING HIS HANDS ON EACH SIDE OF THE HELMET WITH THE FINGERS ON THE PATIENT'S MANDIBLE. THIS POSITION PREVENTS SLIPPAGE IF THE STRAP IS LOOSE.

2 A SECOND RESCUER CUTS OR LOOSENS THE STRAP AT THE D-RINGS WHILE MAINTAINING STABILIZATION.

3 A SECOND RESCUER PLACES ONE HAND ON THE MANDIBLE AT THE ANGLE, THE THUMB ON ONE SIDE, THE LONG AND INDEX FINGERS ON THE OTHER. WITH HIS OTHER HAND, HE HOLDS THE OCCIPITAL REGION. THIS MANEUVER TRANSFERS THE STABILIZATION RESPONSIBILITY TO THE SECOND RESCUER.

4 THE RESCUER AT THE TOP REMOVES THE HELMET.
THREE FACTORS SHOULD BE KEPT IN MIND.
(a) THE HELMET IS EGG-SHAPED AND THEREFORE MUST BE EXPANDED LATERALLY TO CLEAR THE EARS.
(b) IF THE HELMET PROVIDES FULL FACIAL COVERAGE, GLASSES MUST BE REMOVED FIRST.
(c) IF THE HELMET PROVIDES FULL FACIAL COVERAGE, THE NOSE WILL IMPEDE REMOVAL. TO CLEAR THE NOSE, THE HELMET MUST BE TILTED BACKWARD AND RAISED OVER IT.

5 THROUGHOUT THE REMOVAL PROCESS, THE SECOND RESCUER MAINTAINS IN-LINE STABILIZATION FROM BELOW IN ORDER TO PREVENT HEAD TILT.

6 AFTER THE HELMET HAS BEEN REMOVED, THE RESCUER AT THE TOP REPLACES HIS HANDS ON EITHER SIDE OF THE PATIENT'S HEAD WITH HIS PALMS OVER THE EARS, TAKING OVER STABILIZATION.

7 STABILIZATION IS MAINTAINED FROM ABOVE UNTIL A CERVICAL COLLAR AND A SPINE BOARD ARE IN PLACE.

SUMMARY:
THE HELMET MUST BE MANEUVERED OVER THE NOSE AND EARS WHILE THE HEAD AND NECK ARE HELD RIGID.
(a) STABILIZATION IS APPLIED FROM ABOVE.
(b) STABILIZATION IS TRANSFERRED BELOW WITH PRESSURE ON THE JAW AND OCCIPUT.
(c) THE HELMET IS REMOVED.
(d) STABILIZATION IS RE-ESTABLISHED FROM ABOVE.

Figure 9-31 Helmet removal from injured patient.

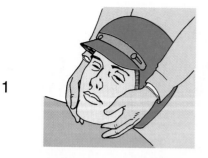

1

THE FIRST EMT POSITIONS HIMSELF ABOVE OR
BEHIND THE VICTIM AND PLACES HIS HANDS ON
EACH SIDE OF THE NECK AT THE BASE OF THE
SKULL. HE MAINTAINS STEADY IMMOBILIZATION
WITH THE NECK IN A NEUTRAL POSITION. HE
MAY USE HIS THUMBS TO PERFORM A MODIFIED
JAW THRUST WHILE DOING THIS.

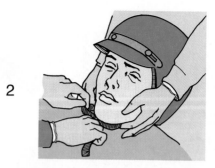

2

THE SECOND EMT POSITIONS HIMSELF OVER
TO THE SIDE OF THE VICTIM AND REMOVES OR
CUTS THE CHIN STRAP.

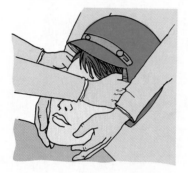

3

THE SECOND EMT NOW REMOVES THE HELMET
BY PULLING OUT LATERALLY ON EACH SIDE TO
CLEAR THE EARS AND THEN UP TO REMOVE.
FULL FACE HELMETS WILL HAVE TO BE TILTED
BACK TO CLEAR THE NOSE (TILT THE HELMET,
NOT THE HEAD). IF THE VICTIM HAS GLASSES
ON, THE SECOND EMT SHOULD REMOVE THEM
THROUGH THE VISUAL OPENING BEFORE
REMOVING THE FULL FACE HELMET. THE FIRST
EMT MAINTAINS STEADY IMMOBILIZATION
DURING THIS PROCEDURE.

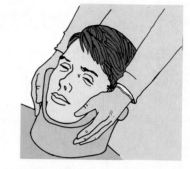

4

THE SECOND EMT NOW APPLIES A RIGID
EXTRICATION COLLAR. THE FIRST EMT
MAINTAINS IMMOBILIZATION UNTIL THE VICTIM
IS TRANSFERRED TO A BACKBOARD AND A
PADDED IMMOBILIZATION DEVICE IS APPLIED.

Figure 9-32 *Alternate method for removal of helmet.*

3. Your partner then assumes the stabilization by placing one
hand under the neck and the occiput and the other hand on
the anterior neck with the thumb pressing on one angle of
the mandible and the index and middle fingers pressing on
the other angle of the mandible.

4. You now remove the helmet by pulling out laterally on each
side to clear the ears and then up to remove. Tilt full-face
helmets back to clear the nose (tilt the helmet, not the head).

If the patient is wearing glasses, remove them through the visual opening before removing the full-face helmet. Your partner maintains steady immobilization of the neck during this procedure.

5. After removal of the helmet, you again assume immobilization of the neck by grasping the head on either side with your fingers holding one angle of the jaw and the occiput.

6. Your partner now applies a suitable cervical immobilization device.

ALTERNATE PROCEDURE FOR REMOVING A HELMET

This has the advantage of one person maintaining immobilization of the neck throughout the whole procedure. This procedure does not work well with full-face helmets.

1. Position yourself above or behind the patient and place your hands on each side of the neck at the base of the skull. Immobilize the neck in a neutral position. If necessary, you may use your thumbs to perform a modified jaw thrust while doing this.

2. Your partner positions himself over or to the side of the patient and removes the chin strap.

3. Your partner now removes the helmet by pulling out laterally on each side to clear the ears and then up to remove. You maintain immobilization of the neck during the procedure.

4. Your partner now applies a suitable cervical immobilization device.

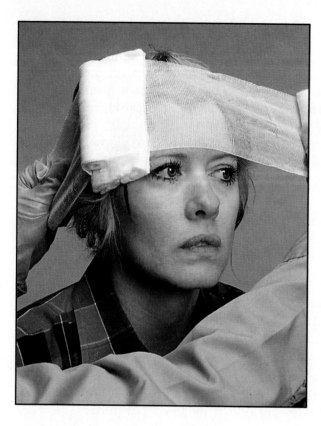

Head Trauma

John E. Campbell, M.D., F.A.C.E.P.

OBJECTIVES

Upon completion of this chapter you should be able to:

1. Describe the anatomy of the head and brain.
2. Describe the process of brain swelling and explain the need for immediate hyperventilation.
3. Describe the assessment of the patient with a head injury.
4. Describe the management of the patient with a head injury.
5. Identify potential problems in the management of the patient with a head injury.

Approximately 40% of multiple-trauma patients have central nervous system (CNS) injuries. This group has a death rate twice as high (35% versus 17%) as that of patients without CNS injuries. Head injuries account for an estimated 25% of all trauma deaths and up to one-half of all motor vehicle fatalities. As with other injuries, prompt and organized evaluation and treatment give the patient the greatest chance for complete recovery. To manage the head-injured patient most effectively, you should have a working knowledge of the basic anatomy and physiology of the head and brain. Head injuries may represent bruising of the brain tissue with swelling and increased intracranial pressure, injury to blood vessels with bleeding and increased intracranial pressure, or penetrating injuries of the skull that directly damage brain tissue. *You must always assume that a serious head injury is accompanied by an injury to the cervical spine and spinal cord.*

ANATOMY OF THE HEAD

The head (excluding the face and facial structures) includes the following (see Figure 10-1):

1. Scalp
2. Skull
3. Fibrous coverings of the brain (meninges)
4. Brain tissue
5. Cerebrospinal fluid
6. Vascular compartments

The scalp is very vascular and bleeds freely when lacerated. Because many of the small blood vessels are suspended in an inelastic matrix of supporting tissue, the normal protective vasospasm that would limit bleeding is inhibited, which may lead to prolonged bleeding and significant blood loss. The skull is like a closed box; the only significant opening through which pressure can be released is the foramen magnum at the base where the brainstem becomes the spinal cord. The rigid and unyielding bony skull contributes to several injury mechanisms in head trauma. Because of the way the brain is situated in the skull, there is greater movement at the top of the brain than at the base. This is a factor upon impact. The temporal bone (temple) is quite thin and easily fractured. The fibrous coverings of the brain include the dura mater ("tough mother"), which covers the entire brain; the thinner pia arachnoid (called simply the arachnoid), which lies underneath the dura and in which are suspended both arteries and veins; and the very thin pia mater ("soft mother"), which lies underneath the arachnoid and is adherent to the surface of the brain. The cerebrospinal fluid is found beneath the arachnoid and pia mater.

The brain fills the entire skull, which virtually excludes any adaptation to swelling. This is of great importance in the pathophysiology of head tissue.

Cerebrospinal fluid ("spinal fluid") is a nutrient fluid that bathes the brain and spinal cord. Spinal fluid is continually created within the ventricles of the brain at a rate of 1/3 mL/min. It is reabsorbed by the arachnoid membrane that covers the brain and spinal cord. Anything obstructing the flow of spinal fluid will cause an accumulation of spinal fluid within the brain (hydrocephalus) and will cause an increase in intracerebral pressure.

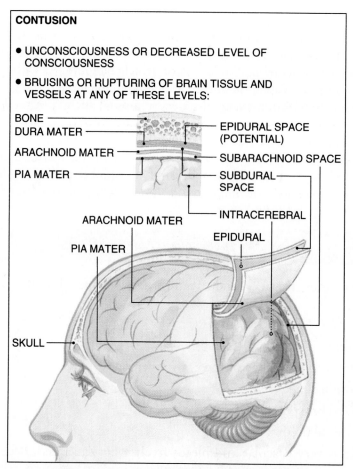

Figure 10-1 *Coverings of the brain.*

PATHOPHYSIOLOGY OF HEAD TRAUMA

Most brain injuries are not from direct injury to brain tissue, but occur either as a result of external forces applied against the exterior of the skull or from movement of the brain inside the skull. In deceleration injuries the head usually strikes an object such as the windshield of an automobile, which causes a sudden deceleration of the skull. The brain continues to move forward, impacting first against the skull in the original direction of motion and then rebounding to hit the opposite side of the inner surface of the skull. Thus, injuries may occur to the brain in the area of original impact ("coup") or on the opposite side ("contrecoup").

The interior base of the skull is rough. Movement of the brain over this area may cause various degrees of injury to the brain tissue or to blood vessels supporting the brain (see Figure 10-2).

The initial response of the bruised brain is swelling. Bruising causes vasodilatation with increased blood flow to the injured area and thus an accumulation of blood that takes up space and exerts pressure on surrounding brain tissue. There is no extra space inside the skull so swelling of the injured area exerts pressure upon and thus decreases blood flow to the uninjured areas of the brain. The increase in cerebral water (edema) does not occur immediately but develops over the next 24 to 48 hours. Your early efforts to decrease the initial vasodilatation in the injured areas of the brain can be life saving.

The blood level of carbon dioxide (CO_2) has a critical effect on cerebral blood vessels. The normal level of CO_2 is 40 mm Hg. An *increase* in the level of CO_2 promotes cerebral *vasodilatation*, while *lowering* the level of CO_2 causes *vasoconstriction*. If a head-injured patient is poorly ventilated, the rise in CO_2 causes vasodilatation and contributes to brain swelling, thereby increasing the intracerebral pressure. Conversely, hyperventilation (more than 24 breaths per minute) can decrease the CO_2 to about 25 mm Hg, causing rapid cerebral vasoconstriction. Prompt definitive airway management along with hyperventilation helps to minimize the development of cerebral edema and allows better perfusion of the entire brain. Early in the course of the injury, hyperventilation is more important than the administration of mannitol or furosemide (Lasix[R]). Because mannitol and furosemide are diuretics (stimulate urination), they require more time for full effect and should not be relied upon to replace vigorous oxygenation and hyperventilation. Any victim who shows signs of increasing intracranial pressure or decreasing level of consciousness should have *immediate hyperventilation.*

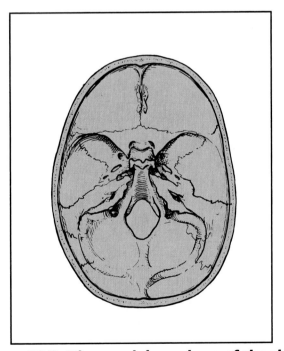

Figure 10-2 *The rough inner base of the skull.*

INTRACRANIAL PRESSURE

Within the skull and fibrous coverings of the brain are the brain tissue, cerebrospinal fluid, and blood. An increase in the volume of one of these components must be at the expense of the other two because the adult skull (a "rigid box") cannot expand. Although there is some "give" to the volume of cerebrospinal fluid, it accounts for little space and cannot offset rapid brain swelling. Blood supply cannot be compromised, for the brain requires a constant supply of blood (oxygen and glucose) to survive. Thus, since none of the supporting components of the brain can be compromised, an increase in brain swelling rapidly becomes catastrophic.

The pressure of the brain contents within the skull is termed intracranial pressure. The pressure of the blood flowing through the brain is termed the cerebral perfusion pressure. Its value is obtained by subtracting the intracranial (intracerebral) pressure from the mean arterial blood pressure. If the brain swells or if there is bleeding inside the skull, intracranial pressure increases and the perfusion pressure decreases. The body has protective reflex (Cushing response or reflex) that attempts to maintain a constant perfusion pressure: as the intracerebral pressure increases, the systemic blood pressure increases to try to preserve blood flow to the brain. As the situation becomes more critical, the pulse rate drops (bradycardia), and eventually the respiratory rate declines. The pressure within the skull continues in an upward spiral until a critical point at which time the head injury becomes overwhelming and all vital signs deteriorate, ending in the patient's death.

HERNIATION SYNDROME

When the brain swells, particularly after a blow to the head, a sudden rise in intracranial pressure may occur. This may force portions of the brain downward, obstructing the flow of cerebrospinal fluid and applying great pressure to the brainstem. This is a life-threatening situation characterized by decreasing level of consciousness that rapidly progresses to coma, dilation of the pupil and outward-downward deviation of the eye on the side of the injury, paralysis of the arm and leg on the side opposite the injury, and decerebrate posturing (described shortly). The patient may soon cease all movement, stop breathing, and die. This syndrome often follows an acute subdural hemorrhage.

ANOXIC BRAIN INJURY

Injuries to the brain from lack of oxygen (e.g., cardiac arrest, airway obstruction, near-drowning) affect the brain in a serious fashion. If the brain is without oxygen for a period greater than 4 to 6 minutes, irreversible damage almost always occurs. Following a nontraumatic anoxic episode, spasm develops in the small cerebral arteries so that blood cannot flow to the cortex, and the patient will ultimately die from brain failure. One theory is that this arterial spasm is related to the flow of calcium into arterial muscle cells; complete spasm does not occur for approximately 90 minutes. While it is currently accepted that the brain cannot be effectively resuscitated after 4 to 6 minutes of anoxia, there are exceptions to the rule, notably the condition of hypothermia. There are cases of hypothermic patients being resuscitated after almost an hour of anoxia. Current research is directed toward finding a medication that will prevent the arterial spasm. In the future, there may be hope of brain recovery if resuscitation is accompanied by specific drug therapy within 90 minutes of anoxic injury.

HEAD INJURIES

SCALP WOUNDS

The scalp is very vascular and often bleeds briskly when lacerated, rapidly resulting in significant blood loss. This can be very important in children who bleed as freely as adults but do not have the same blood volume. Though an uncommon cause of shock in an adult, a child may develop shock from a briskly bleeding scalp wound. As a general rule, if you have an adult patient with a scalp injury who is in shock, look for another cause for the shock (such as internal bleeding). However, do not underestimate the blood loss from a scalp wound. Most bleeding from the scalp can be easily controlled in the field with direct pressure.

SKULL INJURIES

Skull injuries can be linear nondisplaced fractures, depressed fractures, or compound fractures (see Figure 10-3). Suspect an underlying skull fracture in adults with a large contusion or darkened swelling of the scalp. There is very little that can be done for these injuries in the field except to avoid placing direct pressure upon an obvious depressed or compound skull fracture. Penetrating objects in the skull should be left in place *(not removed)* and the patient transported immediately to the emergency department. If your patient has a gunshot wound to the head, unless there is a clear entrance and exit wound in a perfectly linear path, assume that the bullet may have ricocheted and be lodged in the neck near the spinal cord.

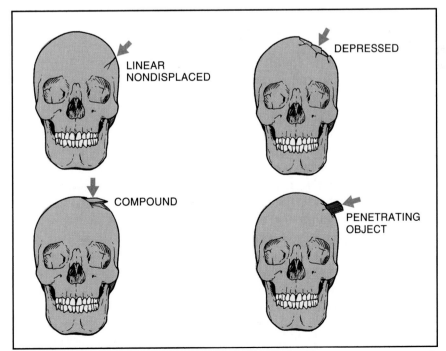

Figure 10-3 *Skull fracture—linear nondisplaced, depressed, compound, and penetrating object.*

Suspect child abuse when you find a child with a head injury and no clear explanation of its cause. Pay particular attention to the setting from which you rescued the child and request police or social service assistance if the circumstances suggest child abuse.

BRAIN INJURIES

CONCUSSION: A concussion implies no significant injury to the brain. There is usually a history of trauma to the head with a variable period of unconsciousness or confusion and then a return to normal consciousness. There may be amnesia from the injury. This amnesia usually extends to some point before the injury (retrograde short-term amnesia) so that often the patient will not remember the events leading to the injury. Short-term memory is often affected and the patient may repeat questions over and over as if he hasn't been paying attention to your answers. There may be dizziness, headache, ringing in the ears, and/or nausea.

CEREBRAL CONTUSION: A patient with cerebral contusion (bruised brain tissue) will have a history of prolonged unconsciousness or serious alteration in state of consciousness (e.g., profound confusion, persistent amnesia, abnormal behavior). Brain swelling may be rapid and severe. The patient may have focal neurological signs or appear to have suffered a cerebrovascular accident (stroke). Depending upon the location of the cerebral contusion, the victim may have personality changes such as inappropriately rude behavior. Any injured patient with an altered level of consciousness should be hyperventilated and rapidly transported to a trauma center.

INTRACRANIAL HEMORRHAGE: Hemorrhage can occur between the skull and dura (the fibrous covering of the brain), between the dura and the arachnoid, between the arachnoid and the brain, or directly into the brain tissue.

> 1. *Acute Epidural Hematoma.* This injury is most often caused by a tear in the middle meningeal artery that runs along the inside of the skull in the temporal region. The arterial injury is often caused by a linear skull fracture in the temporal or parietal region (see Figure 10-4). Because the bleeding is arterial (although it may be venous from one of the dural sinuses), the bleeding and pressure can occur rapidly, so death may occur quickly. Surgical removal of the blood and ligation of the ruptured blood vessel often allows full recovery if the underlying brain tissue is not injured. Symptoms of an acute epidural hematoma include a history of head trauma with initial loss of consciousness followed by a period during which the patient is conscious and coherent (the "lucid interval"). After a period of 30 minutes to 2 hours, the patient will develop signs of increasing intracranial pressure (vomiting, headache, altered mental status), lapse into unconsciousness, and develop body paralysis on the side opposite from the head injury. There is often a dilated and fixed (no response to bright light) pupil on the side of the head injury. Usually, this is followed

rapidly by death. The classic example is the boxer who is knocked unconscious, wakes up, and is allowed to go home, only to be found dead in bed the next morning.

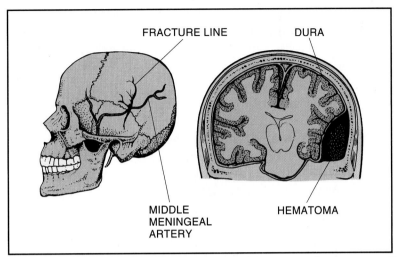

Figure 10-4 *Acute epidural hematoma. This hemorrhage may follow injury to the extradural arteries. The blood collects between the fibrous dura and the periosteum.*

2. *Acute Subdural Hematoma.* This is caused by bleeding between the dura and the arachnoid and is associated with injury to the underlying brain tissue (see Figure 10-5). Because the bleeding is venous, pressure increases more slowly and often the diagnosis is not apparent until hours or days after the injury. The signs and symptoms include

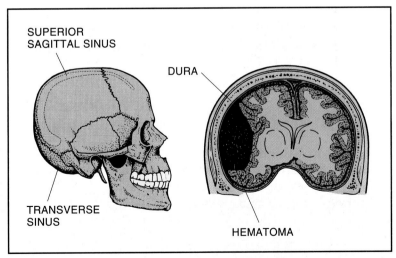

Figure 10-5 *Acute subdural hematoma. This usually occurs following the rupture of dural veins. Blood collects and often severely compresses the brain.*

headache, fluctuations in the level of consciousness, and focal neurological signs (e.g., weakness of one extremity or one side of the body, altered deep tendon reflexes, slurred speech). Because of underlying brain tissue injury, prognosis is often poor. Mortality is very high (60–90%) in victims who are comatose when found. Always suspect a subdural in an alcoholic with any degree of altered mental status following a fall.

3. *Intracerebral Hemorrhage.* This is bleeding within the brain tissue (see Figure 10-6). Traumatic intracerebral hemorrhage is always associated with penetrating injuries of the head and often associated with blunt head trauma. Unfortunately, surgery is usually not helpful. The signs and symptoms depend upon the regions involved and the degree of injury, in patterns similar to those that accompany a stroke.

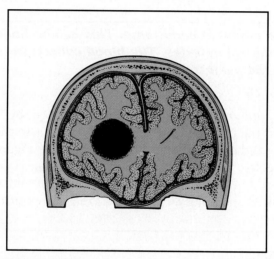

Figure 10-6 *Intracerebral hemorrhage.*

EVALUATION OF THE HEAD TRAUMA PATIENT

Head-injured patients may be difficult to manage because they will rarely be cooperative and are often under the influence of alcohol or drugs. As a rescuer, you must pay extraordinary attention to detail and never lose your patience with an uncooperative patient. Remember that every trauma victim is initially evaluated in the same sequence:

1. Make a total overview of the patient situation as you approach to begin your assessment.

2. Secure the *airway* as you stabilize the cervical spine and check initial level of consciousness.

3. Assess *breathing*.

4. Assess *circulation* and control major *bleeding*.

5. Determine transport decision and critical interventions

6. Perform secondary survey:

   a. Vital signs

   b. Sample history

   c. Head-to-toes exam (including neurological)

   d. Further bandaging and splinting

   e. Continuous monitoring

7. Perform reassessment surveys.

PRIMARY ASSESSMENT

Control of the airway cannot be overemphasized. The supine, restrained, and unconscious patient is prone to airway obstruction from the tongue, blood, vomit, or other secretions. Vomiting is very common within the first hour following a head injury. Protect the airway by placement of an oral or nasal airway and positioning the patient on his side (in the absence of suspicion for a cervical fracture). Be prepared for immediate suctioning.

In general, begin evaluation for head injury by speaking to the patient to obtain the initial level of consciousness. You will perform a much more detailed neurological exam during the secondary survey. Obviously, a patient with a history and physical examination that indicates an epidural hematoma should be transported in greater haste than would be an alert postconcussion victim. It is very important that you record all observations because the treatment is often dictated by detection of the deterioration of clinical stability. The goals of the evaluation are to determine quickly if the patient is brain injured, and if so, is his condition deteriorating? Level of consciousness is the most sensitive indicator of brain function.

It is essential to obtain as thorough a history about the event as possible. The circumstances of the head injury may be extremely important for management of the victim, and may be of prognostic importance with regard to the ultimate outcome. Pay particular attention to reports of near-drowning, electrocution, lightning strike, drug abuse, smoke inhalation, hypothermia, and seizures. Always inquire about the patient's behavior from the time of the head injury until the time of your arrival.

All patients with head or facial trauma have a cervical spine injury until proven otherwise. Stabilization of the cervical spine should accompany airway and breathing management. During the primary survey your neurological exam is limited to level of consciousness and any obvious paralysis. A change in the level of consciousness is the first indicator of a brain injury or increase in intracranial pressure. Keep your evaluation and report simple so that everyone can understand you. The AVPU method is quite adequate:

A— Patient is alert

V— Patient responds to vocal (voice) stimuli

P— Patient responds to painful stimuli

U— Patient is unresponsive

SECONDARY ASSESSMENT

Once the primary survey is completed and recorded, begin with the scalp and quickly, but carefully, examine for obvious injuries such as lacerations or depressed or open skull fractures. The size of a laceration is often misjudged because of the difficulty in assessment through hair matted with blood. Feel the scalp gently for obvious unstable areas of the skull. If none are present, you may safely apply a pressure dressing or hold direct pressure upon a bandage to stop scalp bleeding.

A basilar skull fracture (see Figure 10-7) may be indicated by bleeding from the ear or from the nose, clear fluid running from the nose, swelling and/or discoloration behind the ear (Battle's sign), and/or swelling and discoloration around both eyes (raccoon eyes).

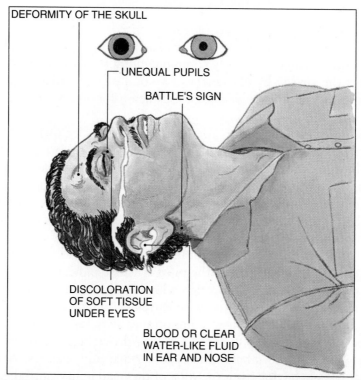

DEFORMITY OF THE SKULL

UNEQUAL PUPILS

BATTLE'S SIGN

DISCOLORATION
OF SOFT TISSUE
UNDER EYES

BLOOD OR CLEAR
WATER-LIKE FLUID
IN EAR AND NOSE

Figure 10-7 *Signs of basilar skull fracture—Battle's sign, raccoon eyes, and fluid from the nose or ears.*

PUPILS: The pupils (see Figure 10-8) are controlled in part by the third cranial nerve. This nerve takes a long course through the skull and is easily compressed by brain swelling, so it may be affected by increasing intracranial pressure. Following a head injury, if both pupils are dilated and do not react to light, the patient probably has a brainstem injury and the prognosis is grim. If the pupils are dilated but still react to light, the injury is often still reversible, so every effort should be made to quickly get the patient to a facility capable of treating a head injury. A unilaterally dilated pupil that remains reactive to light may be the earliest sign of increasing intracranial pressure. The development of a unilaterally dilated pupil ("blown pupil") while you are observing the patient is an extreme emergency and mandates rapid transport. Other causes of dilated pupils that may or may not react to light include hypothermia, lightning strike, anoxia, optic nerve injury, drug effect (e.g., atropine), or direct trauma to the eye. Fixed and dilated pupils signify head injury only in patients with decreased level of consciousness. If the patient has a normal level of consciousness, the dilated pupil is not from head injury.

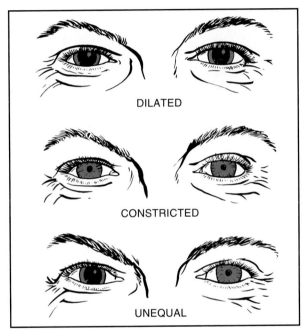

DILATED

CONSTRICTED

UNEQUAL

Figure 10-8 *Pupils of the eyes.*

Fluttering eyelids are often seen with hysteria. Slow lid closure (like a curtain falling) is rarely seen with hysteria. If the brainstem is intact, the eyes will remain synchronized (conjugate gaze) when the head is turned from side to side. The eyes turn in the opposite direction from the way the head is turned. Since this resembles the way a toy doll's eyes move, this test is called the doll's eye reflex (oculocephalic reflex). *This test is never done on a trauma patient* who may have a neck injury, since turning the head from side to side may cause irreversible spinal cord injury.

Testing for a blink response (corneal reflex) by touching the cornea, applying overly noxious stimuli to a patient to test for response to pain are techniques that are unreliable and do *not* contribute to prehospital care.

EXTREMITIES: Note sensation and motor function in the extremities. Can the patient feel you touch his hands and feet? Can he wiggle his fingers and toes? If the patient is unconscious, note his response to pain. If he withdraws or localizes to the pinching of his fingers and toes, he has grossly intact sensation and motor function. This usually indicates that there is normal or minimally impaired cortical function.

Both decorticate posturing or rigidity (arms flexed, legs extended) and decerebrate posturing or rigidity (arms and legs extended) are ominous signs of deep cerebral hemispheric or upper brainstem injury (see Figure 10-9). *Flaccid paralysis usually denotes spinal cord injury.*

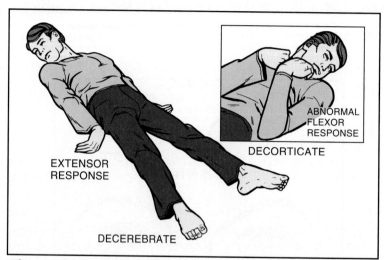

ABNORMAL
FLEXOR
RESPONSE

DECORTICATE

EXTENSOR
RESPONSE

DECEREBRATE

Figure 10-9 *Decerebrate and decorticate posturing.*

To be consistent with the revised trauma score and other field triage scoring systems, you should be familiar with the Glasgow Coma Scale, which is simple, easy to use, and has good prognostic value as to eventual outcome (see Appendix F).

VITAL SIGNS: Vital signs are extremely important in following the course of a patient with head trauma. Most important, they can indicate changes in intracranial pressure (see Table 10-1). You should observe and record vital signs during the secondary survey and each time you perform the reassessment survey.

1. Blood pressure: Increasing intracranial pressure causes increased blood pressure. Other causes of hypertension include fear and pain. *Hypotension* associated with head injury is usually caused by spinal or hemorrhagic shock and should be treated as if caused by hemorrhage. Low blood pressure caused by a head injury is usually a terminal event.

2. Pulse: Increasing intracranial pressure causes the pulse rate to decrease.

3. Respirations: Increasing intracranial pressure causes the respiratory rate to increase, to decrease, and/or to become irregular. Unusual respiratory patterns may reflect the level of brain/brainstem injury. Just before death the patient may develop a rapid, noisy respiratory pattern called central neurogenic hyperventilation. Because respiration is affected by so many factors (e.g., fear, hysteria, chest injuries, spinal cord injuries, diabetes), it is not as useful an indicator as are the other vital signs in monitoring the course of head injury.

	SHOCK	**HEAD INJURY WITH INCREASED INTRACRANIAL PRESSURE**
BLOOD PRESSURE	DECREASED	INCREASED
PULSE	INCREASED	DECREASED
RESPIRATION	INCREASED	VARIES BUT FREQUENTLY DECREASED
LEVEL OF CONSCIOUSNESS	DECREASED	DECREASED

Table 10-1 *Comparison of Vital Signs in Shock and Head Injury*

REASSESSMENT SURVEY

Each time you perform the reassessment survey, record the level of consciousness and the pupil size and reaction to light. This, along with the vital signs, gives enough information to monitor the condition of the head-injured patient.

Decisions on the management of the head trauma patient are made on the basis of changes in all parameters of the physical and neurological examination. You are establishing the baseline from which later judgments must be made; record your observations.

MANAGEMENT OF THE HEAD TRAUMA PATIENT

There is not a great deal that you can do for the head trauma patient in the prehospital setting. It is extremely important to make a rapid assessment and then transport the victim to a facility capable of managing head trauma. The important points of management in the prehospital phase are:

1. *Secure the airway and provide good oxygenation.* The brain does not tolerate hypoxia, so good oxygenation is mandatory. *The head trauma patient should be hyperventilated* (more than 24 breaths per minute). This decreases intracranial pressure. Because head-injured patients are prone to vomiting, be prepared to log-roll the immobilized patient and to suction the oropharnyx, particularly if an airway protective device has not been inserted.

2. Stabilize the patient on a spineboard. The neck should be immobilized in *a semirigid* collar and a padded head-immobilization device.

3. Record baseline observations. Record the blood pressure, respirations (rate and pattern), pupils (size and reaction to light), sensation, and voluntary motor activity. Also record the Glasgow Coma Scale. If the patient develops hypotension, suspect hemorrhage or spinal injury.

4. Frequently monitor and record the observations listed above.

POTENTIAL PROBLEMS

Always anticipate a cervical spine injury in the head-injured patient.

1. *Seizures.* Head trauma, particularly intracranial hemorrhage, may cause seizures. The seizing patient becomes hypoxic and hyperthermic, so persistent seizure activity may worsen his condition. It is not uncommon for seizures to be related to poor airway control, so remember that oxygenation and ventilation are of extreme importance.

2. *Vomiting.* A patient with head trauma almost always vomits. You must remain alert to prevent aspiration. If you are trained to do so and your protocols allow, you should protect the airway of the unconscious patient (with no gag reflex) with an airway protective device such as a BIAD. Otherwise, keep mechanical suction available and be prepared to log-roll the patient onto his side (maintaining immobilization of the cervical spine).

3. *Rapidly deteriorating condition.* A patient who shows rapid deterioration of vital signs or rapid progression of his brain injury (e.g., dilated pupil, decorticate or decerebrate posturing) should be transported rapidly to a trauma center. There is nothing definitive you can do in the field. Attempt to decrease intracranial pressure by hyperventilation. Radio ahead so that a neurosurgeon can be available and the operating room prepared by the time you arrive at the hospital. A rapid field response and transport will not compensate for the time lost in the emergency department or a delay to the operating room.

4. *Shock.* Think spinal cord injury or bleeding.

5. *Metabolic abnormalities.* Remember to administer oral glucose to any patient with altered mental status who is diabetic or alcoholic or who might otherwise be suffering from hypoglycemia. Do not attempt to do this if the patient is unconscious.

SUMMARY

Head injury is a serious complication of trauma. To give your patient the best chance of recovery, you should be familiar with the important anatomy of the head and central nervous system and understand how trauma to the various areas presents clinically. The most important points in management of the head injured patient are rapid assessment, treatment of decreased level of consciousness by hyperventilation and good airway management, rapid transport to a trauma center, and frequent reassessment surveys. In no other area of trauma care is the recording of repeated assessments so important to future management decisions.

BIBLIOGRAPHY

1. Committee on Trauma, American College of Surgeons. "Head Trauma." In *Advanced Trauma Life Support Program,* pp. 133–155. Chicago: The College, 1989.

2. LaHaye, P. A., G. F. Gade, and D. P. Becker. "Injury to the Cranium." In *Trauma,* eds. K. L. Mattox, E. E. Moore, and D. V. Feliciano, pp. 237–249. Norwalk, CT: Appleton & Lange, 1988.

3. Rimel, R. W., J. A. Jane, and R. F. Edlich. "An Injury Severity Scale for Comprehensive Management of Central Nervous System Trauma." *Annals of Emergency Medicine* (December 1979), pp. 64–67.

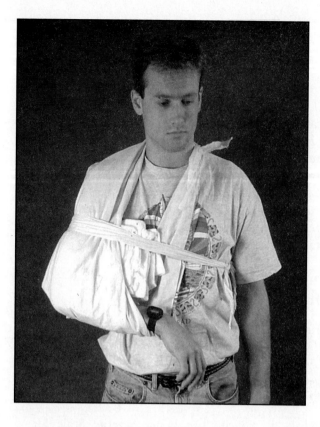

CHAPTER 1

Extremity Trauma

John E. Campbell, M.D., F.A.C.E.P.

OBJECTIVES

Upon completion of this chapter you should be able to:

1. Prioritize extremity trauma in the assessment and management of life-threatening injuries.

2. Discuss the major complications and treatment of the following extremity injuries:

   a. Fractures

   b. Dislocations

   c. Amputations

   d. Open wounds

   e. Neurovascular injuries

   f. Sprains and strains

   g. Impaled objects

   h. Compartment syndrome

3. Estimate blood loss from pelvic and extremity fractures.

4. Discuss major mechanisms of injury, associated trauma, potential complications, and management of injury to the following specific areas:

   a. Pelvis

   b. Femur

Continued on next page

> c. Hip
> d. Knee
> e. Tibia/fibula
> f. Clavicle and shoulder
> g. Elbow
> h. Forearm and wrist
> i. Hand or foot

You must never let distorted or wounded extremities occupy your attention when there may be more life-threatening injuries present. These dramatic injuries are easy to identify upon first encountering the patient and may be disabling, but are rarely immediately life threatening. It is important to remember that the movement of air through the airway, the mechanics of breathing, the maintenance of circulating blood volume, and the appropriate treatment of shock always come before the splinting of any fracture.

Hemorrhagic shock is a potential danger of very few musculoskeletal injuries. Only direct lacerations of arteries or fractures of the pelvis or femur are commonly associated with enough bleeding to cause shock. Injuries to the nerves or vessels that serve the hands and feet are the most common complications of fractures and dislocations. Such injuries cause the loss of function that we lump under the term *neurovascular compromise*. Thus, evaluation of sensation and circulation (PMS: pulse, motor, and sensation) distal to fractures is very important.

INJURIES TO EXTREMITIES

FRACTURES

Fractures may be open (compound) with the broken end of the bone still protruding or having once protruded through the skin, or they may be closed (simple) with no communication to the outside (see Figure 11-1). Fractured bone ends are extremely sharp and are quite dangerous to all the tissues that surround the bone. Since nerves and arteries frequently travel near the bone, across the flexor side of joints, or very near the skin (hands and feet), they are frequently injured. Such neurovascular injuries may be due to lacerations from bone fragments or from pressure due to swelling or hematomas.

Closed fractures can be just as dangerous as open fractures because injured soft tissues often bleed profusely. It is important to remember that any break in the skin near a fractured bone may be considered to be an opening for contamination.

A closed fracture of one femur can cause the loss of up to a liter of blood and thus two fractured femurs can cause life-threatening hemorrhage (see Figure 11-2).

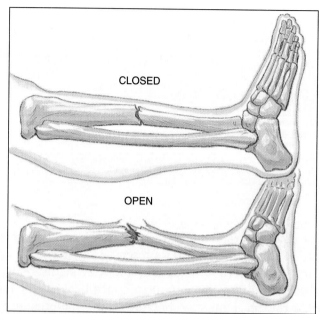

Figure 11-1 *Basic types of fractures.*

A fractured pelvis can cause extensive bleeding into the abdomen or the retroperitoneal space. The pelvis usually fractures in several places and may have 500 cc of blood loss for each fracture. Pelvic fractures may lacerate the bladder or the large pelvic blood vessels. Either of these structures can cause fatal hemorrhage into the abdomen. Remember, multiple fractures can cause life-threatening hemorrhage without any *external* blood loss.

Open fractures add the dangers of contamination as well as loss of blood outside the body. If protruding bone ends are pulled back into the skin when the limb

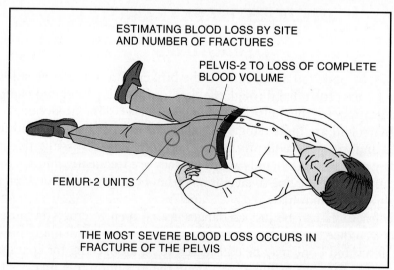

Figure 11-2 *Internal blood loss from fractures.*

is aligned, bacteria-contaminated debris will be pulled into the wound. Infection from such debris may prevent healing of the bone and may even cause death from septic complications.

DISLOCATIONS

Joint dislocations are extremely painful injuries. They are almost always easy to identify because of distortion of the normal anatomy. Major joint dislocations, though not life-threatening, are often true emergencies because of the neurovascular compromise that can, if not treated quickly, lead to amputation. It is impossible to know whether or not a fracture exists in combination with a dislocation. It is very important to check for PMS distal to major joint dislocations. Ordinarily, you splint injuries in the position you find them. There are certain exceptions to this rule. It is universally true, however, that one can apply only *gentle* traction to any distorted extremity in an effort to straighten it. In the few instances that you would use traction to straighten, use no more than 10 pounds of force. Most often the best treatment for the patient is padding and splinting the extremity in the most comfortable position and rapidly transporting to a facility that has orthopedic care available.

AMPUTATIONS

These are disabling and sometimes life-threatening injuries. They have the potential for massive hemorrhage, but most often, the bleeding will control itself quite readily with ordinary pressure applied to the stump. The stump should be covered with a damp sterile dressing and an elastic wrap that will apply uniform, reasonable pressure across the entire stump. If bleeding absolutely cannot be controlled with pressure, a tourniquet may be used. In general, a tourniquet is to be avoided whenever possible.

You should make an effort to find the amputated part and bring it with you. This sometimes neglected detail can have serious implications for the patient in the future, since parts can frequently be used for graft material. Reimplantation is attempted only in very limited situations. For this reason, you should not suggest to the patient that reimplantation will be done. Small amputated parts should be placed in a plastic bag (see Figure 11-3). If ice is available, place the bag in a larger bag or container containing ice and water. Do not use ice alone and *never* use dry ice. Cooling the part slows the chemical processes and will increase the viability from four hours to several times that length of time. It is important to bring amputated parts even if reimplantation appears to you to be impossible.

WOUNDS

Cover wounds with a sterile dressing and bandage carefully. Gross contamination such as leaves or gravel should be removed from the wound and smaller pieces of contamination can be irrigated from the wound with a normal saline drip in the same manner that you would irrigate a chemically contaminated eye. Bleeding can almost always be stopped with pressure dressings or pneumatic splints. Tourniquets

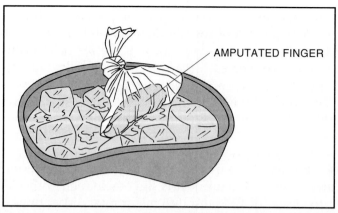

AMPUTATED FINGER

Figure 11-3 *Transportation of amputated part. If ice and time are available, seal part in small container and place this in larger container of ice and water. Do not use dry ice. Do not place amputated part directly on ice. If no ice is available, place part in plastic bag and seal so that the part will not lose moisture. Do not wrap the part in a moistened dressing.*

should almost never be used to stop bleeding from a wound if amputation is not present. If necessary, a blood pressure cuff or pressure on a larger artery proximal to the injury may be appropriate.

NEUROVASCULAR INJURIES

The nerves and major blood vessels generally run beside each other, usually in the flexor area of the major joints. They may be injured together, and loss of circulation and/or sensation can be due to disruption, swelling, or by compression by bone fragments or hematomas. Foreign bodies or broken bone ends may well impinge on delicate structures and cause them to malfunction. PMS is always checked before and after any extremity manipulation, application of splint, or traction.

SPRAINS AND STRAINS

These injuries cannot be differentiated from fractures in the field. Treat them as though they are fractures.

IMPALED OBJECTS

Do not remove impaled objects. Apply a very bulky type of padding to hold the object in place and transport the patient with the object in place. The skin is a pivot point in these cases, and any motion outside the body is translated or magnified within the tissues where the end of the object may lacerate or harm sensitive structures. The cheek of the face is the exception to this rule.

COMPARTMENT SYNDROME

The extremities contain muscle tissue in closed spaces surrounded by tough membranes that will not stretch. Trauma (crush injuries, closed or open fracture, or sustained compression) to these areas may cause bleeding and swelling within the closed spaces. As the area swells, pressure is transmitted to the blood vessels and nerves. This pressure may compress the blood vessels in such a manner that circulation is impossible. The nerves may also be compromised. These injuries usually develop over a period of hours. Late symptoms are the five *P*s: *p*ain, *p*allor, *p*ulselessness, *p*aresthesia, and *p*aralysis. The early symptoms are usually pain and paresthesia. As with shock, you should think of this diagnosis before the later symptoms develop.

ASSESSMENT AND MANAGEMENT

HISTORY

It is especially important to get a history in extremity trauma, because the apparent mechanism of injury and the condition of the extremity when you first arrive may give you important information about how severe the injury actually is. If you have enough rescuers, one can obtain the history while you are performing the primary survey. If not, you should not attempt to elicit a detailed verbal history until you have assessed the status of the airway, breathing, and circulation. In the conscious patient, you should obtain most of the history during the secondary survey. The history becomes especially important in extremity trauma, because certain mechanisms will cause extremity injuries that may not be obvious during your initial exam.

Foot injuries from long jumps (falls landing on the feet) often have lumbar spine injuries associated with them. Any injury to the knee when the patient is in the sitting position may have associated injuries to the hip. In a like manner, hip injuries may refer pain to the knee, so the knee and the hip are intimately connected and must be evaluated together rather than separately. Falls onto the wrist frequently injure the elbow, and so wrist and elbow must be evaluated together. The same is true of the ankle and the proximal fibula of the outside of the lower leg.

Any injury that appears to be in the shoulder must be carefully examined because it may easily involve either the neck, chest, or shoulder. Fractures of the pelvis are usually associated with very large amounts of blood loss. Whenever a fracture in the pelvis is identified, shock must be suspected and proper treatment begun.

ASSESSMENT

During the primary survey, you are concerned with obvious fractures to the pelvis and large bones of the extremities. You also find and control major bleeding from the extremities.

During the secondary survey, you should quickly assess the full length of each extremity, looking for DCAP-BLS and feeling for TIC (see Chapters 2 and 3). Check the joints for pain and movement. Check and record distal PMS. Pulses may be marked with ballpoint pen to identify the area in which the pulse is best felt (see Figure 11-4). *Crepitation or grating of bone ends is a definite sign of fracture, and once identified, the bone ends should be immediately immobilized to prevent further soft tissue injury.* Checking for crepitation should be done *very gently,* especially when checking the pelvis. Crepitation means bone ends are grating on one another, and this means you are causing further tissue injury.

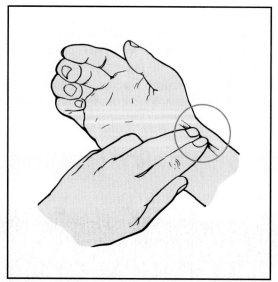

Figure 11-4a *Palpation of radial pulse.*

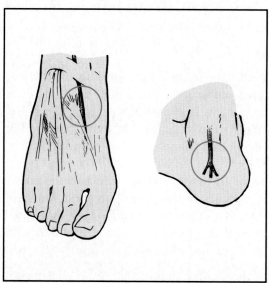

Figure 11-4b *Location of posterior tibial and dorsalis pedis pulses.*

GENERAL MANAGEMENT OF EXTREMITY INJURIES

Proper management of fractures and dislocations will decrease the incidence of pain, disability, and serious complications. Treatment in the prehospital setting is directed at proper immobilization of the injured part by the use of an appropriate splint.

PURPOSE OF SPLINTING: The objective is to prevent motion in the broken bone ends (see Figure 11-5). The nerves that cause the most pain in a fractured extremity lie in the membrane surrounding the bone. The broken bone ends irritate these nerves, causing a very deep and distressing type of pain. Splinting not only decreases pain, but also eliminates further damage to muscles, nerves, and blood vessels by preventing further motion of the broken bone ends.

WHEN TO USE SPLINTING: There is no simple rule that will determine the precise sequence to follow in every trauma patient. In general, the seriously injured patient will be better off if only major (spinal) immobilization is done before transport. The patient who requires a "load-and-go" type of approach can be adequately immobilized by careful packaging on the long spineboard. This does not mean that you have no responsibility to identify and protect extremity fractures, but rather implies that it is better to do some splinting in the vehicle en route to the hospital. It is never appropriate to sacrifice time immobilizing a limb to prevent *disability*, when that time may be needed to save the patient's *life*. Conversely, if the patient appears to be stable, extremity fractures should be splinted before moving the patient.

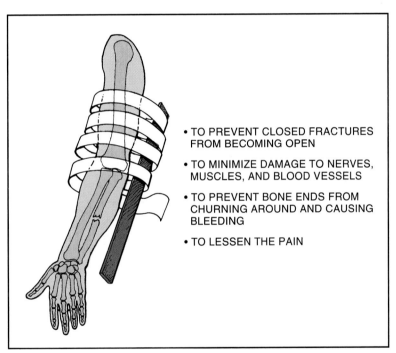

- TO PREVENT CLOSED FRACTURES FROM BECOMING OPEN

- TO MINIMIZE DAMAGE TO NERVES, MUSCLES, AND BLOOD VESSELS

- TO PREVENT BONE ENDS FROM CHURNING AROUND AND CAUSING BLEEDING

- TO LESSEN THE PAIN

Figure 11-5 *Reasons for splinting.*

GENERAL RULES OF SPLINTING

1. You must adequately visualize the injured part. Clothes should be cut off, not pulled off unless there is only an isolated injury that presents no problem with maintaining immobilization.

2. Check and record distal sensation and circulation before and after splinting. Check movement distal to the fracture if possible (for example, ask the conscious patient to wiggle his fingers or observe the motion of the unconscious patient

with the application of painful stimulus). Pulses may be marked with a pen to identify where they were last discovered.

3. If the extremity is severely angulated and pulses are absent, you should apply gentle traction in an attempt to straighten it (see Figure 11-6). This traction should never exceed 10 pounds of pressure. If resistance is encountered, splint the extremity in the angulated position. It is very important when you are attempting to straighten an extremity to be honest with yourself with regard to resistance. It takes very little force to lacerate the wall of a vessel or to interrupt the blood supply to a large nerve. If the trauma center is near, always splint in the position found.

4. Open wounds should be covered with a sterile dressing before you apply the splint. Splints should always be applied on the side of the extremity away from open wounds to prevent pressure necrosis.

5. Use the splint that will immobilize one joint above and below the injury.

6. Pad the splint well. This is particularly true if there is any skin defect or if bony prominences may press against a hard splint.

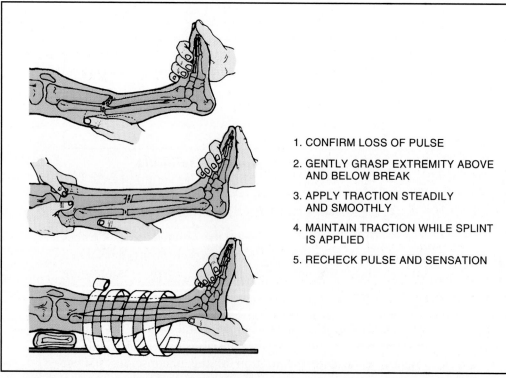

1. CONFIRM LOSS OF PULSE

2. GENTLY GRASP EXTREMITY ABOVE AND BELOW BREAK

3. APPLY TRACTION STEADILY AND SMOOTHLY

4. MAINTAIN TRACTION WHILE SPLINT IS APPLIED

5. RECHECK PULSE AND SENSATION

Figure 11-6 *Straightening angulated fractures to restore pulses.*

7. Do not attempt to push bone ends back under the skin. If you apply traction and the bone end retracts back into the wound, do not increase the amount of traction. You should not use your hands or any tools to try to pull the bone ends back out, but be sure to notify the receiving physician. Bone ends should be carefully padded by bandages prior to the application of pneumatic splints to the lower extremities. The healing of bone is improved if the bone ends are kept moist when transport time is prolonged.

8. When there is a life-threatening situation, injuries may be splinted as the patient is being moved. In cases where the injury is less severe, splint all injuries before moving the patient.

9. If in doubt, splint a possible injury.

TYPES OF SPLINTS

RIGID SPLINT: This type of splint can be made from many different materials and includes all the cardboard, hard plastic, metal, or wooden types of splints. The type of splint that is made rigid by evacuating air from a moldable splint (vacuum splint) is also classified as a rigid splint. Rigid splints should be padded well and always extend one joint above and below the fracture.

SOFT SPLINT: This type includes air splints, pillows, and sling and swathe type splints.

Air splints are good for fractures of the lower arm and lower leg. The pneumatic antishock garment (PASG or MAST) is an excellent air splint. Air splints have the advantage of compression which helps to slow bleeding, but they have the disadvantage of increasing pressure as the temperature rises or the altitude increases. They *should not* be put on angulated fractures since they will automatically apply straightening pressure.

Other major disadvantages of air splints include the fact that the extremity pulses cannot be monitored while the splint is in place; also the splints often stick to the skin and are painful to remove.

Inflating the splints requires you to blow the splints up by mouth or by hand or foot pump (never by compressed air) until they give good support and yet can easily be dented with slight pressure from a fingertip. When using air splints, you must constantly check the pressure to be sure that the splint is not getting too tight or too loose (they often leak).

Remember that if air splints are applied in a cold environment and the patient is moved into the warm environment of the ambulance, the pressure will increase as the splints warm up. Where air ambulances are available, it must be remembered that the pressure in air splints increases if they are applied on the ground and then subsequently the patient is air-lifted to the hospital. Also remember that if pressure is released while in flight, the pressure will be too low when the patient is returned to the ground.

Pillows make good splints for injuries to the ankle or foot. They are also helpful along with a sling and swathe to stabilize a dislocated shoulder.

Slings and swathes are excellent for injuries to the clavicle, shoulder, upper arm, elbow, and sometimes the forearm. They utilize the chest wall as a solid foundation and splint the arm against the chest wall. Some shoulder injuries cannot be brought close to the chest wall without significant force being applied. In these instances, pillows are used to bridge the gap between the chest wall and the upper arm.

TRACTION SPLINT: This device is designed for fractures of the lower extremities. It holds the fracture immobile by the application of a steady pull on the extremity by applying countertraction to the ischium and the groin. This steady traction overcomes the tendency of the very strong thigh muscles to spasm. If traction is not applied, there is worse pain because the bone ends tend to impact or override. Traction also prevents free motion of the ends of the femur that could lacerate the femoral nerve, artery, or vein. There are many designs and types of splints available to apply traction to the lower extremity, but each must be carefully padded and applied with care to prevent excessive pressure on the soft tissues around the pelvis. It is also necessary to use a great deal of care in applying the ankle hitch so as not to interfere with the circulation of the foot. Many of these devices can be used with a Buck's boot as an alternative to the ankle hitch.

MANAGEMENT OF SPECIFIC INJURIES

SPINE: This is covered elsewhere in the book but included here to remind you that if there is any chance of spinal injury proper immobilization must be done to prevent life-long paralysis or even death from a spinal cord injury (see Figure 11-7). In the most urgent cases, careful packaging of the patient on the long spineboard may be adequate splinting for a number of different extremity injuries. Remember that certain mechanisms of injury such as a fall from a height in which a victim lands on both feet may cause lumbar spine fracture because forces are transmitted all the way up the body.

PELVIS: It is practical to include injuries to the pelvis with extremities because they are frequently associated. Pelvic injuries are usually caused by motor vehicle accidents or by severe trauma such as falls from heights. They are identified by *gentle* pressure being placed on the iliac crests, hips, and pubis during patient survey.

There is always the potential for serious hemorrhage in pelvic fractures, so shock should be expected and the patient rapidly transported. The patient with a pelvic injury should always be transported on a spineboard.

FEMUR: The femur usually fractures at the midshaft, although hip fractures are quite common. These fractures may have open wounds in association with them, and if so, they must be presumed to be open fractures. There is a lot of muscle tissue surrounding the femur and a great deal of bleeding can occur into the tissue of the thigh. Bilateral femur fractures can be associated with a loss of up to 50% of the circulating blood volume. Pneumatic splints such as the PASG are useful to decrease internal bleeding around femur fractures.

HIP: Hip fractures are most often in the narrow "neck" of the femur where strong ligaments may occasionally allow this type of fracture to bear weight. The liga-

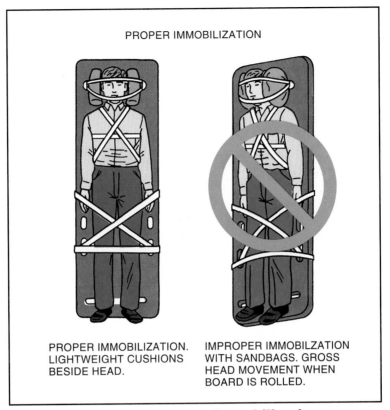

PROPER IMMOBILIZATION

PROPER IMMOBILIZATION. LIGHTWEIGHT CUSHIONS BESIDE HEAD.

IMPROPER IMMOBILZATION WITH SANDBAGS. GROSS HEAD MOVEMENT WHEN BOARD IS ROLLED.

Figure 11-7 *Proper immobilization.*

ments are very strong, and there is very little movement of the bone ends in the most frequent type of hip fracture.

You must consider hip fractures in any elderly person who has fallen and has pain in the knee, hip, or pelvic region. This type of presentation and pain should be considered a fracture until an X-ray proves otherwise. In this age group, pain is frequently well tolerated and sometimes even ignored or denied. In general, the tissues in the elderly patient are more delicate and less force is required to disrupt a given structure.

Always remember that isolated knee pain may well be coming from damage to the hip in the child and in the elderly patient.

Hip dislocation is a different story. Most hip dislocations are a result of the knees being struck by the dashboard, forcing the relatively loose, relaxed hip out of the posterior side of its cup in the pelvis (see Figure 11-8). Thus, any patient in a severe automobile accident with a knee injury must have the hip examined very carefully. Hip dislocation is an orthopedic emergency and requires reduction as soon as possible to prevent sciatic nerve injury or necrosis of the femoral head due to interrupted blood supply. This is a very difficult reduction to perform because the amount of force required is very great and the movement must be quite precise.

The dislocated hip will usually be flexed and the victim will not be able to tolerate having the leg straightened. The leg will almost invariably be rotated toward the midline. A hip dislocation should be supported in the most comfortable position by the use of pillows and by splinting to the uninjured leg (see Figure 11-9). This patient requires rapid transport.

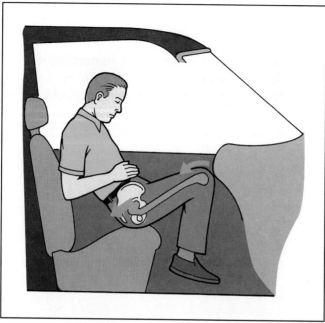

Figure 11-8 *Mechanism of posterior dislocation of the hip, "down and under."*

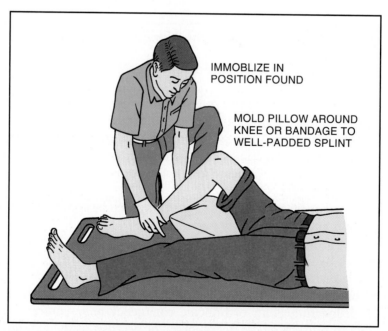

IMMOBLIZE IN
POSITION FOUND

MOLD PILLOW AROUND
KNEE OR BANDAGE TO
WELL-PADDED SPLINT

Figure 11-9 *Splinting posterior dislocation of the hip.*

KNEE: Fractures or dislocation here are quite serious because the arteries are bound down above and below the knee joint and are often bruised or lacerated if the joint is in an abnormal position. There is no way to know whether or not a fracture exists in an abnormally positioned knee, and in either case, the decision must be based on the circulation and neurological function below the knee in the foot.

Some authorities state that about 50% of knee dislocations have associated injuries to the vessels, and many knee injuries later require amputation. It is important to restore the circulation below the knee whenever possible.

Prompt reduction of knee dislocation is very important. If there is loss of pulse or sensation, you should apply gentle traction that may be by hand or with a traction splint. You must be careful to apply *no more than 10 pounds* of force, and this force must be applied along the long axis of the leg. If there is resistance to straightening the knee, splint it in the most comfortable position and transport the patient rapidly. This may be considered to be a true orthopedic emergency.

TIBIA/FIBULA: Fractures of the lower leg are often open due to thin skin over the front of the tibia and often have significant internal and/or external blood loss. Internal blood loss can interrupt the circulation to the foot if a compartment syndrome develops. It is rarely possible for patients to bear weight on fractures of the tibia. Fractures of the lower tibia/fibula may be splinted with a rigid splint, air splint, or pillow (see Figure 11-10). Pneumatic splints will adequately splint upper tibia fractures. Here again it is important to dress any wound and pad any bone ends that may be put under an air splint or PASG.

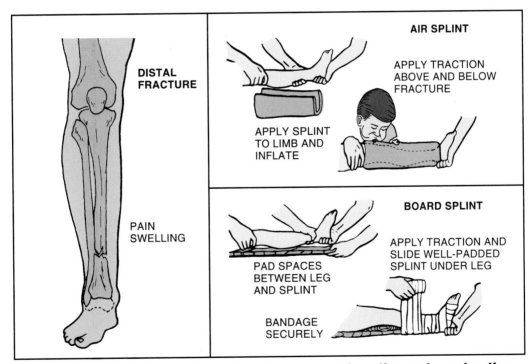

Figure 11-10 *Splinting lower leg fractures. Air splint or board splint.*

CLAVICLE: This is the most frequently fractured bone in the body but rarely causes problems (see Figure 11-11). It is best immobilized with a sling and swathe. Rarely there may be injuries to the subclavian vein and artery or to the nerves of the arm when this area is injured. It is also very important that the ribs and chest be very carefully evaluated whenever an injury to the shoulder or clavicle is discovered.

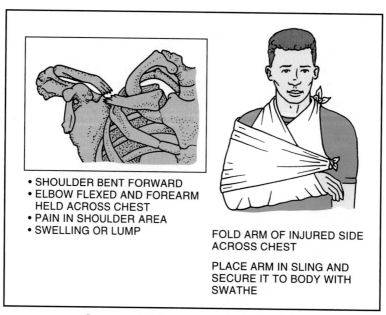

- SHOULDER BENT FORWARD
- ELBOW FLEXED AND FOREARM HELD ACROSS CHEST
- PAIN IN SHOULDER AREA
- SWELLING OR LUMP

FOLD ARM OF INJURED SIDE ACROSS CHEST

PLACE ARM IN SLING AND SECURE IT TO BODY WITH SWATHE

Figure 11-11 *Fractured clavicle.*

SHOULDER: Most shoulder injuries are not life threatening, but they may be associated with severe injuries of the chest or of the neck. Many shoulder injuries are dislocations or separations of joint spaces and may show as a defect at the upper outer portion of the shoulder. The upper humerus is fractured with some degree of frequency, however. The radial nerve travels quite close around the humerus and may be injured in humeral fractures. Injury to the radial nerve results in an inability of the patient to lift the hand (wrist drop). Dislocated shoulders are very painful and quite often require a pillow between the arm and body to hold the upper arm in the most comfortable position. Shoulders that are held in abnormal positions should never be forced into a more anatomic alignment (see Figure 11-12).

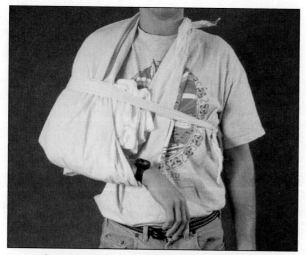

Figure 11-12 *Dislocated shoulder.*

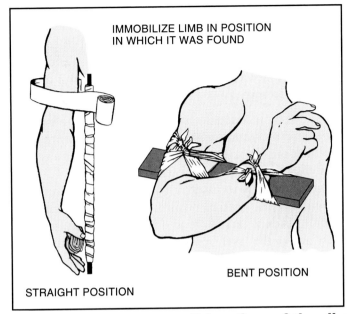

Figure 11-13 *Fractures or dislocations of the elbow.*

ELBOW: It is often difficult to tell whether there is a fracture or dislocation; both can be serious because of the danger of damage to the vessels and nerves that run across the flexor surface of the elbow. Elbow injuries should always be splinted in the most comfortable position and the distal function clearly evaluated (see Figure 11-13). Never attempt to straighten or apply traction to an elbow injury because the tissues are quite delicate and the structure is very complicated.

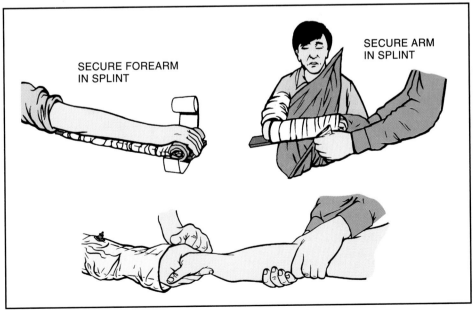

Figure 11-14 *Fractures of the forearm and wrist.*

FOREARM AND WRIST: This a very common fracture, usually as a result of a fall on the outstretched arm. Usually it is best immobilized with a rigid splint or an air splint (see Figure 11-14). If a rigid splint is used, a roll of gauze in the hand will hold the arm in the most comfortable position of function. The forearm is also subject to internal bleeding that can interrupt the blood supply to the fingers and the hand (compartment syndrome).

HAND OR FOOT: Many industrial accidents involving the hand or the foot produce multiple open fractures and avulsions. These injuries are often gruesome in appearance but are seldom associated with life-threatening bleeding. A pillow may be used to support these injuries very effectively (see Figure 11-15). An alternative method of dressing the hand is to insert a roll of gauze in the palm, then arrange the fingers and thumb in their normal position. The entire hand is then wrapped as though it were a ball inside a very large and bulky dressing. Elevating the isolated hand or foot injury above the level of the heart will almost always reduce bleeding dramatically during transport.

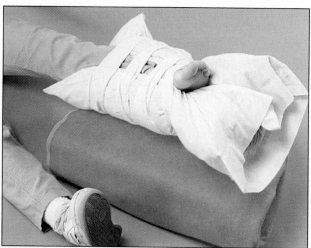

Figure 11-15 *Pillow splinting an injured foot.*

SUMMARY

While usually not life-threatening, extremity injuries are often disabling. These injuries may be more obvious than more serious internal injuries, but do not let extremity injuries distract you from following the usual steps of the primary and secondary survey. Pelvic and femur fractures can be associated with life-threatening internal bleeding so patients with these injuries are in the "load-and-go" category. Proper splinting is important to protect the injured extremity from further injury. Dislocations of elbows, hips, and knees require careful splinting and rapid reduction to prevent severe disability to the affected extremity.

REVIEW OF IMPORTANT POINTS

1. Be very alert to the mechanism of injury so that you know what fractures to suspect and so that you can predict possible complications.
2. Remember the ABCs.
3. Visualize the injured part.
4. Be prepared for hemorrhagic shock when major bones are fractured.
5. Always record sensation and circulation initially and after any manipulation, particularly splinting.
6. Pad joints and hard spots very carefully. Be sure all splints are padded well.
7. Examine and immobilize one joint above and below any suspected fracture.
8. Splint the patient at an appropriate time. The axial skeleton is splinted after the primary survey, but extremities should be splinted en route if a critical situation exists.
9. If in doubt, splint a potential fracture. In major trauma, the axial skeleton is always splinted on a long spineboard.
10. Do not waste the "golden hour." Be cautious but be rapid.

BIBLIOGRAPHY

1. Bledsoe, B. E., R. S. Porter, and B. R. Shade. "Musculoskeletal Injuries." In *Paramedic Emergency Care*, 5th ed., pp. 473–493. Englewood Cliffs, NJ: Prentice Hall, 1991.
2. Committee on Trauma, American College of Surgeons. "Extremity Trauma." In *Advanced Trauma Life Support Program*, pp. 181–196. Chicago: The College, 1989.
3. Grant, H. D., R. H. Murray, and J. D. Bergeron. "The Upper Extremities" and "The Lower Extremities." In *Emergency Care*, 6th ed., pp. 258–323. Englewood Cliffs, NJ: Prentice Hall, 1994.

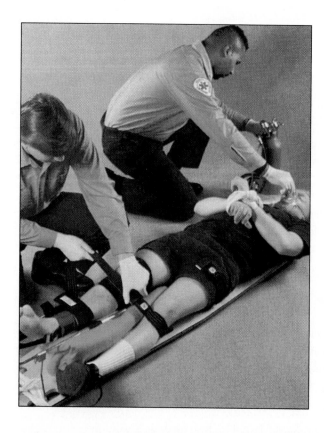

12

Extremity Trauma Skills

Donna Hastings, EMT-P

USE OF TRACTION SPLINTS

OBJECTIVES

Upon completion of this chapter you should be able to:

1. Explain when to use a traction splint.
2. Describe the complications of using a traction splint.
3. Apply the most common traction splints:
   a. Thomas splint
   b. Hare splint
   c. Klippel splint
   d. Sager splint

Traction splints are designed to immobilize fractures of the lower extremities. They are useful for fractures of the femur. They are *not* useful for fractures of the hip, knee, or lower leg. Applying firm traction to a fractured or dislocated knee may tear the blood vessels behind the knee. If there appears to be a pelvic fracture, you cannot use a traction splint because it may cause further damage to the pelvis. Fractures below the midthigh that are not angulated or severely shortened may just as well be immobilized by air splints or the antishock garment. Traction splints work by applying a padded device to the back of the pelvis (ischium) or to the groin. A hitching device is then applied to the ankle and countertraction is applied until the limb is straight and well immobilized. Apply the splints to the pelvis and groin very carefully to prevent excessive pressure on the genitalia. Also use care when attaching the hitching device to the foot and ankle so as not to interfere with circulation. To prevent any unnecessary movement, do not apply traction splints until the victim is on a long backboard. If the splint extends beyond the end of the backboard, be very careful when moving the victim and when closing the ambulance door. You must check the circulation in the injured leg, so remove the shoe before attaching the hitching device. In every case at least two people are needed. One must hold steady, *gentle* traction on the foot and leg while the other applies the splint. When dealing with "load-and-go" situations, do not apply the splint until the victim is in the ambulance (unless the ambulance has not arrived).

APPLYING A THOMAS SPLINT (HALF-RING SPLINT)

See Figure 12-1.

1. The first rescuer supports the leg and maintains gentle traction while the second rescuer cuts away the clothing and removes the shoe and sock to check the pulse and sensation at the foot.

2. Position the splint under the injured leg. The ring goes down and the short side goes to the inside of the leg. Slide the ring snugly up under the hip, where it will be pressed against the ischial tuberosity.

3. Position two support straps above the knee and two below the knee.

4. Attach the top ring strap.

5. Apply padding to the foot and ankle.

6. Apply the traction hitch around the foot and ankle (see Figure 12-2).

7. Maintain gentle traction by hand.

8. Attach the traction hitch to the end of the splint.

9. Increase traction by Spanish windlass action using a stick or tongue depressors.

10. Release manual traction and reassess circulation and sensation.

11. Support the end of the splint so that there is no pressure on the heel.

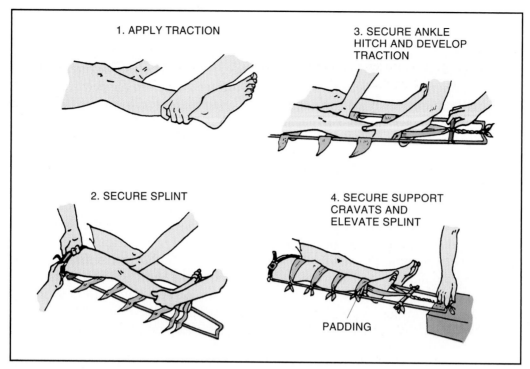

Figure 12-1 *Applying a traction (Thomas) splint.*

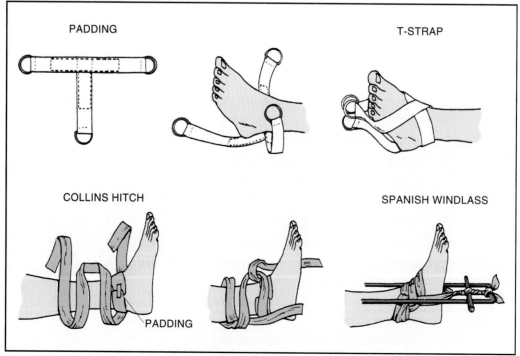

Figure 12-2 *Applying a traction hitch to the ankle.*

APPLYING A SAGER SPLINT

See Figure 12-3.

This splint is different in several ways. It works by providing countertraction against the pubic ramus and the ischial tuberosity medial to the shaft of the femur; thus it does not go under the leg. The hip does not have to be slightly flexed as with the Hare and Klippel. The Sager splint is also lighter and more compact than other traction splints. You can also splint both legs with one splint if needed. The current Sager splints are significantly improved over older models and may represent the "state of the art" in traction splints.

1. Position the victim on a long backboard or stretcher.

2. The first rescuer supports the leg and maintains gentle traction while the second rescuer cuts away the clothing and removes the shoe and sock to check the pulse and sensation at the foot.

3. Using the uninjured leg as a guide, pull the splint out to the correct length.

4. Position the splint to the inside of the injured leg with the padded bar fitted snugly against the pelvis in the groin. The splint can be used on the outside of the leg, using the strap to maintain traction against the pubic. Be very careful not to catch the genitals under the bar (or strap).

5. While maintaining gentle manual traction, attach the padded hitch to the foot and ankle.

6. Extend the splint until the correct tension is obtained.

7. Release manual traction and recheck circulation and sensation.

8. Apply elastic straps above and below the knee.

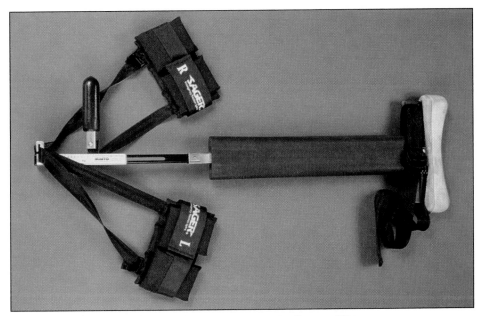

Figure 12-3 *Sager traction splint.*

APPLYING A HARE SPLINT

See Figure 12-4.

1. Position the victim on the backboard or stretcher.
2. The first rescuer supports the leg and maintains gentle traction, while the second rescuer cuts away the clothing and removes the shoe and sock to check pulse and sensation at the foot.
3. Using the uninjured leg as a guide, pull the splint out to the correct length.
4. Position the splint under the injured leg. The ring goes down and the short side goes to the inside of the leg. Slide the ring up snugly under the hip against the ischial tuberosity.
5. Position two support straps above the knee and two below the knee.
6. Attach the heel rest.
7. Attach the top strap.
8. Apply the padded traction hitch to the ankle and foot.
9. Maintain gentle manual traction.
10. Attach the traction hitch to the windlass by way of the S-hook.
11. Turn the ratchet until the correct tension is applied.
12. Release manual traction and recheck circulation and sensation.
13. Attach support straps around the leg with Velcro^R straps.
14. To release traction, pull the ratchet knob outward and then slowly turn to loosen.

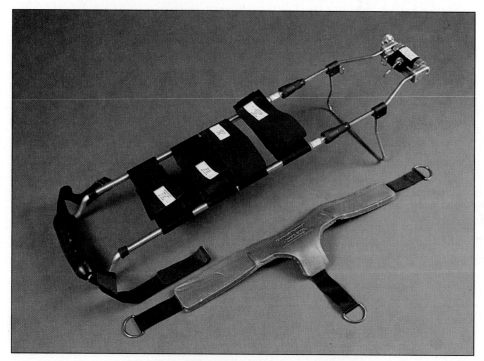

Figure 12-4 *Hare traction splint.*

APPLYING A KLIPPEL SPLINT

1. Position the victim on the long backboard or stretcher.

2. The first rescuer supports the leg and maintains gentle traction, while the second rescuer cuts away the clothing and removes the shoe and sock to check the pulse and sensation at the foot.

3. Using the uninjured leg as a guide, pull the splint out to the correct length.

4. Turn the footplate up by pushing to the side and then turning.

5. Turn the heel rest down by pushing in both knobs simultaneously and then turning.

6. While maintaining gentle traction and support, slide the splint under the leg (ring turned down) until the ring is snugly under the hip against the ischial tuberosity.

7. Position two support straps above the knee and two below the knee.

8. Attach the top ring strap.

9. Push the footplate up against the sole of the foot. Push the two release levers to shorten the splint.

10. Apply padding to the foot and ankle.

11. Bring the traction hitch up under the ankle and then cross the two straps over the foot, around the footplate, and back over the foot, where they attach by Velcro[R] fasteners.

12. While maintaining manual traction, extend the splint by pulling on the two rails until correct tension is obtained.

13. Release manual traction and recheck circulation and sensation.

14. Attach support straps around the leg with Velcro[R] fasteners.

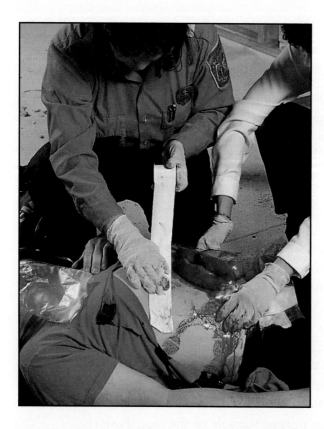

Abdominal Trauma

Gail V. Anderson, Jr., M.D.,
F.A.C.E.P., and Arthur H. Yancey II,
M.D., F.A.C.E.P.

OBJECTIVES

Upon completion of this chapter you should be able to:

1. Identify the basic anatomy of the abdomen and explain how abdominal and chest injuries may be related.

2. Relate how injuries apparent on the exterior of the abdomen can damage underlying structures.

3. Differentiate between blunt and penetrating injuries and identify complications associated with each.

4. Describe possible intraperitoneal injuries based on findings of history, physical examination, and mechanism of injury.

5. List treatment required for the patient with protruding viscera.

Injury to the abdomen can be a difficult condition to evaluate even in the hospital. In the field it is usually more so. Penetrating abdominal injuries obviously need immediate surgical attention; blunt injuries may be more subtle, but potentially just as deadly. Whether the result of blunt or penetrating trauma, abdominal injury presents two life-threatening dangers: hemorrhage and infection. Hemorrhage has immediate consequences, and thus you must be alert to the danger of early shock in all abdominal injury patients. Infection may be just as deadly, but does not require field intervention.

The role of prehospital management of abdominal trauma has been the subject of some controversy. Studies in the mid-1980s demonstrated that appropriate and timely intervention by well-trained paramedics could improve the hemodynamic status of critically injured patients with wounds to the abdomen. More recent studies have suggested that pneumatic antishock garment (PASG) application and vigorous intravenous fluid resuscitation in the prehospital setting may do more harm than good for patients with penetrating abdominal trauma (see the Bibliography and Chapter 7). The effects in blunt trauma are less well studied.

In the field, you need to remember only rapid patient assessment and shock management to manage the patient with abdominal trauma. These procedures are important, because blood loss from an abdominal injury can be fatal if appropriate care is not rendered in a rapid and efficient fashion.

ANATOMY

The abdomen is traditionally divided into three regions: the thoracic abdomen, the true abdomen, and the retroperitoneal abdomen (see Figure 13-1). The thoracic portion of the abdomen is located underneath the diaphragm and the lower ribs and contains the liver, gallbladder, spleen, and stomach. Injury to the liver and spleen can result in life-threatening hemorrhage.

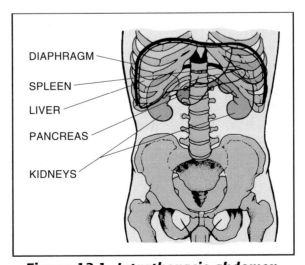

Figure 13-1 *Intrathoracic abdomen.*

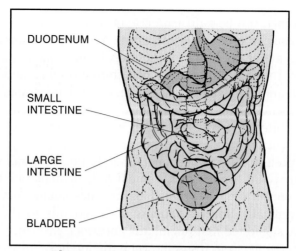

Figure 13-2 *True abdomen.*

The true abdomen contains the large and small intestines and the bladder (see Figure 13-2). Damage to the intestines can result in infection, peritonitis, and shock. In the female, the uterus, fallopian tubes, and ovaries are considered to be part of the pelvic portion of the true abdomen.

The retroperitoneal region lies behind the thoracic and true portions of the abdomen (see Figure 13-3). This area includes the kidneys, ureters, pancreas, posterior duodenum, abdominal aorta, and the inferior vena cava. Because of location, injuries here are difficult to evaluate. While hemorrhage in the true abdomen may cause the anterior abdominal wall to become distended, extensive bleeding in the retroperitoneal space may go undetected.

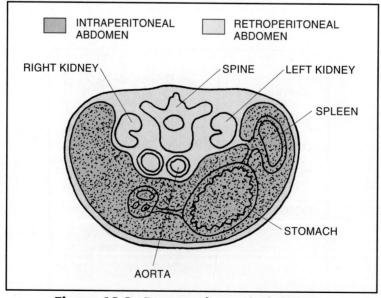

Figure 13-3 *Retroperitoneal abdomen.*

TYPES OF INJURY

Injuries to the abdomen are usually described as being blunt or penetrating. The penetrating group is subdivided into gunshot and stab wound categories. Blunt abdominal injuries have relatively high mortality rates of 10–30%, usually because of the frequency of accompanying injuries to other parts of the body. Blunt abdominal injury may be from direct compression of the abdomen, with fracture of solid organs and blowout of hollow organs, or from deceleration, with tearing of organs or their blood vessels. This is the most common mechanism of abdominal injury, but there has been little research on the best methods of prehospital management. As mentioned previously, the patient who has suffered blunt trauma may have no pain and little external evidence of injury, which may create a false sense of security in the examiner.

Gunshot wounds to the abdomen, as a rule, will be treated in the operating room. These patients have mortality rates of between 5% and 15%. These rates are much higher than those of stab wounds because of greater tendency of injury to abdominal viscera from the gunshot(s).

The mortality rate from abdominal stab wounds is relatively low (1–2%). Unless the knife penetrates a major vessel or organ, such as the liver or spleen, the patient may not initially appear to be in shock at the scene. However, some of these patients can develop life-threatening peritonitis over the next few hours. These wounds need to be carefully evaluated in the hospital.

You should remember that the path of the penetrating object may not be readily apparent from the wound location. A stab to the chest may penetrate the abdomen, and vice versa. The course of a bullet may pass through numerous structures in different body locations. In the prehospital phase, you must be most concerned about intra-abdominal bleeding with hemorrhagic shock.

EVALUATION AND STABILIZATION

HISTORY AND MECHANISMS

You can glean much important information from the scene by noting the circumstances surrounding the patient's injury. An accurate but rapid assessment of circumstances surrounding a victim will usually tip you off as to the possibility of abdominal trauma. Do circumstances on the scene suggest that the victim has fallen from a height or been hit by a passing vehicle? Has there been an explosion that would hurtle the victim against immobile objects or transmit blast pressure to organs inside the abdomen? Has the passenger of an automobile crash had the shoulder strap under the arm rather than over the shoulder? Any of these accident mechanisms can lead to penetrating or blunt abdominal trauma.

If the patient was involved in a motor vehicle crash, as you do your scene survey, quickly observe the damage to the vehicle such as passenger compartment intrusion, broken windows, bent steering wheel, and so on. If the patient needs to be extricated, note the location of the safety belts; although they certainly save lives, incorrectly worn safety belts can cause blunt abdominal injuries.

The person who is stabbed or shot may be able to give you some idea as to the size of the instrument or trajectory of the bullet. With gunshot wounds, it is also important to know the caliber, the range from which it was fired, and the number of times it was fired. Often a bystander may be able to provide such information. When you arrive at the hospital, be sure to report any mechanism that would suggest abdominal injury. However, while at the scene, it is important not to spend a great deal of time attempting to obtain a history. The major cause of preventable mortality in abdominal trauma is *delayed diagnosis and treatment.*

EXAMINATION

As in treating any other traumatic condition, the patient should first have the BTLS Primary Survey. The essence of the prehospital abdominal examination in the primary survey is rapid visual evaluation and palpation. Observe for wounds (DCAP), evisceration, and distension. Note any tenderness or tenseness. The chest is only one thin muscle sheet (the diaphragm) away from the abdominal cavity, so injury to both is not uncommon. Distension of the abdomen should be interpreted as a sign of severe hemorrhage as should tenderness or tenseness over the abdominal wall. Signs of intra-abdominal injury usually don't appear early. If signs of intra-abdominal injury are present in the prehospital phase, there is usually significant injury; shock may be imminent (see Chapter 7). Tenderness or abdominal distention is an indication for immediate transportation to the hospital. Little is gained and critical time is lost by auscultation or percussion in the field.

If clothing must be removed to visualize injury, try to preserve important potential legal evidence by cutting around (rather than through) areas that have signs of possible penetration.

STABILIZATION

Interventions should follow the protocol outlined in Chapter 2. They should proceed in the same order in which evaluation occurred: airway (A), breathing (B), and circulation (C). In critically injured patients, evaluation and treatment should occur simultaneously in the foregoing order. This means that even if a victim has only an abdominal injury, supplemental oxygen by mask or nasal cannula should be delivered through a confirmed open airway. Breathing should be verified to be adequate or the patient treated to ensure adequate ventilation. Then, and only then, should the consequences of any abdominal injury be addressed as part of the circulation assessment.

The patient should be readied for rapid transport. Should the system in which the rescuer practices allow the use of the pneumatic antishock trousers, these may be placed on the patient but inflated only after consultation with Medical Direction (see Chapter 7). The more critically ill the patient, the more important it is to apply the PASG en route. Gently cover, with gauze moistened with saline or water, any organ or viscera protruding from a wound (see Figure 13-4); if the intestines are allowed to dry, they may become irreversibly damaged. Do not *ever* push back into the abdomen any abdominal contents protruding from a wound. Similarly, if a foreign body (e.g., knife, glass shard) is impaled in the abdomen, do not attempt removal or manipulation. Carefully stabilize the object in place without moving it.

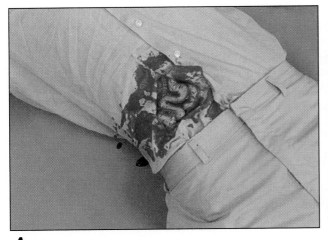

A.

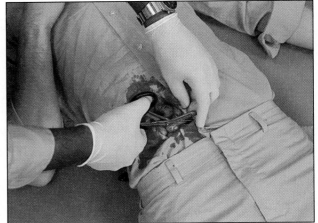

B.

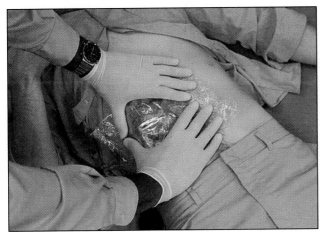

C.

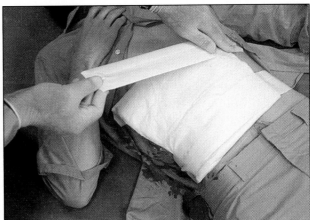

D.

Figure 13-4 *Protruding intestines.*

SUMMARY

Effective prehospital management of the patient with abdominal trauma entails

1. Scene survey for mechanisms and pertinent history from the patient and/or witnesses
2. Rapid patient assessment
3. Rapid transport to the appropriate hospital
4. Other interventions as needed (usually performed en route)

The enemies of the abdominal trauma patient are bleeding and time. If you can minimize on-scene delays, you will help to maximize the patient's chance for survival.

BIBLIOGRAPHY

1. Bickell, W. H., M.J. Wall, Jr., P.E. Pepe, and others. "Immediate Versus Delayed Fluid Resuscitation for Hypotensive Patients with Penetrating Torso Injuries. "*New England Journal of Medicine,* Vol. 331 (1994), pp. 1105–1109.

2. Martin, R. R., W. H. Bickell, P. E. Pepe, and others. "Prospective Evaluation of Preoperative Fluid Resuscitation in Hypotensive Patients with Penetrating Truncal Injury: A Preliminary Report." *Journal of Trauma,* Vol. 33 (1992), pp. 354–362.

3. Mattox, K. L., W. H. Bickell, P. E. Pepe, and others. "Prospective MAST Study in 911 Patients." *Journal of Trauma,* Vol. 29 (1989), pp. 1104–1112.

4. Pons, P. T., B. Honigman, C. E. Moore, and others. "Prehospital Advanced Trauma Life Support for Critical Penetrating Wounds to the Thorax and Abdomen." *Journal of Trauma,* Vol. 25 (1985), pp. 828–832.

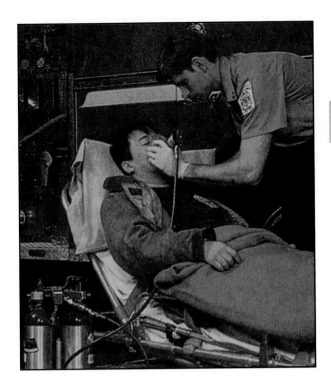

14

Burns

Richard C. Treat, M.D., F.A.C.S.

OBJECTIVES

Upon completion of this chapter you should be able to:

1. Identify the basic anatomy of the skin including the epidermal and dermal layers and structures found within.
2. List the basic functions of the skin.
3. Identify the three severities of burns.
4. Identify complications and describe the management of
   a. Thermal burns
   b. Chemical burns
   c. Electrical burns
5. List situations and physical signs that may indicate upper airway injury.
6. List signs of inhalation injury.
7. List signs and symptoms of carbon monoxide poisoning and discuss why carbon monoxide causes hypoxia.
8. Describe the treatment for carbon monoxide poisoning.
9. Estimate depth of burn based on skin appearance.
10. Estimate extent of burn using the "Rule of Nines."
11. Identify which patients may require transport to a burn center.

There are about 2 million burn injuries per year in the United States with more than 12,000 deaths as a result of these injuries. Many who survive their burns are severely disabled and/or disfigured. Following the basic principles taught here is very important in order to decrease death, disability, and disfigurement from burn injuries. The rescue and treatment of burn patients can be your most dangerous job; following the rules of scene safety is extremely important. Multiple agents (see Table 14-1) can cause burn injuries, but in general, pathologic damage to the skin is similar. Differences among the types of burns will be discussed in later sections.

A. FLAME

B. ELECTRICAL

C. CHEMICAL

D. STEAM

E. RADIATION

F. SCALD

Table 14-1 *Types of Burn Injuries*

ANATOMY AND PATHOLOGY

The largest organ of the body, the skin, is made up of two layers. The outer layer that we can see on the surface is called the *epidermis*. It serves as a barrier between the environment and our body. Underneath the thin epidermis is a thick layer of collagen connective tissue called the *dermis*. This layer contains the important sensory nerves and also the support structures such as hair follicles, sweat glands and oil glands (see Figure 14-1). The skin has many important functions that include acting as a mechanical barrier between the body and the outside world and acting as a protective barrier to seal fluids inside and prevent bacteria and other microorganisms from readily entering the body. The skin is also a vital sensory organ that provides input to the brain on general and specific environmental data and serves a primary role in temperature regulation.

Burn damage to the skin occurs when heat or caustic chemicals come in contact with the skin and damage its chemical and cellular components. In addition to actual tissue injury, there is the body's inflammatory response to the skin damage. Burns are characterized as first, second, or third degree, based on the depth of tissue damage and skin response. First-degree burns result in minor tissue damage to the outer epidermal layer only, but do cause an intense and painful inflammatory response. Although no medical treatment is usually required, various medications can be prescribed that significantly speed healing and reduce the painful inflammatory response. Second-degree burns cause damage through the epidermis and into a vari-

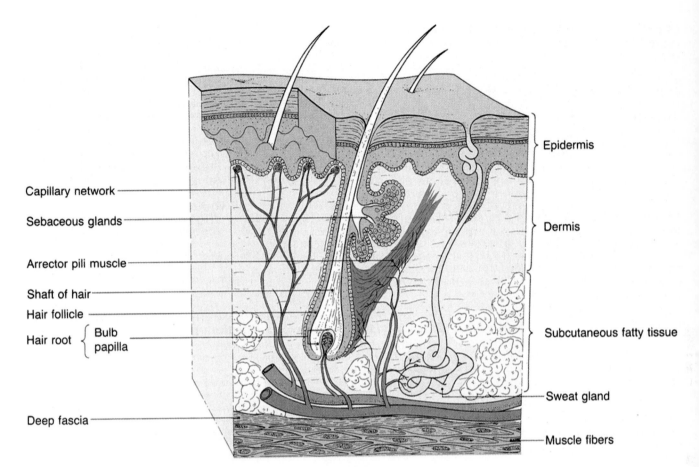

Figure 14-1 *The skin.*

Capillary network

Sebaceous glands

Arrector pili muscle

Shaft of hair

Hair follicle

Hair root { Bulb / papilla

Deep fascia

Epidermis

Dermis

Subcutaneous fatty tissue

Sweat gland

Muscle fibers

able depth of the dermis. These injuries will heal (usually without scarring) because the cell lining at the deep level of the epidermis (which also lines the deeper hair follicles) will multiply and result in the growth of new skin for healing. Antibiotic creams or various specialized types of dressings are standardly used to treat these burns, and, therefore, appropriate medical evaluation and care should be provided for patients with these injuries. Flash burns are virtually always first- or second-degree burns. A flash burn occurs when there is some type of explosion, but no actual fire. The single heat wave traveling out from these explosions results in such short patient–heat contact that only more superficial burns occur. Only areas directly exposed to the true heat wave will be injured. *In situations of possible flash explosion risk, you should ALWAYS wear proper protective clothing.* Other injuries (fractures, internal injuries, blast chest injuries, etc.) may well occur as a result of explosion. Third-degree burns cause damage to all layers of the epidermis and dermis. No more skin cell layers are left, so healing is impossible except in small third-degree burns that usually scar in from the sides. All third-degree burns leave scars. Deeper third-degree burns usually result in skin protein becoming denatured and hard, leaving a firm leatherlike covering that is referred to as eschar. Characteristics of these burns are listed in Table 14-2 and the depth levels are shown in Figure 14-2.

	1ST DEGREE	2ND DEGREE	3RD DEGREE
Cause	SUN OR MINOR FLASH	HOT LIQUIDS, FLASHES, OR FLAME	CHEMICALS, ELECTRICITY, FLAME, HOT METALS
Skin color	RED	MOTTLED RED	PEARLY WHITE AND/OR CHARRED TRANSLUCENT AND PARCHMENTLIKE
Skin surface	DRY WITH NO BLISTERS	BLISTERS WITH WEEPING	DRY WITH THROMBOSED BLOOD VESSELS
Sensation	PAINFUL	PAINFUL	ANESTHETIC
Healing	3 -- 6 DAYS	2-4 WEEKS DEPENDING ON DEPTH	REQUIRES SKIN GRAFTING

Table 14-2 *Characteristics of Various Depths of Burns*

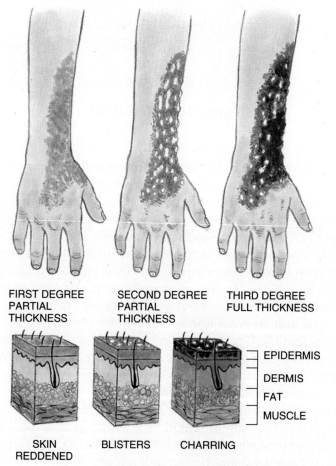

FIRST DEGREE PARTIAL THICKNESS   SECOND DEGREE PARTIAL THICKNESS   THIRD DEGREE FULL THICKNESS

EPIDERMIS
DERMIS
FAT
MUSCLE

SKIN REDDENED   BLISTERS   CHARRING

Figure 14-2 *Degrees of burns.*

The inflammatory response to the burn injury results in progressive tissue damage for a day or two following burn injury; this may well result in an increase in burn depth. Any condition that either reduces circulation to this damaged tissue or itself causes further tissue damage will lead to burn progression with increasing burn depth. Because of the process of burn progression, it is not essential to be able to exactly determine the burn depth in the field. You should, however, be able to clearly discern between superficial and deep burns.

First-degree and second-degree burns are commonly referred to as partial-thickness burns because there are still some layers of skin cells left that can multiply with resultant healing. Third-degree burns are referred to as full thickness burns because all layers of the skin have been destroyed and no skin cells are left to allow healing. The magnitude of burn injury depends on the extent and depth of the burn. Initial care that is directed specifically toward the burn concentrates on limiting any progression of these two factors.

INITIAL FIELD CARE

SCENE SAFETY

Removing the burn source is your number one step, and the most important concept in removing the burn source is the maintenance of safety. This involves both maintaining patient safety *and* maintaining your safety. There are specific and significant dangers in removing the burn source in all type of burn injuries. In the progression of a building fire, there is a point at which "flash-over" occurs. Flash-over is the *sudden* explosion into flame of everything in the room with the temperature rising instantaneously to over 3,000 degrees. There is no warning before this happens; thus *removal of victims from burning buildings takes priority over all other treatment.* Chemicals are not always easy to detect, either on patients or on other objects in the environment. Severe chemical burns to rescuers have occurred because of the inability to note sources of toxic and caustic chemicals. Special training in hazardous materials management is recommended for all rescuers. Electricity is exceptionally dangerous, and handling of high voltage wires is extremely hazardous. Specialized training and knowledge are required to appropriately deal with these situations, and you should not attempt to remove wires unless specifically trained to do so. Even objects commonly felt to be safe, such as wooden sticks, manila rope, and firefighters gloves, may not be protective and may result in electrocution. If at all possible, the source of electricity should be turned off before any attempt at rescue is made.

PATIENT CARE

People do not actually die rapidly from burn injuries. Even though the burn is highly visible and makes an intense impression at the scene, care of the burn itself has low priority. You should manage burn patients routinely as *trauma* patients and perform a primary survey immediately upon arrival in a safe staging area. Primary survey should follow the standard format as described in Chapter 2.

Once you determine that the patient is stable and no load-and-go situations are present, you may turn your attention to the burn wound itself. You should try to specifically limit burn wound progression as much as possible. Rapid cooling early in the course of a surface burn injury may help limit progression. Immediately following removal from the source of the burn, the skin is still hot and heat continues to radiate away from the patient and to some degree deeper into the tissues. This will cause increase in burn depth and increase the seriousness of the injury. Cooling halts this process and, if done appropriately, is beneficial. Cooling should be done with any source of water, but this should be undertaken for a *maximum of one minute* since the burn is only 1 or 2 millimeters thick. Cooling for longer periods of time is actually detrimental to patients because it will induce hypothermia and subsequent shock. Following the brief period of cooling, manage the burn by the use of clean, dry sheets and blankets to keep the patient warm and prevent hypothermia. (It is not necessary to have *sterile* sheets.) The patient should be covered even when the environment is not cold because damaged skin loses temperature regulation capacity. Patients should never be transported on wet sheets, wet towels, or wet clothing, and *ice is absolutely contraindicated*. Ice will positively worsen the injury because it causes vasoconstriction and thus reduces the blood supply to already damaged tissue. It is better not to cool the burn wound at all rather than cool the burn wound improperly and cause hypothermia or additional tissue damage. Initial management of chemical and electrical burn injuries will be described in the sections on those injuries.

In your assessment of the burn patient, note and record the type of burn mechanism and the particular circumstances such as entrapment, explosion, mechanisms for other possible injuries, smoke exposure, chemical/electrical details, and so forth. An appropriate past medical history should also be documented in writing.

Perform a standard secondary survey on stable patients. This survey should specifically include an evaluation of the burn with an estimate of the depth based on appearance and a rough calculation of the burn size. These findings are important in determining the level of medical care that would be appropriate for the burn victim. The burn size is best judged by using the rule of nines (see Figure 14-3). The body is divided into areas that are assigned either 9% or 18% of total body sizes, and by roughly drawing in the burned areas, the size can be estimated. There are some differences in body size proportionality in children. For smaller or irregular burns, the size can be estimated using the surface of the victim's hand as about 1% of the total body surface area.

Even small burns are serious if they involve certain parts of the body (see Figure 14-4).

Next remove the patient's loose clothing and jewelry. Cut around burned clothing that is adherent.

It is appropriate that nearly all burn injuries be seen by a physician. This is important since we now have specialized forms of therapy that offer specific advantages to the treatment of first-degree, second-degree, and third-degree burns. We have all seen second-degree burns become infected and progress to third-degree burns because of poor care. The sooner that specialized burn therapy can be initiated, the more rapid and satisfactory the results will be. Table 14-3 lists conditions that would benefit from care at a burn center.

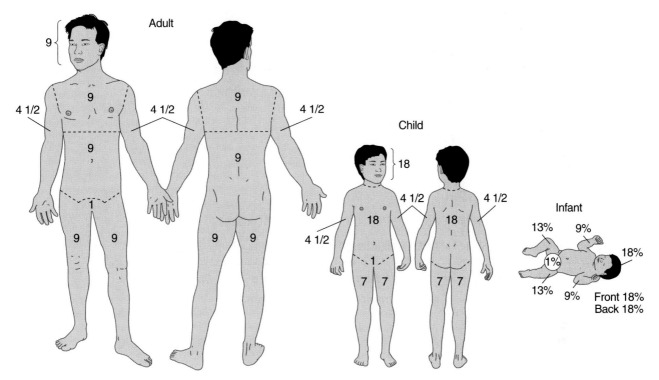

Figure 14-3 *"The rule of nines."*

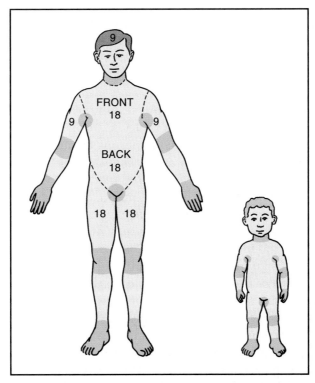

Figure 14-4 *Areas in which small burns are more serious. Second- or third-degree burns in these areas (shaded portions) should be treated in the hospital.*

1. SECOND- AND THIRD-DEGREE BURNS, 10% BODY SURFACE AREA IF AGE <10 OR >50
2. SECOND- AND THIRD-DEGREE BURNS, 20% BODY SURFACE AREA, ANY AGE
3. BURNS OF FACE, HANDS, FEET, GENITALIA, PERINEUM, MAJOR JOINTS
4. THIRD-DEGREE BURNS, 5% BODY SURFACE AREA

5. SPECIALIZED BURN TYPES
   a. ELECTRICAL, INCLUDING LIGHTNING
   b. CHEMICAL
   c. INHALATION INJURY
   d. CIRCUMFERENTIAL CHEST OR EXTREMITY INJURY

6. PRESENCE OF SIGNIFICANT PREEXISTING MEDICAL DISORDERS
7. PRESENCE OF SIGNIFICANT OTHER INJURIES

Table 14-3 *Injuries That Benefit From Care at a Burn Center*
Source: American Burn Association.

SPECIAL PROBLEMS IN BURN MANAGEMENT

INHALATION INJURIES

Inhalation injuries account for more than half of the 12,000 burn-related deaths per year and are classified as carbon monoxide poisoning, heat inhalation injuries, or smoke inhalation injuries. Most frequently, inhalation injuries occur when a patient is injured in a confined space or is trapped; however, even victims of fires in open spaces may have inhalation injuries. Flash explosions (no fire) practically never cause inhalation injuries.

Carbon monoxide poisoning and asphyxiation are by far the most common cause of early death associated with burn injury. Carbon monoxide is simply a by-product of combustion and is one of the numerous chemicals in common smoke. It is present in high concentrations in auto exhaust fumes and fumes from some types of home space heaters. Since it is colorless, odorless, and tasteless, its presence is virtually impossible to detect. Carbon monoxide binds to hemoglobin (257 times stronger than oxygen), resulting in the hemoglobin being unable to transport oxygen. Patients quickly become hypoxic even in the presence of very small concentrations of carbon monoxide, and alteration in their level of consciousness is the most predominant sign of hypoxia (see Table 14-4). A cherry-red skin color or cyanosis is virtually *never* present as a result of carbon monoxide poisoning and, therefore, cannot be used in the assessment of patients for carbon monoxide poisoning. Death usually occurs because of myocardial ischemia and myocardial infarction due to progressive cardiac hypoxia. Treat patients suspected of having carbon monoxide poisoning with high-flow oxygen by mask. If such a patient has lost consciousness, begin ventilation using 100% oxygen. If a patient is simply removed from the source of the carbon monoxide and allowed to breath fresh air, it takes up to seven hours to reduce the carbon monoxide–hemoglobin complex to

CARBOXYHEMOGLOBIN LEVEL (%)	SYMPTOMS
20	HEADACHE COMMON, THROBBING IN NATURE; SHORTNESS OF BREATH ON EXERTION
30	HEADACHE PRESENT; ALTERED CENTRAL NERVOUS SYSTEM (CNS) FUNCTION WITH DISTURBED JUDGMENT; IRRITABILITY, DIZZINESS; DECREASED VISION
40–50	MARKED CNS ALTERATION WITH CONFUSION, COLLAPSE, ALSO FAINTING WITH EXERTION
60–70	CONVULSIONS; UNCONSCIOUSNESS; APNEA WITH PROLONGED EXPOSURE
80	RAPIDLY FATAL

Table 14-4　*Symptoms Associated with Increasing Levels of Carboxyhemoglobin Binding*

a safe level. Having a patient breath 100% oxygen decreases this time to about 90–120 minutes, and use of hyperbaric oxygen (100% oxygen at 2.5 atmospheres) will decrease this time to about 30 minutes (see Figure 14-5).

Heat inhalation injuries selectively damage the upper airway since breathing in flame and hot gases does not result in heat transport down to the lung tissue itself. The water vapor in the air in the tracheal–bronchial tree effectively absorbs this heat. Steam inhalation causes an exception to this rule (since it is already super-heated water vapor). As a result of the heat injury, tissue swelling occurs just as it does with surface burns. The vocal cords themselves do not swell because they are

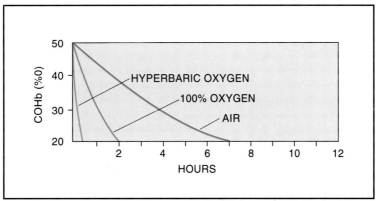

Figure 14-5　*Decay curve for disappearance of carboxyhemoglobin from 50% lethal level to 20% acceptable level in air, 1 atm. O2 (100% oxygen) and 2.5 atm. O2 (hyperbaric oxygen—100% at 2.5 atmospheres).*

dense fibrous bands of connective tissue. The loose mucosa in the supraglottic area (the hypopharynx) is where the swelling occurs, and this can easily progress to complete airway obstruction and death (see Figure 14-6). Airway swelling, like surface burn swelling, usually does not occur until after I.V. fluids have been running for some time, and, therefore, heat airway injury compromise is very uncommon in prehospital burn care. During secondary transport to a burn center, however, airway swelling can become significant and cause airway obstruction as volume resuscitation I.V. fluids are being administered. Figure 14-7 lists signs that should alert

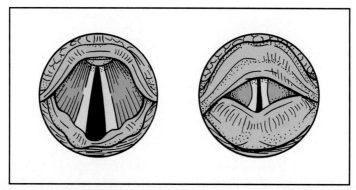

Figure 14-6 *Heat inhalation can cause complete airway obstruction by swelling of the hypopharynx. Left side: normal anatomy; right side: swelling proximal to cords.*

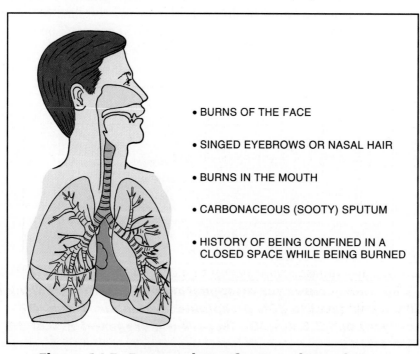

- BURNS OF THE FACE
- SINGED EYEBROWS OR NASAL HAIR
- BURNS IN THE MOUTH
- CARBONACEOUS (SOOTY) SPUTUM
- HISTORY OF BEING CONFINED IN A CLOSED SPACE WHILE BEING BURNED

Figure 14-7 *Danger signs of upper airway burns.*

you to the danger of your patient having upper airway burns. Swollen lips indicate the presence of hot gases and burn injury at the airway entry, and hoarseness (indicating altered airflow through the larynx area) is a warning of early airway swelling. Stridor (high-pitched breathing, seal-bark cough) indicates severe airway swelling with more than 85% obstruction and *represents an immediate emergency*. The only appropriate treatment is immediate transport to the appropriate hospital for airway stabilization.

Smoke inhalation injuries (see Figure 14-8) are the result of inhaled toxic chemicals that cause structural damage to lung cells. Smoke may contain hundreds of toxic chemicals that damage the delicate alveolar cells. Smoke from plastic and synthetic products is the most damaging. Damage from smoke inhalation usually takes days to develop and is virtually never a problem in initial field management. These patients are also treated with 100% oxygen.

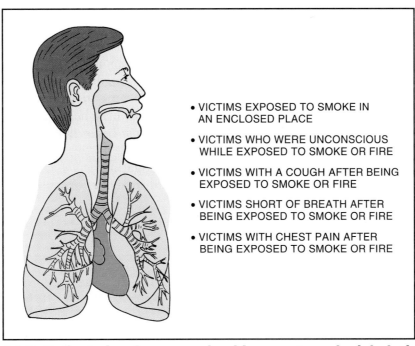

- VICTIMS EXPOSED TO SMOKE IN AN ENCLOSED PLACE

- VICTIMS WHO WERE UNCONSCIOUS WHILE EXPOSED TO SMOKE OR FIRE

- VICTIMS WITH A COUGH AFTER BEING EXPOSED TO SMOKE OR FIRE

- VICTIMS SHORT OF BREATH AFTER BEING EXPOSED TO SMOKE OR FIRE

- VICTIMS WITH CHEST PAIN AFTER BEING EXPOSED TO SMOKE OR FIRE

Figure 14-8 Patients in whom you should suspect smoke inhalation injury.

CHEMICAL BURNS

There are virtually thousands of different types of chemicals that can cause burn injuries. Chemicals may not only injure the skin, but also may be absorbed into the body and cause internal organ failure (especially liver and kidney damage). Volatile forms of chemicals may be inhaled and cause lung tissue damage with subsequent severe life-threatening respiratory failure. Chemical injuries are frequently deceiving in that initial skin changes may be minimal even when a severe injury is present.

This may cause a secondary problem in that such burns may not be obvious but you can get these chemicals on your own skin unless appropriate precautions are taken. Tissue damage factors include chemical concentration, quantity, manner and duration of skin contact, and the mechanism of action. The pathologic process causing the tissue damage continues until the chemical is either consumed in the damage process or until it is removed. Attempts at inactivation with specific neutralizing chemicals are dangerous because neutralizing chemicals generate other chemical reactions that may worsen the injury. Therefore, you should aim treatment at chemical removal by following these four steps:

1. Wear protective gloves, eyewear, and so on.
2. Remove all clothing with chemicals on it.
3. Flush most chemicals off the body by irrigating copiously with any source of available water or other irrigant.
4. Remove any retained agent adherent to the skin by any appropriate physical means such as wiping or scraping. Follow this by further irrigation.

In all but the most trivial injuries, continue flushing for 15 minutes, unless a critical or unstable situation warrants transport sooner (see Figure 14-9a). Irrigation of caustic chemicals in the eye is exceptionally important since irreversible damage will occur in a very short period of time (less than the transport time to get to the hospital). Irrigation of injured eyes may be difficult because of pain associated with eye opening. However, you must begin irrigation to prevent severe and permanent damage to the corneas (see Figure 14-9b). Check for contact lenses and, if present, remove them early during irrigation.

If dry chemicals are on the skin, they should first be thoroughly brushed off before performing copious irrigation.

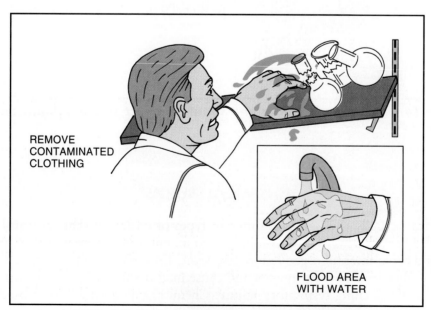

REMOVE CONTAMINATED CLOTHING

FLOOD AREA WITH WATER

Figure 14-9a *Chemical burns of the skin.*

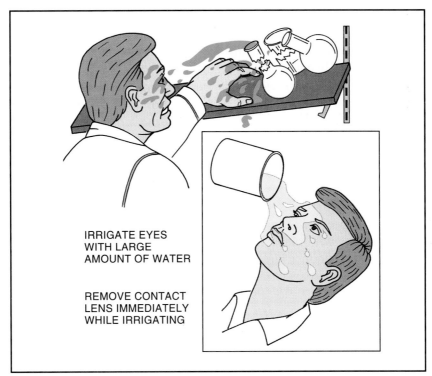

IRRIGATE EYES
WITH LARGE
AMOUNT OF WATER

REMOVE CONTACT
LENS IMMEDIATELY
WHILE IRRIGATING

Figure 14-9b *Chemical burns of the eye.*

ELECTRICAL BURNS

In cases of electrical burns, damage is caused by electricity entering the body and traveling through the tissues. Extremities usually have more significant tissue damage because their small size results in higher local current density. The factors that determine severity of electrical injury include

1. The type and amount of current

2. Path of the current

3. Duration of contact with the current

The most serious injury that occurs due to electrical contact is immediate cardiac dysrhythmias. *Any patient involved with an electric current injury, regardless of how stable he or she looks, should have a careful immediate evaluation of his or her cardiac status and continuous monitoring of cardiac activity.* The most common life-threatening dysrhythmias are premature ventricular contractions, ventricular tachycardia, and ventricular fibrillation. Automated defibrillators are very useful in this situation since these patients usually have normal healthy hearts and the chances for resuscitation are excellent. For a patient in ventricular fibrillation with only basic life support available, start cardiopulmonary resuscitation (CPR) and transport immediately to a hospital facility. Most of these victims do not have pre-existing cardiovascular disease, and their heart muscle tissue is usually not damaged as a result of the electricity. Even under circumstances of prolonged CPR, resuscitation is often possible. Once those efforts at managing cardiac status are complete, provide field care as previously described for thermal burns.

Additional electrical injuries include skin burns at entrance and exit sites because of high temperatures generated by the electric arc (2,500 degrees centigrade) at the skin surface. Additional surface flame burns may be present as a result of the patient's clothing being ignited. Fractures and/or dislocations may be present due to the violent muscle contractions that electrical injuries cause. Internal injuries usually involve muscle damage, nerve damage, and possible intravascular blood coagulation due to electrical current passage. *Internal chest or abdominal organ damage is exceedingly rare.*

At the scene of an electrical injury your first priority in determining scene safety is to determine if the patient is still in contact with the electrical current. If so, you must remove the patient from contact without becoming a victim yourself (see Figure 14-10). Handling high-voltage electrical wires is extremely hazardous. Special training and special equipment are needed to deal with downed wires; never attempt to move wires with makeshift equipment. Tree limbs, pieces of wood, and even manila rope may conduct high-voltage electricity. Even firefighter's gloves and boots do not protect one in this situation. If possible, leave the handling of downed wires to power company employees, or develop a special training program with your local power company to learn how to use the special equipment needed to handle high-voltage lines.

Initially, it is impossible to tell the total extent of the damage in electrical burns; all electrical burn patients should be transported for hospital evaluation.

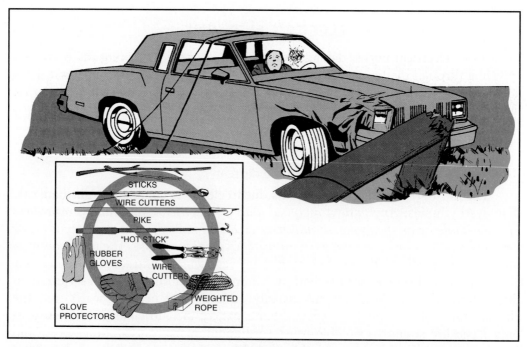

Figure 14-10 *Removal of high-voltage electrical wires. Do not try to remove wires with the safety equipment (or with sticks) unless specially trained. Turn off the electricity at the source or call the power company to remove the wires.*

SECONDARY TRANSPORT

Major burns usually do not occur in locations where immediate transport to one of the major burn centers is possible. As a result, transport from a primary hospital to a burn center is commonly necessary. After the initial stabilization (which should require between one and three hours), immediate movement to a major burn center is best for the patient. During this transport, it is important to be able to continue resuscitation.

Prior to secondary transports, the transferring physician should have completed the following:

1. Obtain Advanced Life Support personnel (nurse or advanced EMT) to help you

2. Stabilization of respiratory and hemodynamic function. This may necessitate intubation, and certainly two large-bore I.V.s for fluid administration are standard

3. Assessment and management of associated injuries

4. Review of appropriate lab data (specifically blood gas analysis)

5. Placement of a nasogastric tube in all burns covering more than 20% of the body surface area

6. Assessment of peripheral circulation and appropriate wound management

7. Proper arrangements with the receiving hospital and physician

You should specifically discuss the transport with either the referring or the receiving physician to determine what special functions may need monitoring. It is important for you to maintain careful records indicating patient condition and treatment during the transport. You should also make an in-depth report to the receiving facility.

SUMMARY

Burn injuries are potentially deadly for both you and your patient. You must never forget the rules of scene safety. Half of all burn deaths are from inhalation injuries; do not forget the airway. Give 100% oxygen if there is any chance of inhalation injury. Cool the burn to halt the burning process, but do not cause hypothermia. You must begin irrigating chemical burns in the field, or the burn damage will continue during transport. This is one of the few instances in trauma care when extra time spent in the field may be beneficial to the patient. Electrical burns are commonly associated with cardiac arrest but rapid evaluation and management is usually life saving. High-voltage electricity is extremely dangerous; get trained personnel to turn it off. Do not begin secondary transfer of a burn patient until the patient has been properly stabilized.

IMPORTANT POINTS TO REMEMBER

1. Maintain appropriate safety when removing patients from the source of a burn injury.

2. Treat burn patients as trauma patients—primary survey, critical interventions, and transport decision, and secondary survey, critical care and reassessment survey.

3. Properly cool the surface thermal injury if early after burn event.

4. Almost all types of burns may have some degree of inhalation injury.

5. Chemical injuries, in general, require prolonged and copious irrigation.

6. Immediately check cardiac status of victims of electrical injury.

7. Plan all secondary transports to major burn centers and effectively continue resuscitation during such transports.

BIBLIOGRAPHY

1. Committee on Trauma, American College of Surgeons. "Injuries due to Burns and Cold." *Advanced Trauma Life Support*. Chicago: The College, 1989.

2. Committee on Trauma, American College of Surgeons. *Advanced Burn Life Support*. Chicago: The College, 1988.

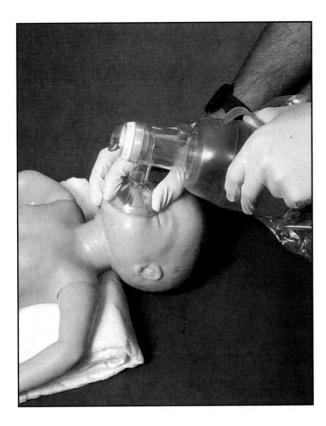

Trauma in Children

Carden Johnston, M.D., F.A.C.E.P.,
F.A.A.P, and Lisa Santer, M.D, F.A.A.P.

OBJECTIVES

Upon completion of this chapter you should be able to:

1. Describe effective techniques for gaining the confidence of children and their parents.

2. Demonstrate understanding of the need for immediate transport in potentially life-threatening circumstances, regardless of lack of immediate parental consent.

3. Differentiate equipment needs of pediatric patients from those of adults.

4. Describe the primary and secondary surveys in the pediatric patient.

5. Describe the various ways to immobilize a child and how this differs from an adult.

6. Predict pediatric injuries based on common mechanisms of injury.

7. Discuss the need for involvement of EMS personnel in prevention programs for parents and children.

COMMUNICATING WITH THE CHILD AND FAMILY

Because children come with parents, you have at least two patients, even if the adult is not injured. Parents can be your greatest asset or hindrance in caring for an injured child. Parents are anxious, upset, and often feeling guilty. They can transfer these feelings, along with unreasonable expectations, to the child and even to you. The good news is that if you can gain the parents' confidence, this also can be transferred to the child and to you. Parents generally want you to help their child, and they want to help you do so.

The best way to get the parents' confidence is to demonstrate your competence in managing the child. Parents are more likely to be cooperative if they see that you are confident and organized and are using equipment that is designed for children. Show the parents you know how important they are by involving them in the care of their child. Whenever possible, keep parents in physical and verbal contact with the child. They can perform simple tasks such as holding a pressure dressing or just comforting the child. They can explain what is going on, even sing nursery rhymes. Show your concern for the child—but don't freeze. One technique is to pretend that the parent is one of your examiners. You can then talk your way through the examination using language that is understandable both to the child and family. You will also be able to better assess mental status. A child who can be consoled or distracted by a person or a toy has a brain that is being adequately perfused with oxygen and nutrients. On the other hand, a child who cannot be consoled or distracted may have a head injury, be in shock, be experiencing hypoxia, or be in severe pain. Changes in distractibility and consolability are important observations about the level of consciousness of a child. Record and report them just as you would report changes in level of consciousness of an adult.

A child less than 9 months old likes to hear "cooing" sounds, the tinkle and sight of keys, and often feels more comfortable when swaddled. For the child less than age 2, the flashlight is a good distractor. As the child knows many "ah" sounds, like "mama" and "papa," try to use those. The 2-year-old child is typically negative, and often difficult to distract or comfort. Expect all questions to be answered by "no." Try making faces and word sounds, and smile a lot. The toddler and young child can benefit from a toy or doll. If the child had one in the car or nearby, ask the parent to get it. It will make the trip to and through the hospital easier. You can make an airplane out of two tongue blades or a doll out of a rubber glove (if child is over 3 years old and won't choke on the rubber).

A quick trick to help patients to be calm and still is to suggest "blow out your hurt and scared, like you are blowing up a balloon." If you blow with them, children will physically and mentally relax, and often describe the color of the balloon. Also remember to watch your language. Say "this might bother you now" or "now you'll feel squeezing," not "now I'll poke you, and it will hurt." Calm words decrease fear.

Don't get caught in the trap of asking the child if he wants to take a trip in the ambulance or to be placed in a cervical collar. The child will answer "no" most of the time. Tell the child what you are doing with a smile on your face. Show it does not hurt, perhaps by doing it to a parent or yourself. Size is intimidating. When approaching a child, try to make yourself small by getting on the child's level. In the care of the child, it is appropriate that paramedics spend much field time on their knees. Frightened children, especially around the age of 2 to 4, may try to defend themselves by biting, spitting, or hitting. They are acting out of fear. Stay calm, recognize that the behavior is normal, reassure the child, and use firm, not painful, physical control of the patient as needed. Parents and children do not understand packaging, which makes them more likely to resist it. Explain why packaging is necessary. Most parents will understand if you explain that even though the chances are low there is anything seriously wrong with the spine, the stakes are high if there is. Make a game of packaging with the child. If the parent refuses to let you package, write it down on your run report and get the parent to sign it.

Many states do not allow transport or treatment of the pediatric patient without the consent of the parent or legal guardian, unless there are extenuating circumstances. You have to make a decision whether it will take too long to find a parent to obtain consent. In a situation of a child needing emergency care (e.g., an asphyxiated infant where the mother is unconscious), you must treat that child appropriately. Transport before you receive permission, document why you are transporting without permission, and notify Medical Direction of this action. If the parents or legal guardians do not want you to transport or treat, try to persuade them. If you cannot, document your actions on the written report and try to get them to sign it. If you suspect abuse, notify authorities.

Before you leave the scene with the child, be sure to ask the parent about other children. Sometimes they are so concerned about one they forget other small children who may be in a high-risk situation, such as alone in the house.

EQUIPMENT

Table 15-1 contains a list of suggested pediatric equipment for the prehospital provider. The Broselow tape (see Figure 15-1) is a commercial tape measure that, when used to measure the length of a child, gives you the estimated weight of the child, precalculated doses of fluid and medications, and estimated sizes of common equipment needed. Simply put the end of the tape that says "measure from head" at the top of the child's head. Stretch the tape the length of the child and put your other hand on the tape at the level of the child's heel. You can call ahead to the

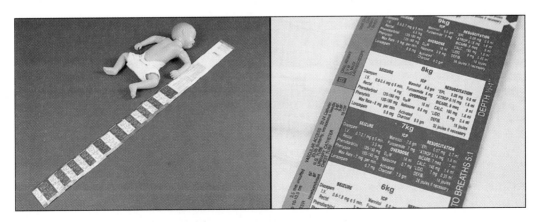

Figure 15-1 *Broselow tape.*

PEDIATRIC FEMUR TRACTION SPLINT
PEDIATRIC BACKBOARD
PEDIATRIC CERVICAL COLLARS (RIGID)
PEDIATRIC BAG-VALVE-MASK (BVM) RESUSCITATOR WITH NEWBORN AND CHILD-SIZE MASKS
BLOOD PRESSURE CUFF, INFANT AND CHILD
HEAD IMMOBILIZER
KID (IMMOBILIZATION DEVICE)
ORAL AIRWAYS, 0 TO 5
BROSELOW TAPE

Table 15-1 *Prehospital Pediatric Equipment and Supplies*

receiving hospital and give them the colored section of the child. The emergency department can then have all of the appropriately sized equipment ready when you arrive.

PATIENT ASSESSMENT

The approach to the injured child is the same as for the adult:

1. Total overview of patient situation while approaching the patient
2. Airway with C-spine stabilization
3. Breathing
4. Circulation
5. Briefly examine abdomen, pelvis, and extremities
6. Control major bleeding
7. Critical interventions and transport decision
   a. Critical situation present
      Backboard
      Immediate transport
      Life-saving interventions en route
      Secondary survey en route
   b. Critical situation not present
      Backboard
      Secondary survey
      Transport

8. Notification of Medical Direction
9. Critical care and reassessment surveys

AIRWAY WITH C-SPINE STABILIZATION AND INITIAL LEVEL OF CONSCIOUSNESS

This aspect of assessment is easier in the child than in the adult. It is true that the child's tongue is large, the tissue is soft, and the airway is easy to obstruct, but other characteristics make it easier to manage the child's airway. For example, neonates are obligatory nose breathers, so just opening the mouth or clearing the nose with a bulb syringe can be life saving. To use the bulb syringe, collapse the bulb end of the syringe, put the point end in the nose of the child, and release the bulb. Remove the syringe from the nose; recollapse the bulb to empty the mucus, blood, or vomit, and repeat. The bulb syringe can be used to remove secretions from the posterior pharynx of infants as well.

Be sure to stabilize the neck in a neutral position with your hands. Do not take time to apply a cervical collar until you have finished the primary survey. So that the neck does not have to be moved, the jaw thrust should be the first airway maneuver in the unconscious child who has sustained trauma. In small children, the occiput is so big that it will flex the neck and may occlude the airway when the child is lying flat. It is often necessary to place a pad underneath the torso to keep the neck in a neutral position (see Figure 15-2 and Chapter 9). Hyperextension of the neck also may cause airway occlusion. For the unconscious child, an oral airway is very helpful to get the tongue out of the way and keep the airway open (see Chapter 5). If a tooth is loose, be sure to remove it from the mouth so that the child does not choke on it. The oral airway can stimulate a gag reflex, which is very sensitive in the conscious child, thus limiting the use of this airway to unconscious children. Nasopharyngeal airways are too small to work predictably in children; do not use them. Give ventilation instructions as soon as you complete your evaluation of breathing.

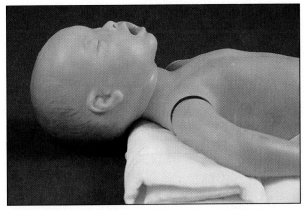

Figure 15-2 *Child with pad under shoulders to keep neck in neutral position.*

Check the neck for signs of injury, carotid pulse, and distended neck veins, and feel for a deviated trachea. What appears to be minor blunt trauma to the neck can be life threatening. A deviated trachea is difficult to detect in a small child, but has the same significance as in adults. Make a mental note of the child's initial level of consciousness as you begin your survey. A sleeping preschool child can look unconscious; young children can even sleep through a gentle pupillary check with a flashlight. However, they will usually awaken with pain. In the trauma situation, decreased level of consciousness suggests shock, head trauma, or seizure. Remember to hyperventilate children with decreased LOC.

ASSESSMENT OF BREATHING

Look at the chest rise, listen for air going in and out, and feel the air coming out of the nose. If there is no movement or if ventilation is inadequate, you must breathe for the child. When performing mouth-to-mouth ventilation for a small child, you may cover both the child's nose and mouth with your mouth. If the face mask does not fit well when performing bag-valve-mask ventilation, try turning the mask upside down for a better seal. Pay attention to your hand placement (see Figure 15-3). Your large hands can easily obstruct the airway or injure the child's eyes. Give the breaths slowly at low pressure, less than 20 cm H_2O, to keep from inflating the stomach or causing a pneumothorax. The rates are 40 per minute for a child less than a year of age, 20 per minute for greater than 1 year of age, and 15 per minute for an adolescent. Most important, watch for chest rise. If the chest is rising, air is getting into the lungs. Check air entry on both sides of the chest with your stethoscope. *Gentle* cricoid pressure (Sellick maneuver, see Chapter 3) is useful and rec-

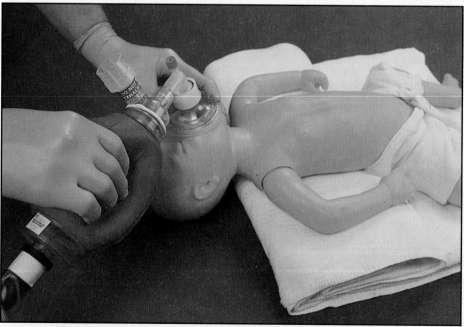

Figure 15-3 *Bag-valve-mask ventilation in a child.*

ommended in a child. Some self-inflatable bag-valve masks have a pop-off valve at about 40 cm H_2O pressure. The pressure generated by these devices is more than adequate most of the time. However, lungs are sometimes stiff from a near-drowning, bronchospasm, or aspiration, and more pressure is needed. Be familiar with your equipment. Make sure that your BVM does not have a pop-off valve.

ASSESSMENT OF CIRCULATION

Early shock is more difficult to diagnose in a child than an adult. Capillary refill may be used along with other methods to assess the circulation but do not depend on it alone to diagnose shock. At the present time the capillary refill test is considered controversial. To test capillary refill, compress the nailbed, the entire foot, or the skin over the sternum for 2 seconds, and release to see how quickly the blood returns. Skin color should return to the precompressed state within two seconds. If it does not, the child has vasoconstriction, which can be a sign of shock. You must be aware that the signs of shock in a child may also be caused by other conditions. Mottled skin is a normal finding in an infant less than six months of age, but it also may be a sign of poor circulation, so note it. Extremities can be cold because of nervousness, cold weather, or poor perfusion. Heart rate increases for many reasons in children, including shock, fear, and fever. Comparing carotid and radial pulses is not useful in a child. As pulses may be difficult to find and judge in a child, practice feeling them on most of your pediatric runs and on your children. In a child, the brachial pulse is usually easy to feel, whereas the carotid is not. Feeling a dorsalis pedis pulse causes less anxiety, and may be easier than a femoral pulse. A weak, rapid pulse with a rate over 130 is usually a sign of shock in all children except neonates (see Table 15-2, Ranges for Vital Signs). The child's level of consciousness is also a useful indicator of circulatory status, yet note that circulation can be poor even though the child appears awake. As mentioned earlier, if the child is consolable by the parent or member of the EMS team, there is enough circulation to allow the child's brain to be

AGE	WEIGHT (KG)	RESPIRATIONS	PULSE	SYSTOLIC BLOOD (KG) PRESSURE
NEWBORN	3–4	30–50	120–160	>60
6 MO–1 YR	8–10	30–40	120–140	70–80
2–4 YR	12–16	20–30	100–110	80–95
5–8 YR	18–26	14–20	90–100	90–100
8–12 YR	26–50	12–20	80–100	100–110
>12 YR	>50	12–16	80–100	100–120

Table 15-2 *Ranges for Vital Signs*

working. Though not proven by scientific study, yawning is considered a good sign that shock is not imminent. Low blood pressure is a sign of late shock, but measuring BP in a frightened child can be time consuming, especially for the inexperienced. To make it easier and more reliable to obtain blood pressure in an emergency, practice taking it at every opportunity. The rule of thumb for cuff size is to use the largest one that will fit snugly on the patient's arm. If there is too much noise, you can perform a blood pressure by palpation. Find the radial pulse, pump up the blood pressure cuff until you no longer feel the pulse, and allow air to leak slowly while observing the dial on the BP cuff. Record the pressure at which you first feel the pulse and label it "p" for palpation. This will be a systolic blood pressure only and will be slightly lower than a blood pressure that can be auscultated. A systolic blood pressure less than 80 in children, less than 70 in young infants, is a sign of shock.

A common cause of shock secondary to occult bleeding is a femur fracture. Also, although we teach that patients don't go into shock from intracranial blood loss, this can happen in the young infant. Thus, if you see an infant in shock with no obvious source of bleeding, consider intracranial blood loss or femur fracture.

The antishock garment (MAST or PASG) is no longer recommended for treatment of shock except in special circumstances (see Chapter 7). Remember, older children wearing tight-fitting pants are already wearing a form of antishock garment. Cutting these off, like deflating traditional antishock garments, may produce a drop in perfusion. Thus, in children with signs of shock, it is wise to delay cutting off tight pants until after vascular accesshas been established.

CONTROL OF BLEEDING

Obvious bleeding sources must be controlled to maintain circulation. Remember, the child's blood volume is about 80 to 90 cc per kilogram, so a 10 kg child has less than 1 L of blood. Three or four lacerations can cause a 200 cc blood loss, which is about 20% of the child's total volume. Therefore, pay closer attention to blood loss in a child than you do in an adult. Use pressure firm enough to control arterial bleeding if necessary. If you ask the parent or a bystander to help hold pressure, monitor them to be sure they are applying enough pressure to stop the bleeding. Use a bandage tight enough to control venous bleeding, not one that will just soak up the blood so that you do not see it. Elevating an injured extremity also can help to control bleeding.

DECISION: IS THERE A CRITICAL TRAUMA SITUATION PRESENT?

If you have found a critical trauma situation, the child needs rapid transport. Log-roll the child onto a pediatric spineboard and go. Remember to use a pad under the torso to align the neck in a neutral position. While appropriately sized rigid cervical collars are useful and can help remind the patient and the providers not to move the head, they often do not fit small children well. Do not depend on the cervical collar alone; immobilize the head with tape and a head immobilizer. Children are portable and they can (and should) be transported rapidly. *There are very few procedures that should be done in the field.* Minutes count, especially in children. On-scene times of less than 5 minutes are desirable. Administer maximal oxygen to all critical pediatric patients. Assist ventilations if necessary. Not all emergency departments have the equipment or personnel to handle pediatric emergencies. Transfer arrangements for more severe problems should be worked out in advance so that when the injury occurs, confusion will be minimized and time will be saved. See Table 15-3 for a partial list of mechanisms of injury that are criteria for transport to an emergency department approved for pediatrics or a pediatric trauma center. These, plus pediatric burns, near-drowning, and head injuries with loss of consciousness, should go to facilities qualified to handle major pediatric trauma. Call ahead so that the emergency department can have the necessary equipment and personnel ready. Perform secondary survey and reassessment surveys en route if there is time.

If, after completing the primary assessment, you find no critical trauma situation, place the child on a backboard and do a methodical secondary survey.

UNCONSCIOUS

DILATED PUPIL

DECREASING LEVEL OF CONSCIOUSNESS

GLASGOW COMA SCORE <10

PEDIATRIC TRAUMA SCORE <8

MECHANISM OF INJURY ASSOCIATED WITH SEVERE INJURIES
1. FALL FROM A HEIGHT OF 15 FEET OR MORE
2. AN ACCIDENT WITH FATALITIES
3. EJECTED FROM AN AUTOMOBILE IN A MOTOR VEHICULAR ACCIDENT
4. IN A MOTOR VEHICULAR ACCIDENT, THE ENGINE ENTERED THE PASSENGER COMPARTMENT
5. HIT BY A CAR AS A PEDESTRIAN OR BICYCLIST
6. FRACTURES IN MORE THAN ONE EXTREMITY
7. SIGNIFICANT INJURY TO MORE THAN ONE ORGAN SYSTEM

Table 15-3 *Suggested Criteria for Transfer to an Emergency Department Approved for Pediatrics or a Pediatric Trauma Center*

SECONDARY SURVEY

As in adults, record accurate vital signs, take a "SAMPLE" history, and perform a complete head-to-toes exam, including a more detailed neurological exam. A brief neurological check such as AVPU, with notation of whether the child is consolable or distractable, is useful. Finish bandaging and splinting, and transport the child with continuous monitoring. Notify Medical Direction. Calculate the Glasgow Coma Scale (GCS) and Pediatric Trauma Score during transport (Tables 15-4 and 15-5).

	>1 YEAR	<1 YEAR
EYES OPENING	4 SPONTANEOUSLY 3 TO VERBAL COMMAND 2 TO PAIN 1 NO RESONSE	SPONTANEOUSLY TO SHOUT TO PAIN NO RESONSE
	>1 YEAR	<1 YEAR
BEST MOTOR RESPONSE	6 OBEYS 5 LOCALIZES PAIN 4 FLEXION-WITHDRAWAL 3 FLEXION-ABNORMAL (DECORTICATE RIGIDITY) 2 EXTENSION (DECEREBRATE RIGIDITY) 1 NO RESPONSE	LOCALIZES PAIN FLEXION-NORMAL FLEXION-ABNORMAL (DECORTICATE RIGIDITY) EXTENSION (DECEREBRATE RIGIDITY) NO RESPONSE

	>5 YEARS	<2–5 YEARS	0–23 MONTHS

BEST VERBAL RESPONSE	5 ORIENTED
	   AND CONVERSES
	4 DISORIENTED
	   AND CONVERSES
	3 INAPPROPRIATE
	   WORDS
	2 INCOMPREHENSIBLE
	   SOUNDS
	1 NO RESPONSE
		APPROPRIATE
		WORDS AND
		PHRASES
		INAPPROPRIATE
		WORDS
		CRIED AND/OR
		SCREAMS
		GRUNTS
		
		NO RESPONSE
			SMILES, COOS, CRIES
			APPROPRIATELY
			CRIES
			
			INAPPROPRIATE CRYING
			AND/OR SCREAMING
			GRUNTS
			
			NO RESPONSE

Table 15-4 *Glasgow Coma Scale*

INJURIES

HEAD INJURY

The head is the primary focus of injury in the child because the child's head is proportionately larger than the adult's. The force of impact does some damage to the brain, but much of the brain damage from head injuries comes after impact, from preventable causes. To avoid this, you must do four things:

1. *Give oxygen.* Head injury increases brain cell metabolic rate and decreases blood flow in at least part of the brain.

2. *Keep blood pressure up.* Blood must get to the brain to carry oxygen, so systolic pressure must be at least 80 mm Hg in the preschool child and 90 mm Hg in older children.

Because of the difficulty in obtaining accurate blood pressure readings in small children, you will have to rely on signs of poor perfusion.

3. *Lower intracranial pressure.* Hyperventilate the patient (see Table 15-6, Approximate Normal Respiratory and Hyperventilation Rates). As a general rule, increase the rate of ventilation about ten breaths per minute above normal. This contracts blood vessels in the brain and lowers the intracranial pressure, allowing blood into the intracranil vault. *If the child is not in shock,* you may elevate the head

PTS	+2	+1	−1
WEIGHT	>44 LB (>20 KG)	22–44 LB (10–20 KG)	<22 LB (<10 KG)
AIRWAY	NORMAL	ORAL OR NASAL AIRWAY	INTUBATED TRACHEOSTOMY INVASIVE
BLOOD PRESSURE	PULSE AT WRIST >90 MMHG	CAROTID OR FEMORAL PULSE PALPABLE 50–90 MMHG	NO PALPABLE PULSE <50 MMHG
LEVEL OF CONSCIOUSNESS	COMPLETELY AWAKE	OBTUNDED OR ANY LOC	COMATOSE
OPEN WOUND	NONE	MINOR	MAJOR OR PENETRATING
FRACTURES	NONE	CLOSED FRACTURE	OPEN OR MULTIPLE FRACTURE

Table 15-5 *Pediatric Trauma Score*

AGE RANGE	APPROXIMATE NORMAL RATE	APPROXIMATE HYPERVENTILATION RATE
INFANT	40	50
CHILD	20–30	30–40
ADOLESCENT	15–20	25–30

Table 15-6 *Approximate Normal Respiratory and Hyperventilation Rates*

of the backboard 15–30 degrees to help lower intracranial pressure (controversial). Do not flex the neck. Let the blood out of the brain. Do not compress jugular veins by pressure, rotation of the neck, or tight-fitting collars.

4. *Be prepared to prevent aspiration.* Head injury patients frequently vomit. You must have suction out and ready in case this happens.

Changing level of consciousness is the best indicator of head trauma. A child entering the emergency department with a GCS of 10, that has come down from 13, will be approached very differently from the child who has a GCS of 10, that has come up from 7. Assessments using vague words like "semiconscious" are not helpful. Instead, note specific points such as whether the child is distractible, consolable, reaches for the parent, or reacts to pain or voice. Pupil assessment is as important in the child as in the adult. Note also whether the eyes are moving both left and right or whether they remain in one position. Do not move the head to determine this!

Children with head injury often fare much better than adults with the same degree of injury. Children with head trauma and low GCS may still recover completely with good care. On the other hand, children with head injury may need immediate surgical intervention to give the brain a maximal chance of complete healing. Transport children with serious head injury to a trauma center equipped to provide definitive care.

CHEST INJURY

Children generally give visible signs of respiratory distress, such as tachypnea, grunting, nasal flaring, and retractions. Be aware that children's normal respiratory rates are higher than adults (Table 15-6). A child breathing faster than 40, or an infant faster than 60, usually has respiratory distress and would benefit from supplemental oxygen. A few grunts are not significant, but persistent grunting indicates a need for ventilatory assistance. A child in respiratory distress often breathes with his nose like a rabbit, which is called flaring. Retractions relate to caving in of the suprasternal, intercostal, or subcostal areas with inspiration. Retractions suggest the child is having to work harder to breathe. If any of these signs are persistent, they should alert you that something is wrong with the respiratory system (pneumo/hemothorax, foreign body, bronchospasm).

Children with blunt chest injury are at risk for pneumothorax. Because the chest is small, a difference in breath sounds from side to side may be more subtle than in the adult. You may not be able to tell a difference, even by listening carefully. It is also difficult to diagnose tension pneumothorax in young children who usually have short fat necks that mask both neck vein distension and tracheal deviation. If a tension pneumothorax develops, the heart and trachea should eventually shift away from the side of the pneumothorax. To help detect a shift of a child's heart, place an "X" over the point of maximum impulse (PMI).

Children in the preadolescent age group have highly elastic chest walls. Pericardial tamponade, flail chest, and aortic rupture are, therefore, seldom seen in this group. However, pulmonary contusion is common.

ABDOMINAL INJURY

The second leading cause of traumatic death in most pediatric centers is internal bleeding secondary to rupture of the liver and/or spleen. In children the liver and spleen both protrude below the ribs, exposing the organs to blunt trauma. This poor protection and the relatively large size of the liver and spleen in children allow easy tearing of these organs. If a child has blunt injury to the chest or abdomen, be prepared to treat for shock. As a child goes into shock, blood flow decreases, as does the rate of blood loss. A delicate clot may then form. Bleeding may restart as perfusion increases from moving the child or from therapy. If a child with blunt trauma is in shock with no obvious source of bleeding, your decision should be to "load and go." Life-saving interventions should be made en route to the hospital. Children with abdominal injury are likely to vomit; be prepared.

SPINAL INJURY

Although children have short necks, big heads, and loose ligaments, C-spine injuries are uncommon before adolescence. Cervical spine injuries do occur, however, and you should immobilize a child's cervical spine using a padded head immobilization device. A C-collar is not necessary if the head is properly immobilized in a padded device. Again, try to make a game of packaging the child. You can promise you will give him a ride in the ambulance as a reward after you get him all wrapped up and ready. Use a parent or other familiar person, if possible. Be sure your packaging does not restrict chest movement. As mentioned before, children up to about 8 years of age will need a pad under the torso to keep the neck in a neutral position.

COMMON MECHANISMS OF INJURY IN CHILDREN

Children are most commonly injured from falls, motor vehicle crashes, auto-pedestrian accidents, burns, airway obstruction from a foreign body, and child abuse. Children who fall from a height usually land on their heads because it is the largest and heaviest part of a small child's body. You should anticipate head injury when a child falls. A child hit by a car will frequently have Waddell's triad—a combination of left femur, spleen, and right head injuries. Because we drive on the right side of the road, the bumper of the car generally hits the child's left femur while the fender hits the spleen area. The child then flies through the air and lands on the right side of the head. Auto accidents and other mechanisms involving blunt trauma to the abdomen may injure the liver and spleen as mentioned earlier.

CHILD RESTRAINT SEATS

A child in a wreck while properly restrained is much less likely to have a serious injury than an unrestrained passenger. If the child is in a car seat, he or she can usually be transported without being removed from the device. Assess the child as you would other trauma patients. Place padding around the child's head and tape the head directly to the car seat. If not in shock the child can be transported in the upright position. If the child is showing early signs of shock, the car seat can be laid on its back, elevating the child's legs (you may prefer to remove the child to a spineboard). Some new-model cars have built-in infant restraint seats. These seats cannot be removed so the child who is restrained in one of these will have to be extricated and placed on a pediatric immobilization device.

SUMMARY

To provide good trauma care for children you must have the proper equipment, know how to interact with frightened parents, know the normal vital signs for various ages (or have them posted in your trauma box), and be familiar with the injuries that are more common in children. Fortunately the assessment sequence is the same for children as for adults. If you perform your assessment well, you will obtain the information needed to make the right decisions in management.

While assessment and management of the injured child are life-saving skills, all of us involved in the care of the seriously injured child also should be concerned about prevention (see Appendix H). Car seats, bicycle helmets, seat belts, all-terrain vehicle injuries, water safety, scald burn injuries, firearm safety, and fire drills are within our area of concern. We should donate our time to teaching safety and we should speak out for laws (infant seat restraints, seat belts, drunk driving) that save lives.

BIBLIOGRAPHY

1. Nypaver, M., and D. Treloar. "Neutral Cervical Spine Positioning in Children." *Annals of Emergency Medicine,* Vol. 23 (February 1994), pp. 208–211.

2. Schriger, D. L., and L. J. Baraff. "Capillary Refill—Is It a Useful Predictor of Hypovolemic States?" *Annals of Emergency Medicine,* Vol. 20 (June 1991), pp. 601–605.

3. American Academy of Pediatrics, Joint Task Force on Advanced Pediatric Life Support. *APLS: The Pediatric Emergency Medicine Course,* 2nd ed. Elk Grove, IL.: The Academy, 1993.

4. American Academy of Pediatrics, Committee on Pediatric Emergency Medicine: *Emergency Medical Services for Children: The Role of the Primary Care Provider.* Elk Grove, IL.: The Academy, 1992.

5. Allhouse, M., T. Rouse, and M. Eichelberger. "Childhood Injury: A Current Perspective." *Pediatric Emergency Care,* Vol. 9, no. 3 (June 1993), p. 159.

6. French, G., E. Painter, and D. Coury. "Blowing Away Shot Pain: A Technique for Pain Management During Immunization." *Pediatrics,* Vol. 93, no. 3 (March 1994), p. 384.

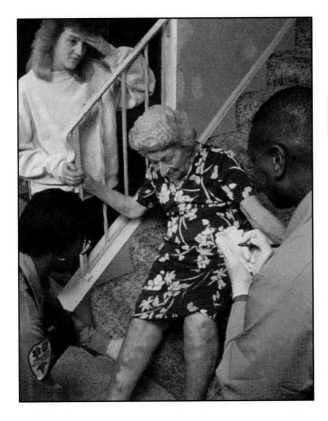

CHAPTER 16

Trauma in the Elderly

Leah J. Heimbach, R.N., NREMT-P, and Jere F. Baldwin, M.D., F.A.C.E.P., F.A.A.F.P.

OBJECTIVES

Upon completion of this chapter you should be able to:

1. Describe the changes that occur with aging, and explain how these changes can affect your assessment of the geriatric trauma patient.
2. Describe the assessment of the geriatric trauma patient.
3. Describe the management of the geriatric trauma patient.

By the twenty-first century, it is estimated that citizens over the age of 65 years will comprise one-fifth of the U.S. population. The geriatric population already comprises a significant number of the patients being transported by ambulance. In the United States, over 30% of all patients transported by ambulance are over the age of 65.

"Elderly" is often understood as being 65 years or older because retirement benefits are usually initiated at this point in life. However, chronological age is not the most reliable definition of "elderly." It is more appropriate to consider the biologic processes that change with time, for example, the fewer number of neurons, the decreased functioning of the kidneys, and the decreased elasticity of the skin and tissues.

As a group, geriatric patients tend to respond to injury less favorably than the younger adult population. Geriatric patients who are injured are more likely to experience fatal outcomes, even if the injury is of a relatively low severity. According to the National Safety Council, falls, thermal injury, and motor vehicular crashes have been identified as common causes of traumatic death in the geriatric population.

Falls account for the majority of injuries in the geriatric population, the most common pathology being fractures of the hip, femur, wrist, and head injuries. Motor vehicular crashes account for approximately 25% of geriatric deaths although the elderly drive fewer miles. The geriatric population have a higher incidence of collision than other age groups, second only to that group under the age of 25. Eight percent of deaths are attributable to thermal injuries. These injuries include inhalation, contact with the heat source resulting in scalding and flame burns, and electrical injury.

Little has been written regarding the response of the geriatric patient to trauma. By gaining an understanding of the normal physiologic changes involved in the aging process, you will be better prepared to provide optimum care to the geriatric trauma victim.

This chapter addresses these processes, highlights illnesses to which the geriatric patient is susceptible, and shows how these processes and illnesses make it difficult to predict the physiological response to trauma in the geriatric patient.

PATHOPHYSIOLOGY OF AGING

Aging is a gradual process whereby changes in bodily functions may occur. These changes are in part responsible for the greater risk of injury in the geriatric population.

AIRWAY: Changes in airway structures of the geriatric patient may include tooth decay, gum disease, and use of dental prosthesis. Caps, bridges, dentures, and fillings all present potential airway obstructions in the geriatric trauma patient.

RESPIRATORY SYSTEM: Changes in the respiratory system begin to appear in the early adult years, and increase markedly after the age of 60. Circulation to the pulmonary system decreases 30%, reducing the amount of carbon dioxide and oxygen exchanged at the alveolar level. There is a decrease in chest wall movement and in the flexibility of the muscles of the chest wall. These changes cause a decreased inhalation time resulting in rapid breathing. There is a decreased vital capacity (or decrease in the amount of air exchanged per breath) because of an increased residual volume (volume of air in the lungs after deep exhalation). Overall breathing capacity and maximal work rate may also decrease. If there is a history of cigarette smoking, or a history of working in an area with pollutants, these changes in breathing are even more significant.

CARDIOVASCULAR SYSTEM: Circulation is reduced due to changes in the heart and the blood vessels. Cardiac output and stroke volume may decrease, and the conduction system may degenerate. The ability of the valves of the heart to operate efficiently may decline. These changes may predispose the patient to congestive heart failure and pulmonary edema. Arteriosclerosis occurs with increasing frequency in the course of the aging process resulting in an increased peripheral vascular resistance (and perhaps systolic hypertension). There may be a normally higher blood pressure in the elderly. Thus a significant change may have occurred in a patient when the normal blood pressure of 160 drops to 120 as a result of trauma. There may be a decreased blood flow to the periphery, making the capillary refill an inaccurate indicator of shock.

NEUROLOGICAL AND SENSORY FUNCTION: Several changes occur in the brain with age. The brain shrinks, and the outermost meningeal layer, the dura mater, remains tightly adherent to the skull. This creates a space or an increased distance between the brain and skull. Instead of protecting the brain during impact, the space allows an increased incidence of subdural hematoma following trauma. There is also a hardening, narrowing, and loss of elasticity of some arteries in the brain. A deceleration injury may cause blood vessel rupture and potential bleeding inside the skull. There is decreased blood flow to the brain. The patient may experience a slowing of sensory responses such as pain perception, a decrease in hearing, in eyesight or in other sensory perception. Many older patients may have a higher pain tolerance from living with conditions such as arthritis, or from being on analgesic medications chronically. This can result in their failure to identify areas where they have been injured. Other signs of decreased cerebral circulation due to the aging process may include confusion, irritability, forgetfulness, altered sleep patterns, and mental dysfunctions such as loss of memory and regressive behavior. There may be a decrease in the ability, or even an absence in the ability, to compensate for shock.

THERMOREGULATION: Mechanisms to maintain normal body temperature may not function properly. The geriatric patient may not be able to respond to an infection with a fever, or the patient may not be able to maintain a normal temperature in the face of injury. The geriatric patient with a broken hip who has been lying on the floor in a room where the temperature is 64 degrees Fahrenheit can experience hypothermia.

RENAL SYSTEM: A decrease in the number of functioning nephrons in the kidneys of the geriatric patient can result in a decrease in the filtration and a reduced ability to excrete urine and drugs.

MUSCULOSKELETAL SYSTEM: The geriatric patient may exhibit signs of changes in posture. There may be a decrease in total height due to the narrowing of the vertebral discs. There may be slight flexion of the knees and hips. There may be decreased muscle strength. This may result in a kyphotic deformity of the spine, resulting in the "S" curvature of the spine often seen in the stooped elderly. The geriatric patient may also have advanced osteoporosis—which is a thinning of the bone with resulting decrease in the density of bone. This renders the bone more susceptible to fractures. Finally, there may be a weakening of the strength of the muscle and bone from the decrease in physical activity; this will also render the geriatric patient more susceptible to fractures with only a slight fall.

GASTROINTESTINAL SYSTEM: Saliva production, esophageal motility, and gastric secretion may decrease. This may result in the decreased ability to absorb nutrients. The liver may be enlarged because of disease processes or may be failing due to disease or malnutrition. This may result in a decreased ability to metabolize medications.

IMMUNE SYSTEM: As the aging process continues, the geriatric patient may have a decreased ability to fight off infection. The patient who has a poor nutritional state will thus be more susceptible to infection from open wounds, I.V. access sites, as well as lung and kidney infections. The geriatric trauma patient who is not severely injured otherwise may die from sepsis from an impaired immune system.

OTHER CHANGES: The total body water and total number of body cells may be decreased and there is an increase in the proportion of the body weight as fat. There may be a loss in the capacity of the systems to adjust to illness or injury.

MEDICATIONS: Many geriatric patients take several medications that can interfere with their ability to compensate after sustaining trauma. Anticoagulants may increase bleeding time. Antihypertensives and peripheral vasodilators can interfere with the body's ability to vasoconstrict blood vessels in response to hypovolemia. Beta-blockers can inhibit the heart's ability to increase the rate of contraction even in hypovolemia shock.

A number of the aging processes contribute to the increased risk of injury to the geriatric patient. The changes that may increase susceptibility to injury include:

1. Slower reflexes
2. Failing eyesight
3. Hearing loss
4. Arthritis
5. Fragile skin and blood vessels
6. Fragile bones

Causative factors related to the aging process have been linked with specific injuries such as tripping over furniture and falling down stairs. Further investigation reveals that often these falls are related as much to a decrease in the function of special senses such as loss in peripheral vision as they are to syncope, postural instability, transient impairment of cerebrovascular perfusion, alcohol ingestion, or medication usage. Alterations in perception and delayed response to stressors may also contribute to injury in the geriatric patient. When treating the geriatric trauma patient, remember that the priorities are the same as for all trauma patients. However, you must give consideration to three important areas:

1. General organ systems may not function as effectively as those in the younger adult, especially the cardiovascular, pulmonary, and renal systems.

2. The geriatric patient may also have a concomitant illness that may complicate the effectiveness of trauma care.

3. Bones may fracture more easily with less force.

ASSESSMENT AND MANAGEMENT OF THE ELDERLY TRAUMA PATIENT

Geriatric patient assessment, as with any assessment, must take into account priorities, interventions, and life-threatening conditions. However, *you must be acutely aware that geriatric patients can die from less severe injuries than younger patients.* In addition, it is often difficult to separate the effects of the aging process or of a concurrent illness from the consequences of the injury. The chief complaint may seem trivial because the patient may not report truly important symptoms. You must search for important signs or symptoms. In the geriatric patient, it is not uncommon for the patient to suffer from more than one illness or injury at the same time. Remember that the elderly patient may not have the same response to pain, hypoxia, or hypovolemia as a young person. Don't underestimate the severity of the patient's condition.

You may have difficulty communicating with the patient. This could result from the patient's diminished senses, hearing or sight impairment, or depression. The geriatric patient nonetheless should not be approached in a condescending manner. Do not allow others to take over the reporting of events from the patient who is able and willing to communicate reliable information. Unfortunately, the patient may minimize or even deny symptoms out of fear of becoming dependent, bedridden, institutionalized, or even losing a sense of self-sufficiency. It is important that you explain any actions, including removing any clothing, before initiating the physical assessment.

There are other considerations in assessing the geriatric trauma patient. Peripheral pulses may be difficult to evaluate. Older patients often wear many layers of clothing, which can impede physical assessment. You must also distinguish between signs and symptoms of a chronic disease and an acute problem; for instance,

1. The geriatric patient may have nonpathologic rales.
2. The loss of skin elasticity and the presence of mouth breathing may not necessarily represent dehydration.
3. Dependent edema may be secondary to venous insufficiency with varicose veins or inactivity rather than congestive heart failure.

Pay attention to deviation from expected ranges in vital signs and other physical assessment findings in the geriatric patient. An injury that is isolated and noncomplicated in the young adult may be debilitating in the older adult. This may be due to the patient's overall condition, lowered defenses, or ability to keep the effects of an injury localized.

When obtaining the past medical history, it is important to note what medications the patient may be taking. Medications cannot only account for an abnormal pulse, but may also mask normal circulatory responses that would indicate deterioration in the circulatory system. The result can be a rapid decompensation without warning. Knowledge of medications being taken can alert you that the patient's condition may be more unstable than that which is presented by current signs and symptoms. Antihypertensives, anticoagulants, beta-blockers, and hypoglycemic agents may profoundly influence the response of the geriatric patient to traumatic injury.

SCENE SURVEY: Survey the scene to decide if it is safe, to determine the number of patients, and to obtain the mechanism of injury. After the primary survey, it may be helpful to obtain further information and verify the patient's history from reliable family members or neighbors. This is best done in an area where the patient is unable to overhear the conversation, otherwise it may suggest that the geriatric patient is less than a competent adult. Observe the surrounding area for indications that the patient is able to provide his or her own care, for signs of alcohol abuse or polydrug ingestion, as well as for signs of violence, abuse or neglect. Abuse and/or neglect of the elderly is common. When your assessment of the patient and surroundings is suspicious for abuse or neglect, do not fail to notify the proper authorities. *Be sure to gather the patient's medications and bring them to the hospital.*

EVALUATE AIRWAY, C-SPINE CONTROL, AND INITIAL LOC: As with any trauma patient, you must evaluate and provide an adequate airway and maintain C-spine control while assessing the initial level of consciousness. The initial level of consciousness has more significance here than with younger patients. Subsequent health care providers may attribute a decreased level of consciousness to a preexisting condition rather than to the trauma. This is more likely to occur if you have not clearly indicated that the patient was clear, lucid, and cooperative at the scene.

If patients respond appropriately to the initial verbal statements, they have an open airway and are conscious. If they do not respond, gently open the airway with a modified jaw thrust while maintaining the neck in a neutral position. This position may be difficult to determine with certainty because of arthritis and kyphosis of the spine. It is important to recognize this and not to forcibly place the occiput flat on the backboard or ground.

The airway is likely to be partially obstructed. Clear the airway, being alert to possible teeth fragments due to decay and gum disease and dental devices such as caps, bridges, dentures, and fillings. Look, listen, and feel for movement of air. Ensure that the rate and volume of air exchange is adequate. The geriatric patient with unresolved airway difficulty or a decreased level of consciousness should be transported immediately. If the level of consciousness is decreased, the patient should be hyperventilated at 24 breaths per minute with 100% supplemental oxygen. In such a case, frequently monitor the respiratory effort and level of consciousness.

BREATHING AND CIRCULATION: Place your face over the patient's mouth to look at the chest rise, to listen to the quality of the breath sounds from the mouth, and to feel the patient's breath against your ear. If the breathing is so fast that there is inadequate air exchange (greater than 24 breaths per minute), or if it is too slow (less than 12 breaths per minute), or if the volume of air being exchanged is inadequate, provide assisted ventilation with 100% supplemental oxygen. As the neck is held in a neutral position by your partner, palpate the carotid pulse with an index finger to note the rate and quality of the pulse. Compare this to the rate and quality of the pulse at the wrist. Evaluate skin color and condition. At this time you should also determine the presence or absence of jugular vein distension, the position of the trachea, and the presence or absence of subcutaneous emphysema.

Look, feel, and listen to the chest. Look for DCAPP-BLS and feel for TIC (see Chapter 2). Listen for breath sounds. Make appropriate interventions for chest injuries. Remember that chest injuries are more likely to cause serious problems in older people with poor pulmonary reserve. Be especially alert to problems in patients with chronic lung disease. They usually have borderline hypoxia even when not injured.

EXAMINE ABDOMEN, PELVIS, AND EXTREMITIES: Look for DCAP-BLS and gently palpate all four quadrants of the abdomen for tenderness. Check the pelvis and extremities for DCAP-BLS and feel for TIC. Control major bleeding.

CRITICAL TRANSPORT DECISIONS: There are a few procedures that may be initiated on scene, but do not delay transport. Examples of critical interventions that may be initiated at the scene are:

1. Airway management
2. Controlling major bleeding
3. Sealing sucking chest wounds
4. Initiation of CPR

Consider whether the time delay in initiating these procedures outweighs the risks of delaying transportation. As mentioned elsewhere, the chance of survival decreases with a corresponding increase in the length of scene time. The same indications for immediate transport apply for the elderly as for younger patients (see Chapters 2 and 19), but remember that you may not have as dramatic a response to injury in the elderly so you should have a low threshold for early transport. If one of the critical conditions is present, immediately transfer the patient to a long backboard with appropriate padding, apply oxygen, load the patient into the ambulance, and transport rapidly to the nearest appropriate emergency facility.

PACKAGING AND TRANSPORT: "Package" or prepare the elderly patient for transport as quickly and gently as possible. Take extra care when immobilizing the geriatric trauma patient. This includes padding void areas that may be exaggerated due to the aging process. The elderly patient with kyphosis will require padding under the shoulders and head to maintain the neck in its usual alignment. Do not force the neck into a neutral position if it is painful to do so, or if the neck is obviously fused in a forward position. Remember to treat and transport the geriatric trauma patient, as all trauma patients, gently and quickly.

SECONDARY AND REASSESSMENT SURVEYS: Perform a complete secondary survey on scene if the patient is stable. If there is any question as to the patient's condition you should transport and perform the secondary survey en route. Perform frequent reassessment surveys. Frequently assess the patient's pulmonary status, including lung sounds and cardiac rhythm. All elderly patients should have cardiac monitoring and also pulse oximetry if available.

SUMMARY

You will be called upon to treat and transport an increasing number of geriatric trauma patients. Although the mechanisms of injury may be different from those of the younger adults, the prioritized evaluation and treatment is the same. As a general rule elderly patients have more serious injuries and more complications than younger patients. The physiologic processes of aging and the frequent concurrent illness make evaluation and treatment more difficult. You must be aware of these differences to provide optimal care to the patient.

BIBLIOGRAPHY

1. Baker, S. P., B. O'Neil, and R. S. Karph. *The Injury Fact Book.* Lexington, MA: Lexington Books, 1985.

2. Spaite, D. W. "Geriatric Injury and Analysis of Prehospital Demographics, Mechanisms, and Patterns." *Annals of Emergency Medicine,* Vol. 19, no. 12 (December 1990), pp. 1419–1421.

3. Hogue, C. C. "Injury in Late Life: Epidemiology." *Journal of the American Geriatric Society,* Vol. 30 (1982), pp. 183–190.

4. Waller, J. A. "Injury in Aged." *New York State Journal of Medicine,* Vol. 74 (1974), pp. 2200–2208.

5. Bobb, J. K. "Trauma in the Elderly." In *Trauma Nursing from Resuscitation Through Rehabilitation,* pp. 692–706. Philadelphia: W. B. Saunders, 1988.

6. Smith, D. P., B. L. Enderson, and K. I. Maull. "Trauma in the Elderly: Determinants of Outcome." *Southern Medical Journal,* Vol. 83, no. 2 (February 1990), pp. 171–176.

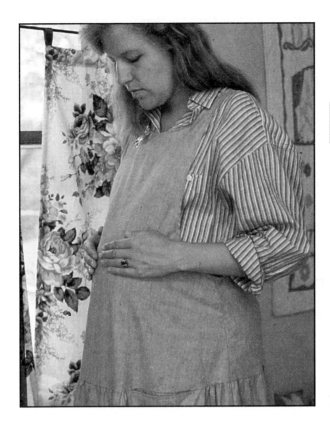

CHAPTER 17

Trauma in Pregnancy

Ron W. Lee, M.D., M.B.A., F.A.C.E.P.

OBJECTIVES

Upon completion of this chapter you should be able to:

1. State the twin goals of managing the pregnant trauma patient.

2. Describe physiological changes to the cardiopulmonary system during pregnancy, and relate them to
   a. Blood volume
   b. Cardiac output
   c. Stroke volume and heart rate
   d. Blood pressure
   e. Respiratory status

3. Describe the major physiological changes in the gastrointestinal and genitourinary systems during pregnancy.

4. Describe uterine response to maternal hypovolemia and relate its implications to assessment and management of the mother.

5. Predict potential injury to the mother and/or fetus based on the following mechanisms of injury:
   a. Motor vehicle collisions, including use of lap and shoulder restraints

Continued

> b. Penetrating abdominal injuries
>
> c. Falls, especially those resulting in pelvic fractures
>
> d. Burns
>
> 6. Compare and contrast evaluation and management of a pregnant to a nonpregnant trauma patient.
>
> 7. Identify transport considerations for a pregnant trauma patient.

The pregnant trauma patient represents a unique challenge for the prehospital provider. It is important to remember that the pregnant patient represents two patients with separate requirements, those of the mother and those of the fetus. Therefore, any intervention must have the twin goals of supporting the mother and identifying the needs of the fetus. The pregnant patient is also often at risk for a higher incidence of accidental trauma. The increase in fainting spells, hyperventilation, and excess fatigue that are common in early pregnancy, as well as the changes in the physiological parameters of the pregnant patient, such as the loosening of the pelvic joints, all add to the risk of minor accidental trauma. It is estimated that accidental injury may complicate 6 to 7% of all pregnancies. The pregnant patient with minor injuries rarely represents a problem for the prehospital provider, and therefore our discussion will be centered on moderate to severe traumatic injuries.

PHYSIOLOGICAL CHANGES DURING PREGNANCY

To understand the unique aspects associated with trauma in pregnancy, it is important to recall certain physiological processes that are peculiar to pregnancy. During the first three months of pregnancy, the fetus is being formed. The fetus is very tiny, so there is little growth of the uterus during this period. After the third month of gestation the fetus and uterus grow rapidly, reaching the umbilicus by the fifth month and the epigastrium by the seventh month (see Figure 17-1). The cardiopulmonary changes that occur during pregnancy are significant (see Figure 17-2). The cardiac output will increase by 20 to 30% during the first 10 weeks of gestation. This increase in cardiac output peaks at term and approximates 6 to 7 L/min. The average maternal heart beat will increase by 10 to 15 beats per minute, while the systolic and diastolic blood pressure will often lessen by 10 to 15 mm Hg when compared to the nonpregnant patient.

The respiratory status of the patient undergoes significant changes because of the enlarging uterus that will elevate the diaphragm and decrease the overall volume of the thoracic cavity. There tends to be some flaring out of the rib margins to compensate for this decrease in capacity. There is also an increase in the amount of gas exchange occurring over each minute. This leads to a relative alkalosis and predisposes the patient to the hyperventilation syndrome. The pregnant

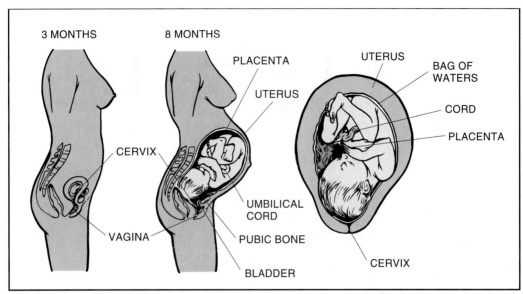

Figure 17-1 *Anatomy of pregnancy: Uterus at 3 months and at 8 months gestation.*

patient also undergoes a change that is described as the "hypervolemia" of pregnancy. This represents an increase of both red blood cells and plasma, yielding an increase in the total blood volume of approximately 45 to 50%. However, since there is a greater increase in plasma over blood cells, the patient tends to manifest a relative anemia.

This enlargement in plasma volume is particularly important since the patient may lose 30 to 35% of the circulating blood volume before developing hypotension. This also means that if the injured pregnant patient has significant hypotension, she has already had a major loss of blood volume and will require large amounts of fluids (preferably blood).

The major physiological changes in the gastrointestinal system are secondary to the enlarging uterus, and lead to:

1. A compartmentalization of the organs within the abdomen. This compartmentalization now displaces most of the small bowels upward, while the uterus becomes the largest organ within the abdominal cavity. This is a major consideration when trying to identify organ systems that are injured from either penetrating or blunt trauma.

2. A general decrease in gastrointestinal motility, with a resulting delay in gastric emptying. This often places the injured pregnant patient in great risk for vomiting and aspiration.

The changes in the urinary system are many; however, the most significant is the displacement of the bladder anteriorly and superiorly, placing it in a position where penetrating or blunt trauma is more likely to do greater harm.

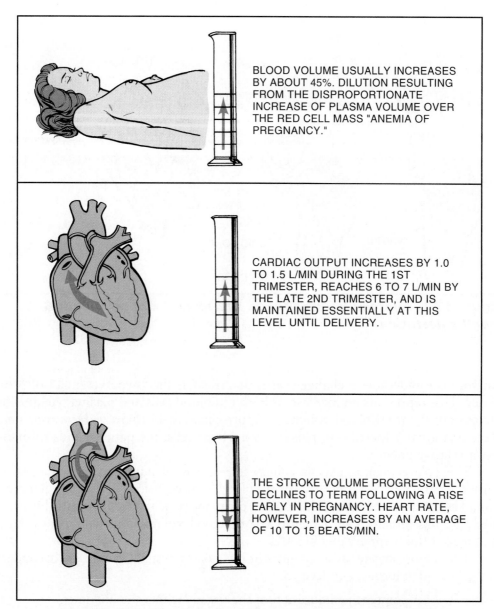

Figure 17-2 *Physiological changes during pregnancy.*

The multiple changes in the reproductive system are significant in that the uterine blood flow, which is normally approximately 2% of the cardiac output, now increases to approximately 20%. It is important to realize that the vessels supplying the uterus are low-resistance vessels that vasoconstrict vigorously in response to the catecholamines produced in early shock. Therefore, under periods of stress there may be significant vasoconstriction with a reduction of blood flow to the uterus. Unfortunately, the uterus is not responsive to vasodilitation and cannot increase blood flow to the uterus in times of placental hypoperfusion. This means that very early in the shock syndrome, the pregnant patient will divert blood away

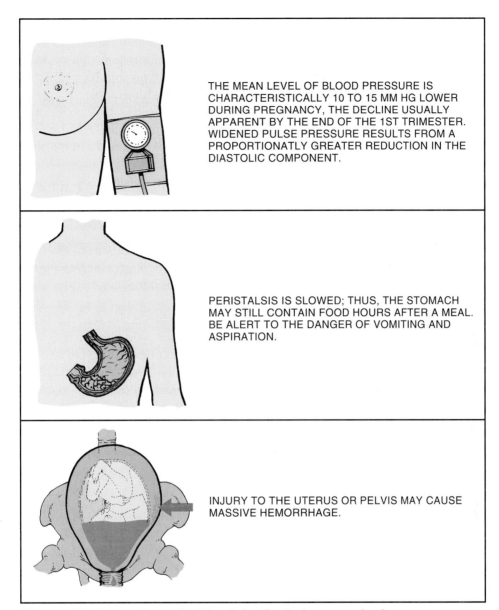

THE MEAN LEVEL OF BLOOD PRESSURE IS CHARACTERISTICALLY 10 TO 15 MM HG LOWER DURING PREGNANCY, THE DECLINE USUALLY APPARENT BY THE END OF THE 1ST TRIMESTER. WIDENED PULSE PRESSURE RESULTS FROM A PROPORTIONATLY GREATER REDUCTION IN THE DIASTOLIC COMPONENT.

PERISTALSIS IS SLOWED; THUS, THE STOMACH MAY STILL CONTAIN FOOD HOURS AFTER A MEAL. BE ALERT TO THE DANGER OF VOMITING AND ASPIRATION.

INJURY TO THE UTERUS OR PELVIS MAY CAUSE MASSIVE HEMORRHAGE.

Figure 17-2 (continued) *Physiological changes during pregnancy.*

from the fetus to save the mother. Thus death of the fetus is more common if the mother has a period of hypotension.

RESPONSES TO HYPOVOLEMIA

Acute blood loss results in a decrease in circulating blood volume. The cardiac output decreases as the venous return falls. This hypovolemia causes the arterial blood pressure to fall, resulting in an inhibition of vagal tone and also the release of catecholamines. The effect of this response is to produce vasoconstriction and tachycardia. This vasoconstriction profoundly affects the pregnant uterus. Uterine vasoconstriction leads to a reduction in uterine blood flow by 20 to 30%. This reduction in uterine blood flow may occur prior to any detectable change in the blood pressure of the maternal system. The fetus reacts to this hypoperfusion by a drop in arterial blood pressure and a decrease in heart rate. The fetus now begins to suffer from a reduction in oxygen concentration in the maternal circulation. It is important to remember that some methods for oxygenation of the maternal patient in hemorrhagic shock may not always provide adequate oxygenation of the fetus. Therefore, it is important to give large amounts of supplemental oxygen to provide sufficient oxygen to the fetus, who suffers from both oxygen starvation and inadequate blood supply.

Another cause of hypotension in the pregnant patient results from the decrease in venous return when the patient is in the supine position. The enlarging uterus can cause significant compression of the vena cava, which reduces venous return to the heart (see Figure 17-3). This effect is particularly evident after the twentieth week of gestation. The reduced venous return has been shown to lead to maternal hypotension, syncope, and fetal bradycardia. Therefore, you should transport all pregnant patients in the left lateral decubitus or decubent position. Do this only if it can be done without risk to the patient. If the type of patient trauma prevents this type of maneuver, you can prevent or alleviate the vena cava obstruction by one of the following methods.

1. Tilt or rotate the backboard 20 to 30 degrees to the left.
2. Manually displace the uterus to the left side during transport.

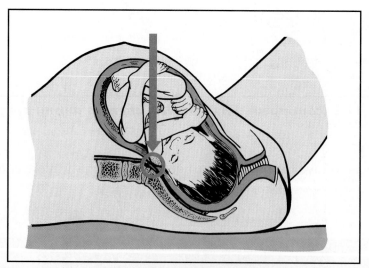

Figure 17-3 *Venous return to the maternal heart may be decreased up to 30% because of uterine compression by the fetus. Transport the patient on her left side or tilt the backboard to the left.*

TYPES OF INJURIES

VEHICULAR COLLISIONS

A pregnant patient is subject to all types of accidental injuries, including vehicular collisions, gunshot wounds, falls, and electrical and thermal injuries.

The most common cause of maternal injury is the blunt injury resulting from vehicular collisions. A review of this type of injury indicates that where there is only minor damage to the vehicle, fewer than 1% of pregnant patients will sustain injury. As with nonpregnant patients, the probability of a major life-threatening injury is directly related to the damage inflicted on the vehicle. To best predict the severity of injury, you need to determine the answers to following questions:

1. How fast was the vehicle traveling at impact?
2. What was the position of the patient in the vehicle at the time of impact?
3. Were any restraints utilized?
4. Which body parts sustained the impact?
5. On what side of the vehicle did the impact occur in relation to the patient?

Head injury is the most common cause of death in pregnant patients in vehicular collisions. The other most common cause of death is internal injuries

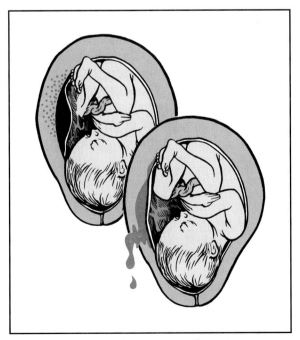

Figure 17-4 *Blunt trauma to the uterus. Blunt trauma may cause separation of the placenta or rupture of the uterus. Massive bleeding may occur, but there may not be visible vaginal bleeding early.*

with uncontrolled hemorrhage. The old concern that an injury to the fetus is likely to occur with the seat belt connected was based on early data, which revealed that with the use of the *lap belt alone,* there was an increased incidence of injury to the uterus and fetus. However, the overall vehicular mortality for pregnant patients was less with the use of only the lap belt. The use of a *lap belt with shoulder restraint* decreases patient mortality and *has not shown any increase in uterine injuries.*

The most common cause of fetal death is maternal death. Fetal death with maternal survival occurs most often in abdominal trauma with placental separation or ruptured uterus (see Figure 17-4). In this case, the patient presents with vaginal bleeding, abdominal pain, and irritable uterus, and often some degree of hypotension.

Pregnant victims of vehicular collisions have associated injuries, such as pelvic injuries, that often result in placental separation and concealed hemorrhage within the retroperitoneal area. The retroperitoneal area, because of its low-pressure venous system, can accomodate a loss of 4 or more liters of blood into that area with few clinical signs. Fetal skull fractures are much more common when maternal pelvic fractures occur.

PENETRATING INJURIES OF THE ABDOMEN

The most common type of penetrating injury to the pregnant patient is the gunshot wound. The probability of any abdominal organ being struck by a bullet is directly related to the size of the organ and the space it occupies within the peritoneal cavity. Therefore, in early pregnancy the likelihood of uterine injury or fetal injury is low. However, as the pregnancy progresses toward term, the chance for injury increases proportionately. The most common organs injured from gunshot wounds to the nonpregnant patient are the small bowel, liver, colon, and stomach, in decreasing order. The mortality and complication rates are related to the number of organs injured. About 19% of women who sustain gunshot wounds to the uterus will also have injuries to other organs. Fetal injuries from gunshot wounds to the uterus vary from 60 to 90%, with mortality of 40 to 70%. Fetal death is secondary to direct injury to the fetus or injuries to the membranes, cord, or placenta.

The second most common cause of penetrating abdominal wounds is the stab wound. Stab wounds to the abdomen have an associated mortality of approximately 1.4% in the nonpregnant individual. The enlarged uterus protects the pregnant patient from serious organ injury when lower abdominal stab injuries occur. However, due to the compartmentalization, stab wounds to the upper abdomen often carry a higher incidence of visceral injury, especially to the small bowel. Fetal mortality in these injuries is related directly to maternal mortality, and when isolated fetal death occurs, it is usually secondary to either direct fetal injury or to prematurity.

FALLS

The incidence of significant injury to the pregnant patient resulting from a fall is proportional to the force of impact and the specific body part that sustains the impact. Injuries associated with pelvic fractures manifest an increase in placental separation and fetal fractures of the skull and long bones. The incidence of falls increases with the progression of the pregnancy. This is secondary to the loosening of ligaments from the hormone relaxin and the added weight gain that alters the patient's center of gravity. These falls may appear minor; however, many cases of minor trauma have resulted in fetomaternal hemorrhage or placental separation. These patients benefit from evaluation and monitoring in an emergency department.

BURNS

The overall mortality and morbidity resulting from thermal injuries to the pregnant patient is not markedly different from the nonpregnant individual. However, it is important to remember that the fluid requirement for the pregnant patient is greater than that in the nonpregnant individual. Fetal mortality increases when the maternal surface burn exceeds 20%.

EVALUATION

The evaluation of the injured pregnant female does not differ from that of the non-pregnant patient. The priorities remain the same.

1. Secure the *airway* and stabilize the cervical spine.
2. Assess *breathing*.
3. Assess *circulation*.
4. Stop the bleeding.
5. Determine transport decision and critical interventions.
6. Transport.
7. Secondary survey (may be done before transport if patient is stable).
8. Critical care and reassessment survey.

THINGS TO REMEMBER: The pregnant patient has a resting pulse that is 10 to 15 beats faster than usual and the blood pressure is 10 to 15 mm Hg lower than usual. Therefore, it is important not to mistake normal vital signs in pregnant individuals as signs of shock. However, it is also important to realize that a blood loss of 30 to 35% can occur in these patients before there is a significant change in blood pressure. Therefore, these patients must be managed expectantly. It is important to realize that trauma to the abdominal compartment can cause occult bleeding in either the intrauterine or retroperitoneal area. Keep in mind that gradual stretching of the abdominal wall during pregnancy, along with hormonal changes within the body, make the peritoneal surface less sensitive to irritable stimuli. Therefore, bleeding can occur intraperitoneally, and the signs of rebound, guarding, and rigidity may not be present.

MANAGEMENT OF THE PREGNANT PATIENT

The management of most injuries to the pregnant patient are the same as discussed in other chapters. However, severe hemorrhagic shock can occur from injuries to the uterus because this very vascular organ can bleed profusely. If your system uses the antishock garment, you may inflate the leg compartments if the patient is in severe shock (BP < 50 mm Hg). Your Medical Director will have to guide you on this.

OXYGEN ADMINISTRATION AND PATIENT TRANSPORT

Oxygen requirements for women in late pregnancy have been reported to be 10 to 20% greater than normal. Maternal shock of *any degree* will cause vasoconstriction of the uterus, with a marked decrease in oxygenation of the fetus. *Any injured pregnant patient should receive high-flow oxygen immediately.*

The transport of any pregnant patient whose pregnancy is greater than 20 weeks should occur with the patient on her back, with the uterus displaced to the left to prevent inferior vena cava obstruction. If there is no danger of spinal injury, you can transport the patient on her left side. If there is a possibility of spinal injury, secure the patient appropriately to the long spineboard, but prop up the board slightly on the right side so that the uterus is tilting to the left (see Figure 17-5). An alternate method is to manually hold the uterus to the left side.

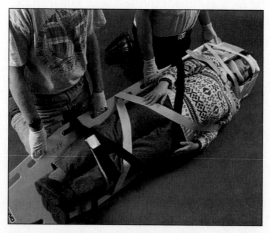

Figure 17-5 *Pregnant patient packaged and turned on her left side.*

SUMMARY

The pregnant patient presents a challenge because of the physiological changes that cause confusing vital signs and the unique uterine response to shock. Anatomical changes also make the patient difficult to extricate and transport. The important points in management of the pregnant patient are summarized as follows:

IMPORTANT POINTS TO REMEMBER

1. It is imperative to recall that you are treating two patients; however, the mortality of the fetus is related to the treatment provided to the mother. The goal of prehospital intervention is to maximize the chances of maternal survival, which will provide the fetus with the best chance for survival.

2. Treat shock expectantly; do not wait for definitive signs or symptoms of classic shock. Rapid transport for surgical treatment to stop the bleeding is the most important treatment.

3. Hypoxemia of the fetus may go unnoticed in the injured pregnant patient. Treatment should include high-flow oxygen.

4. Transport must include appropriate spinal immobilization, extremity splints, and prevention of vena cava compression.

5. Reassessment and constant monitoring are important during transport.

6. If the mother dies, continue CPR and notify the hospital to be prepared for immediate caesarean section.

BIBLIOGRAPHY

1. American College of Surgeons Committee on Trauma. "Trauma in Pregnancy." In *Advanced Trauma Life Support*. Chicago: The College, 1989.

2. Buchsbaum, H. J. *Trauma in Pregnancy*. Philadelphia: W. B. Saunders, 1979.

3. Maull, K. I., G. S. Rozycki, R. E. Pedigo, and others. "Female Reproductive System Trauma." In *Trauma*, eds. E. E. Moore, D. V. Feliciano, and K. L. Mattox, pp 553–560. Norwalk, CT: Appleton-Lange, 1987.

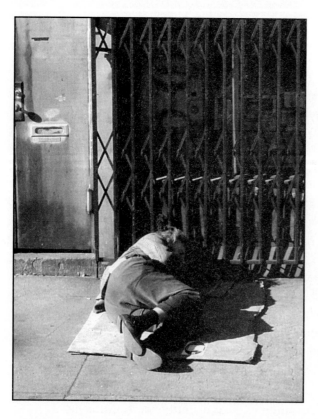

18

Patients under the Influence of Alcohol or Drugs

Jonathan G. Newman, M.D., REMT-P

OBJECTIVES

Upon completion of this chapter you should be able to:

1. List signs and symptoms of patients under the influence of alcohol and/or drugs.

2. Describe the five strategies you would use to best ensure cooperation during assessment and management of a patient under the influence of alcohol and/or drugs.

3. Describe situations in which you would restrain patients and tell how to handle an uncooperative patient.

4. List the special considerations for assessment and management of patients in whom substance abuse is suspected.

The relationship between alcohol and trauma is well documented. For instance, it is reported that car crashes involving alcohol result in injuries to about 500,000 people a year. The involvement of drugs in trauma has not been as well examined. However, substance abuse, which includes individuals who have abused alcohol, drugs, or both, has been associated with a number of traumatic events. The trauma caused by substance abuse often results from accidents, car crashes, suicides, homicides, and other violent crimes. Therefore, it would not be surprising to find that a number of your trauma patients are under the influence of alcohol or some other substance. This group of trauma patients often presents with unique challenges that can require some special patient management techniques along with good BTLS care.

A high index of suspicion, combined with the results of your physical exam, the history obtained from the patient or bystanders, and evidence at the scene, can clue you into whether your patient is under the influence of alcohol or drugs.

Table 18-1 includes some commonly abused drugs along with signs and symptoms of their use.

DRUG CATEGORY	COMMON NAMES	SIGNS AND SYMPTOMS OF USE OR ABUSE
ALCOHOL	BEER, WHISKEY, WINE	ALTERED MENTAL FUNCTION, CONFUSION, POLYURIA, SLURRED SPEECH, COMA
AMPHETAMINES	BENNIES, ICE, SPEED, UPPERS, DEXIES	EXCITEMENT, HYPERACTIVITY, DILATED PUPILS, HYPERTENSION, TACHYCARDIA, TREMORS, SEIZURES, FEVER, PARANOIA, PSYCHOSIS
COCAINE	COKE, CRACK, BLOW, ROCK	SAME AS AMPHETAMINES PLUS CHEST PAIN; LETHAL DYSRHYTHMIA
HALLUCINOGENS	ACID, LSD, PCP	HALLUCINATIONS, DIZZINESS, DILATED PUPILS, NAUSEA, RAMBLING SPEECH PSYCHOSIS
MARIJUANA	GRASS, HASH, POT TEA, WEED	EUPHORIA, SLEEPINESS, DILATED PUPILS, DRY MOUTH
OPIATES	HEROIN, HORSE, BIG H, DARVON, CODEINE, STUFF MORPHINE, SMACK	ALTERED MENTAL STATUS, CONSTRICTED PUPILS, BRADYCARDIA, HYPOTENSION, RESPIRATORY DEPRESSION, HYPOTHERMIA
SEDATIVES	LIBRIUM, VALIUM, XANAX, THORAZINE, BARBITURATES	ALTERED MENTAL STATUS, DILATED PUPILS, BRADYCARDIA, HYPOTENSION, RESPIRATORY DEPRESSION, HYPOTHERMIA

Table 18-1 *Commonly Abused Drugs with Their Associated Signs and Symptoms.*

ASSESSMENT AND MANAGEMENT

While your primary and secondary surveys should follow the BTLS guidelines that have been described in this book (see Chapter 2), there are some particular aspects to be aware of when conducting your exam.

When you suspect the patient has abused substances, pay particular attention to mental status, pupils, speech, and respirations, and note any needle marks you may discover. An altered mental status can be seen in every form of substance abuse. However, remember that an altered level of consciousness is due to a head injury or shock until proven otherwise. Pupils are often constricted in patients who have abused opiates. Dilated pupils are common in patients exposed to amphetamines, cocaine, hallucinogens, and marijuana. Patients who use barbiturates will have pupils that are constricted early on; however, if high doses have been consumed, the pupils can eventually become fixed and dilated. Speech can be slurred when patients use alcohol or sedatives, and patients who are under the influence of hallucinogens may seem to ramble when they talk. Respiration can be significantly depressed with opiates and sedatives.

The history supplied by the patient or bystanders can also help to establish whether substance abuse is involved. Try to find out what was used, when it was taken, and how much was taken. However, be aware that patients often deny that they have used or abused any substance. If possible, inspect the patient's surroundings for clues that drugs or alcohol may have been used. Note any alcohol beverage bottles, pill containers, injection equipment, smoking paraphernalia, or unusual odors.

Trauma patients under the influence of alcohol or drugs can challenge the provider not only by their traumatic injuries but by their attitudes as well. *The way in which you interact with patients who have abused substances can determine if the patient will be cooperative or uncooperative.* How you speak to these patients can be as important as what you are doing for them. Your interaction style, if offensive, can make patients uncooperative and lose them precious minutes of the golden hour. If your interactive style is positive and nonjudgmental, the patient is more likely to be cooperative and allow all the appropriate medical interventions, thus decreasing on-scene time. As noted before, all the substances that are abused can cause an altered mental state. When interacting with patients you must be prepared to deal with euphoria, psychosis, paranoia, or confusion and disorientation. Some strategies to help you gain your patient's cooperation follow.

1. Identify yourself to patients and orient them to their surroundings. Tell them your name and your title, for example, "EMT, Pam Osbush." Ask them their name and how they would like to be addressed. Avoid using generic names like "Bub" or "Honey." With this patient population it may be necessary to orient them to place, date, and what is going on. These patients may need to be reoriented frequently.

2. Treat the patient in a respectful manner and avoid being judgmental. Often a lack of respect can be heard in the tone of your voice or how you say things, not just in what you

say. Never forget that you are there to save lives; this includes *all patients*. You are not a police officer (don't gather or destroy evidence), and you are not there to pass judgment on the patient's worth to society.

3. Acknowledge the patient's concerns and feelings. The patient who is scared or confused may be more comfortable with what is taking place if you recognize and address these feelings. Be gentle but firm. Explain all treatment interventions before they are performed. Be honest. Backboards and extrication collars are uncomfortable.

4. Let your patients know what will be required of them. For instance, they may be confused and not realize that they need to hold still while you are trying to immobilize them.

5. Ask closed-ended questions when getting your history from the patient. These are questions that can be answered with a yes or no. These patients may only be able to concentrate for short periods of time, and they may ramble when asked open-ended questions that require a full answer. Consider getting as much of the history as you can from relatives, friends, or bystanders. This may help improve the reliability of what you discover. Get as much relevant history as you can, *but do not delay transport*.

THE UNCOOPERATIVE PATIENT

A small percentage of your patients may be uncooperative. You must be firm with these patients. Set limits to their behavior, and let them know when their behavior is inappropriate. Consider physical restraint only if you are not able to secure enough cooperation to provide adequate care for your patient. Often a show of force may be enough to convince an uncooperative patient to allow medical care to be provided. First check with your local jurisdiction to determine what protocol you must use when restraining patients against their will. Most municipalities allow police officers to place people in custody if they are a threat to themselves or others. Severely injured trauma patients who refuse or will not cooperate with care can be considered a threat to themselves. Once the decision has been made to restrain the patient, it must be carried out with care. Securely immobilizing a patient with cervical collar, cervical immobilization device, backboard, and straps will serve to restrain most patients. Caution must be taken not to worsen any current injuries or inflict any new ones. There is often no good solution to this predicament. Restrained patients may struggle so hard that spinal immobilization is rendered ineffective. The Reeves sleeve is one of the few pieces of equipment that is very effective in providing both restraint and immobilization (see Figure 18-1). The predispatch stage is the time when crews should plan and practice procedures for restraining patients. The trauma scene is not the place to learn new skills.

The standard BTLS approach to patient care will work well, even with patients under the influence of alcohol or drugs. Assure that the scene is safe, determine the

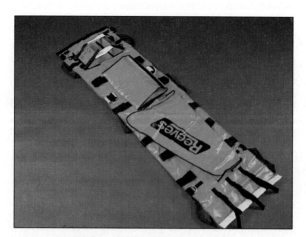

Figure 18-1 *Reeves sleeve*

number of injured, and discover the mechanism of injury. Use universal precautions. This patient population includes people who are at high risk for infection with hepatitis B, hepatitis C, and HIV. Follow the primary and secondary survey as recorded in Chapter 2. Remember to note any mental status changes that might be associated with substance abuse. When performing your secondary survey be sure to include the specific areas that can provide clues to substance abuse. As with all trauma patients, treatment includes the consideration of oxygen, an intravenous line, and cardiac monitoring. Table 18-2 lists some drug categories and associated specific treatments or areas to pay close attention to when substance abuse is suspected.

DRUG CATEGORY	SPECIFIC TREATMENTS AND AREAS TO ASSESS
ALCOHOL	WATCH FOR HYPOTHERMIA
AMPHETAMINES	MONITOR FOR SEIZURES AND DYSRHYTHMIAS
COCAINE	MONITOR FOR SEIZURES AND DYSRHYTHMIAS
HALLUCINOGENS	PROVIDE REASSURANCE
MARIJUANA	PROVIDE REASSURANCE
OPIATES	WATCH FOR HYPOTHERMIA, HYPOTENSION, AND RESPIRATORY DEPRESSION
SEDATIVES	WATCH FOR HYPOTHERMIA, HYPOTENSION, AND RESPIRATORY DEPRESSION

Table 18-2 *Drug Categories and Specific Treatments to Consider or Areas to Assess Closely*

SUMMARY

Knowing the signs and symptoms of alcohol and drug abuse will allow you to recognize the patient who may be impaired from their use. Assessing the patient for signs and symptoms outlined in this section can help you confirm your suspicions. Determining that your patient has abused some substance will allow you to pay attention to specific areas for critical changes as well as provide life-threatening interventions that may be indicated for individual substances. The five interaction strategies for improving patient cooperation are very important when dealing with the patient under the influence of alcohol or drugs, but these strategies should also be used with all patients. Remember that the patient's safety is a primary concern. If you must restrain a patient for his or her safety, do so in a preplanned manner that is most sensitive to your patient's needs.

BIBLIOGRAPHY

1. Hafen, B., and K. Frandsen. *Psychological Emergencies & Crisis Interventions: A Comprehensive Guide for Emergency Personnel,* pp. 256–280. Englewood, CO: Morton, 1985.

2. Bledsoe, B., R. Porter, and B. Shade. *Paramedic Emergency Care,* pp. 795–800. Englewood Cliffs, NJ: Prentice Hall, 1991.

3. Caroline, N. *Emergency Care in the Streets,* 4th ed., pp. 628–637. Boston: Little, Brown, 1991.

4. Bassuk, E., S. Fox, and K. Pendergast. *Behavioral Emergencies: A Field Guide for Paramedics,* p. 82. Boston: Little, Brown, 1983.

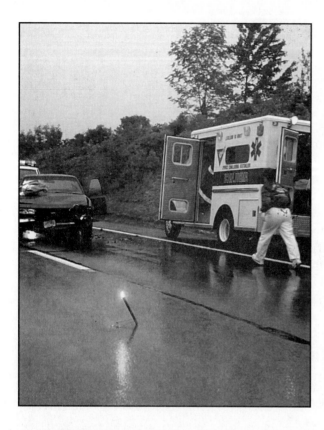

Critical Trauma Situations: "Load and Go"

John E. Campbell, M.D., F.A.C.E.P.

OBJECTIVE

Upon completion of this chapter, you should be able to identify the critical situations in which you should transport the patient immediately.

There are certain situations that require hospital treatment within minutes if the patient is to have any chance for survival. When you recognize these situations, immediately load the patient onto a spineboard, transfer to the ambulance, and transport rapidly with lights and siren. Life-saving procedures may be needed but should be done during transport. Nonlife-saving procedures (such as splinting and bandaging) must not hold up transport. The following are critical situations that require "load and go."

1. Airway obstruction that cannot be quickly relieved by mechanical methods such as suction or digital removal.

2. Traumatic cardiopulmonary arrest

3. Conditions resulting in possible inadequate breathing

   a. Large open chest wound (sucking chest wound)

   b. Large flail chest

   c. Tension pneumothorax

   d. Major blunt chest injury

4. Shock
5. Head injury with unconsciousness, unequal pupils, or decreasing level of consciousness
6. Tender abdomen
7. Unstable pelvis
8. Bilateral femur fractures

PRIMARY SURVEY

The following are assessment findings that should alert you to possible critical trauma situations:

1. Assess the airway, control the C-spine, and note initial level of consciousness.

CRITICAL FINDINGS	POSSIBLE CAUSES
A. NO MOVEMENT OF AIR	AIRWAY OBSTRUCTION OR CARDIAC ARREST
B. POOR MOVEMENT OF AIR	PARTIAL AIRWAY OBSTRUCTION OR CHEST INJURY
C. UNRESPONSIVE OR RESPONSIVE	HYPOXIA, HYPOGLYCEMIA, LATE SHOCK, POORLY HEAD INJURY, CARDIAC ARREST, OR DRUG OVERDOSE

2. Assess breathing and circulation.

CRITICAL FINDINGS	POSSIBLE CAUSES
A. NO RESPIRATION	CARDIAC OR RESPIRATORY ARREST
B. DIFFICULTY WITH RATE OR DEPTH OF RESPIRATION	SLOW OR IRREGULAR—HEAD INJURY, FAST AND SHALLOW—SHOCK OR CHEST INJURY
C. NO PULSE	CARDIAC ARREST OR LATE SHOCK
D. PULSE AT NECK BUT NOT AT THE WRIST	LATE SHOCK
E. RAPID, WEAK PULSE >100 PER MINUTE	SHOCK

3. Examine the neck.

CRITICAL FINDINGS	POSSIBLE CAUSES
A. DISCOLORATION AND SWELLING	DEVELOPING AIRWAY OBSTRUCTION
B. DISTENDED NECK VEINS AND/OR DEVIATED TRACHEA, RESPIRATORY DIFFICULTY AND SHOCK	TENSION PNEUMOTHORAX
C. DISTENDED NECK VEINS AND SHOCK	PERICARDIAL TAMPONADE

4. Examine the chest.

CRITICAL FINDINGS	POSSIBLE CAUSES
A. SUCKING CHEST WOUND	OPEN PNEUMOTHORAX
B. DECREASED BREATH SOUNDS AND HYPERRESONANCE ON ONE SIDE, RESPIRATORY DIFFICULTY, SHOCK, DISTENDED NECK VEINS, TRACHEA DEVIATED AWAY FROM THE SIDE OF DECREASED BREATH SOUNDS	TENSION PNEUMOTHORAX
C. UNSTABLE SEGMENT OF CHEST WALL OR STERNUM, DIFFICULTY BREATHING	FLAIL CHEST
D. DIFFICULTY BREATHING, BREATH SOUNDS DECREASED ON ONE SIDE, CREPITATION	MAJOR BLUNT CHEST INJURY
E. CONTUSION OR PUNCTURE WOUND OF ANTERIOR CHEST, SHOCK, DISTENDED NECK VEINS	CARDIAC TAMPONADE, MYOCARDIAL INJURY
F. PENETRATING CHEST WOUND, SHOCK	HEMOTHORAX, MYOCARDIAL INJURY MAJOR THORACIC VASCULAR INJURY

5. Examine the abdomen.

CRITICAL FINDINGS	POSSIBLE CAUSES
TENDERNESS	INTRA-ABDOMINAL INJURY

6. Examine the pelvis.

CRITICAL FINDINGS	POSSIBLE CAUSES
UNSTABLE PELVIS	PELVIC FRACTURES

7. Examine the legs.

CRITICAL FINDINGS	POSSIBLE CAUSES
SWELLING, TENDERNESS, AND DEFORMITY OF BOTH UPPER LEGS	FEMUR FRACTURES

8. Control active bleeding.

CRITICAL FINDINGS	POSSIBLE CAUSES
MAJOR BLOOD LOSS OR POORLY CONTROLLED BLEEDING	MAJOR VASCULAR INJURY

At this point you should be able to make a decision about critical trauma situations and who should be in the "load-and-go" category. These diagnosis-based criteria can be further simplified to symptom-based criteria. Any patient with the following *signs and symptoms* falls into the "load-and-go" category:

1. Decreased level of consciousness
2. Respiratory difficulty
3. Signs of shock

Also place in the "load-and-go" category any patient who has *injuries that will rapidly lead to shock or respiratory difficulty,* even though they may not demonstrate these signs and symptoms during the primary survey. This includes large flail chest, open pneumothorax, tender abdomen, unstable pelvis, bilateral femur fractures, and poorly controlled major bleeding.

SECONDARY SURVEY

If the patient does not appear to have a critical trauma situation, you may perform the secondary survey before transport. During the secondary survey, the development of any of the foregoing signs or symptoms will change the patient's category to "load and go." Be very suspicious of those patients in whom the mechanisms of injury are such that severe injuries may have occurred. These patients may suddenly deteriorate. It is for this reason that you should perform the secondary survey with the patient on the backboard. If the patient's condition changes you can transport immediately.

REASSESSMENT SURVEY

The reassessment survey is almost always performed during transport. However, if you are still on-scene and the reassessment survey reveals any of the foregoing signs or symptoms, load the patient and go.

SUMMARY

Survival from major trauma is time dependent. Certain conditions may require prompt surgical intervention to save the patient. If you are alert to the clinical signs described in this chapter, you will be aware of those conditions requiring "load and go" and will give your patient the best chance for survival.

In all "load-and-go" situations you should call ahead to have the emergency department and possibly the operating room prepared for your arrival. If specific surgeons are needed, Medical Direction can call them before you arrive. Rapid assessment and transport is not life saving if the necessary staff is not present or the operating room is not available when needed. The true test of an EMS system is whether every phase of emergency care can work together as a team when a life depends on definitive care within a matter of minutes.

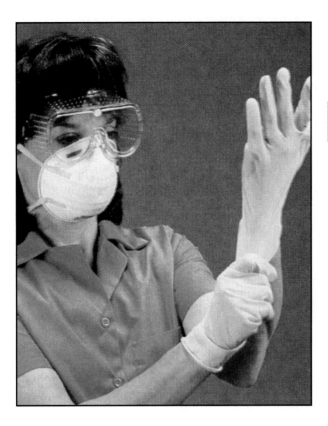

20

Blood and Body Fluid Precautions in the Prehospital Setting

Howard Werman, M.D., F.A.C.E.P., and
Richard N. Nelson, M.D., F.A.C.E.P.

OBJECTIVES

Upon completion of this chapter you should be able to:

1. State the three viral illnesses that EMS providers are most likely to contract from exposure to contaminated blood or body fluids.

2. State the groups of people who are most likely to harbor the virus for the following illnesses:

   a. Hepatitis B

   b. Hepatitis C

   c. Human Immunodeficiency Virus

3. Describe precautions EMS providers can take to prevent exposure to blood and body fluids.

4. Describe procedures for EMS providers to follow if they are accidentally exposed to contaminated blood or body fluids.

EMS personnel have always faced risks when carrying out their jobs. In the past, however, these risks have mostly involved highway hazards, fires, downed electrical wires, toxic substances, and scene security problems. Now you must assume you are also at risk of acquiring certain diseases from the patients you are treating. Fortunately, there are many precautions which may be taken to markedly reduce these risks.

The spectrum of diseases to which you are potentially exposed is beyond the scope of this book. However, three types of viral infections are appropriate to discuss in conjunction with trauma management, since their modes of spread are primarily by contaminated blood and body fluids: hepatitis B, hepatitis C, and acquired immunodeficiency syndrome (AIDS).

HEPATITIS B

The term viral hepatitis is used to describe a group of infections involving the liver. At least four types of viruses have been described: hepatitis A, hepatitis B, delta hepatitis, and non-A, non-B hepatitis. Because of their frequent contact with blood and needles, health care workers are considered at intermediate risk of becoming infected with the hepatitis B virus (HBV). Fortunately, hepatitis B is the one form of hepatitis for which there is an effective vaccine.

HBV is a major cause of acute and chronic hepatitis, cirrhosis, and liver cancer. An estimated 200,000 persons in the United States are infected each year; 12,000 of these are health care workers who acquire the disease through occupational exposure. Following acute infection, 5 to 10% of these patients continue to be chronic carriers of the virus (between 500,000 and 1,000,000 persons are carriers of the virus). These carriers are potentially infectious. HBV is spread by contact with contaminated blood or body fluids. Infection usually occurs from contaminated needle sticks or through sexual contact. It is estimated that 25% of health care workers who are exposed to a needlestick by HBV-contaminated blood will develop hepatitis B infection. Infection can also occur by contacting infectious secretions with skin lesions or mucosal surfaces. Routine testing of donor blood for HBV makes transmission from blood transfusion very rare.

Although HBV infection is uncommon in the general population, members of certain groups are considered much more likely to harbor the virus. High-risk groups are immigrants from areas where HBV is prevalent, institutionalized patients, intravenous drug users, male homosexuals, hemophiliacs, household contacts of HBV patients, and hemodialysis patients.

Two forms of protection are available to prevent infection following HBV exposure. The first, hepatitis B vaccine, produces active immunity against HBV infection. Persons receiving the vaccine are exposed to inactivated surface proteins from the virus and thus develop antibodies that prevent infection. The vaccine is safe and produces immunity in over 90% of persons vaccinated. In the United States the Occupational Safety and Health Administration (OSHA) requires that the vaccine be offered to any health care worker who is at risk of exposure to blood or contaminated body fluids. The second form of protection is hepatitis B immunoglobulin (HBIG). This preparation contains antibodies to HBV and provides temporary, passive protection against HBV. HBIG is used only when there has been a significant exposure to HBV in an unimmunized person.

HEPATITIS C

Recently, the hepatitis C virus (HCV) has been identified. This virus is thought to be responsible for a majority of what had been identified as non-A, non-B hepatitis infections. Antibodies to the HCV have been used to identify patients with previous HCV infection.

HCV is thought to be the leading cause of hepatitis resulting from blood transfusions. Unfortunately, this accounts for only about 5 to 10% of all cases of HCV infection. In addition to spreading by blood transfusion, the virus also appears to be spread by sharing of intravenous needles and sexual contact, much like HBV. Health care workers can acquire infection though needlesticks with contaminated needles, but the likelihood of becoming infected with HCV after a single needlestick is unknown.

HCV infection tends to be less severe than HBV during the initial infection. However, there appears to be a greater likelihood of becoming a chronic carrier of the HCV following infection, placing the health care worker at an increasing risk of exposure. Liver failure and cirrhosis occur in 10 to 20% of chronic HCV carriers.

There is currently no available vaccine to protect against HCV infection. The only available protection is provided by administering immune globulin (IG) following exposure to HCV. This provides the exposed person with temporary, passive immunity.

ACQUIRED IMMUNODEFICIENCY SYNDROME AND HUMAN IMMUNODEFICIENCY VIRUS INFECTION

The acquired immunodeficiency syndrome is the most serious infectious complication caused by the human immunodeficiency virus (HIV). Patients with HIV infection develop a defect in their immune system. This predisposes the AIDS patient to a variety of unusual infections that are not generally seen in healthy patients of similar age. The disease has a uniformly high mortality, and its incidence is increasing. Currently, over 160,000 cases of AIDS have been reported in the United States. At present, there is no effective vaccination or cure for the disease.

Patients infected with HIV can present with a wide spectrum of clinical manifestations. Most commonly, patients with HIV infection are asymptomatic carriers. Any patient who carries HIV, whether he or she manifests symptoms of AIDS or is asymptomatic, can transmit the virus. HIV appears to be transmitted in a manner similar to HBV. Although the virus has been cultured from a variety of body fluids, only blood, semen, and vaginal secretions have been implicated in the transmission of the virus. There is no evidence to suggest that the HIV is transmitted by casual contact. Transmission to health care workers has been documented only after accidental parenteral exposure (needlestick) or exposure of mucous membranes and open wounds to large amounts of infected blood.

HIV appears to be different from the hepatitis B virus in two ways. The virus appears to be easily inactivated by common sterilization methods—Environmental Protection Agency (United States)-approved disinfectants, diluted household bleach, alcohol—and HIV is transmitted far less efficiently than HBV. Several studies have shown that there is a seroconversion rate (demonstrating antibodies to HIV) of approximately 0.3% for health care workers who have experienced an accidental parenteral exposure.

Several groups have been identified as having a high risk of HIV infection. These include male homosexuals or bisexuals, intravenous drug abusers, patients who have received blood transfusions or pooled-plasma products (e.g., hemophiliacs), and heterosexual contacts of HIV carriers. However, because of the difficulty in identifying HIV-infected patients, all contacts with blood and/or body fluids should be considered a potential HIV exposure. In one recent study in an urban emergency department, 5% of patients without an identifiable risk for HIV infection were found to be unsuspected carriers of the virus.

There is currently no available vaccine to protect against HIV infection. Zidovudine (AZT), though not a cure, has been shown to prolong the life of AIDS patients. Recently, AZT has been given to some health care workers immediately following a potential significant exposure to HIV-infected blood or body fluids. It is hoped that AZT may decrease the chance of HIV infection in this setting. Scientific studies are still pending, and the use of AZT in this setting remains controversial.

PRECAUTIONS FOR PREVENTION OF HEPATITIS B, HEPATITIS C, AND HIV TRANSMISSION

"Universal" precautions refers to treating everyone (including yourself) as if they are infectious. Your goal is to prevent the spread of infection from you to the patient and from the patient to you. In today's environment, you must use the following precautions for each and every patient:

A. GENERAL CONSIDERATIONS:

1. You should be knowledgeable about infection from hepatitis B, hepatitis C, and HIV. You should understand their etiologies, epidemiologies, and routes of transmission.

2. If you have open or weeping lesions, take special precautions to prevent exposure of these areas to blood or body fluids. If these lesions cannot be adequately protected, avoid invasive procedures, other direct patient care activities, or handling of equipment used for patient care.

3. Perform routine handwashing before and after all patient contacts. Wash hands as soon as possible following exposure to blood or body fluids.

4. Become immunized against the hepatitis B virus.

B. BARRIER PRECAUTIONS DURING PATIENT EXPOSURES:

1. Wear gloves if exposure to blood or other body fluids is anticipated. This precaution should be taken when performing an invasive procedure or handling any item soiled with blood or body fluid. Almost all trauma patients are risks for blood or body fluid exposure.

2. Disposable gowns, masks, and eye coverings are necessary only when extensive contact with blood or body fluids is anticipated. These precautions are advised when spraying or airborne spread of blood or body fluids is likely (e.g., BIAD insertion, vaginal deliveries, and major trauma).

3. Wear a mask when treating any patient with respiratory complaints to prevent the possible transmission of respiratory infection (such as tuberculosis).

4. Direct mouth-to-mouth ventilation of patients during CPR is to be discouraged. Use disposable mouthpieces when mouth-to-mouth ventilation is indicated.

C. HANDLING OF ITEMS EXPOSED TO BLOOD OR BODY FLUIDS:

1. Consider any sharp instrument potentially infective after patient use. Place disposable syringes, needles, scalpel blades, and other sharp objects directly in puncture-resistant containers. Needles should *not* be recapped, bent, or otherwise manipulated following use. It is strongly recommended that you consider using recently developed exposure-proof parenteral injection sets.

2. Any disposable equipment such as masks, gowns, gloves, mouthpieces, and airways that have been contaminated by blood or body fluids should be collected in an impervious plastic bag. These plastic bags should then be disposed of in proper waste containers available in the hospital emergency departments or other health care locations.

3. Wash, with a low-sudsing detergent with a neutral pH, any surface spills on nondisposable equipment that does not usually come in contact with skin or mucous membranes. The equipment should then be wet down or soaked for 10 minutes in a 1:10 dilution of household bleach (or 70% isopropyl alcohol). Do not use bleach on metal objects because it can cause corrosion.

4. Wash, using a low-sudsing detergent with a neutral pH, nondisposable medical devices that will frequently contact skin or mucous membranes. Then soak them for 30 minutes or more in 2% alkaline glutaraldehyde (e.g., Cidex^R) or similar solution.

D. PROCEDURE AFTER ACCIDENTAL EXPOSURE TO BLOOD OR BODY FLUIDS:

1. Thoroughly wash or irrigate the exposed area immediately following an exposure to blood or contaminated body fluids.

2. Notify the receiving facility of the possible exposure at the time of the incident. Ask the facility to cooperate in determining the serologic status of the source of the blood or contaminated body fluid. In some areas, informed consent need not be obtained to determine serologic status of the source.

3. Write a report of the incident as soon as possible. The minimum information that should be recorded on the report is included in Figure 20-1. The written ambulance report may be used to supplement, but not replace, the incident report. A copy of the report should be forwarded to the EMS coordinator, the EMS medical director, and the infection control committee (or equivalent body) of the receiving institution.

4. Any personnel who has had a significant exposure (e.g., needlestick or mucous membrane or open lesion contact with blood or contaminated secretions) should undergo HIV serology determination at the time of the incident. Repeat testing should be done at one month, three months, and six months following the exposure. If not already immunized, hepatitis B vaccine should be administered. The administration of HBIG or IG should be determined by the serologic testing of both the source (where possible) and the exposed health care provider, as well as by the assessment of the risk of the exposure.

5. In the case where an EMS provider is found to have a positive HBV or HIV serology, restrictions on patient care activities should be determined by the EMS coordinator and EMS medical director.

REPORT OF EXPOSURE TO BLOOD OR BODY FLUID

NAME OF EMS PERSONNEL _____

NAME OF EMS SERVICE _____

ADDRESS OF EMS SERVICE _____

_____

PHONE NUMBER (HOME) _____(WORK) _____

DATE OF EXPOSURE_____TIME OF EXPOSURE _____

NAME OF PATIENT_____

HOSPITAL ID NUMBER _____

PATIENT ADDRESS_____

_____

_____

PHONE NUMBER (WORK) _____(HOME)_____

ROUTE OF EXPOSURE:

(   ) Parenteral exposure (needlestick or sharp instrument)

(   ) Mucous membrane

(   ) Open skin

(   ) Intact skin

(   ) Other _____

TYPE OF FLUID:

(   ) blood   (   ) emesis   (   ) saliva

(   ) stool   (   ) urine   (   ) other _____

SOURCE OF EXPOSURE:

HIV: (   ) Yes   (   ) No   (   ) Unknown

Hepatitis B: (   ) No   (   ) Acute   (   ) Chronic Carrier   (   ) Unknown

Hepatitis C: (   ) No   (   ) Acute   (   ) Chronic Carrier   (   ) Unknown

Figure 20-1 *Sample Report Form*

RISK FACTORS:

( ) Homosexual   ( ) I.V. Drug Abuser

( ) Hemophilia   ( ) Dialysis Patient

( ) Sexual Contact of the Above

( ) Other_____

HIV Test: ( ) Pos.   ( ) Neg.   ( ) Unknown

Date of Test:_____

HBsAg: ( ) Pos.   ( ) Neg.   ( ) Unknown

Date of Test:_____

PERSONNEL DATA:

HBV Vaccine: ( ) No   ( ) Yes

Date Completed:_____

Doses:_____

HIV Test: ( ) Pos.   ( ) Neg.   ( ) Unknown

Date of Test:_____

HBsAg: ( ) Pos.   ( ) Neg.   ( ) Unknown

Date of Test:_____

HBsAb: ( ) Pos.   ( ) Neg.   ( ) Unknown

Date of Test:_____

Description of Circumstances Surrounding the Exposure, Including Measures
Taken after Exposure:_____

_____

_____

_____

INSTITUTION NOTIFIED: _____

PHYSICIAN OR RESPONSIBLE PERSON: _____

DATE OF NOTIFICATION:_____TIME OF NOTIFICATION:_____

NAME OF EXPOSED PERSONNEL_____DATE_____

SIGNATURE _____

Figure 20-1(continued) *Sample Report Form*

SUMMARY

Like most health care workers, you are at risk of exposure to many contagious diseases. Because of the presence of blood and contaminated secretions in many trauma victims, you must take extra precautions to avoid exposure to the viruses that cause hepatitis B, hepatitis C, and AIDS. Knowledge of the modes of exposure, as well as adherence to barrier precautions, will reduce your risk of contracting any of these infections. In the United States, the recent standards released by OSHA make adherence to these precautions mandatory for health care workers at risk for exposure to contaminated blood and body fluids.

BIBLIOGRAPHY

1. Friedland, L. R. "Universal Precautions and Safety Devices Which Reduce the Risk of Occupational Exposure to Blood-borne Pathogens: A Review for Emergency Health Care Workers." *Pediatric Emergency Care*, Vol. 7 (1991), pp. 356–362.

2. Werman, H. A., and G. D. Kelen. "AIDS and Other HIV Infections." In *Emergency Medicine*, Vol. 1, eds. D. Schillinger and A. Harwood-Nus. New York: Churchill-Livingstone, 1989.

3. Fontanarosa, P. B. "Occupational Considerations for the Prehospital Care Provider." *Emergency Medical Clinician*, Vol. 8 (1990), pp. 119–134.

Appendix A

Optional Skills

Donna Hastings, EMT-P

OPTIONAL SKILL 1: ANTISHOCK GARMENT

Also known as military antishock trousers (MAST) or pneumatic antishock garment (PASG).

OBJECTIVES

Upon completion of this skill station you should be able to:

1. Recite the indications and contraindications for the use of the antishock garment.
2. Apply and inflate the antishock garment.
3. Deflate and remove the antishock garment.

INDICATIONS FOR USE OF THE ANTISHOCK TROUSERS

1. Shock secondary to external hemorrhage that can be controlled
2. Spinal shock without evidence of other internal injuries
3. Isolated fractures of legs without evidence of other internal injuries
4. Systolic blood pressure less than 50 mm Hg (controversial)
5. Anaphylactic shock

CONTRAINDICATIONS FOR USE OF ANTISHOCK TROUSERS

1. *Absolute:*
   a. Pulmonary edema
   b. Bleeding that cannot be controlled
2. *Conditional:* Pregnancy: May use leg compartments.

TECHNIQUES

APPLICATION (SEE FIGURE A-1):

1. Evaluate the patient through at least the primary survey. Apply a blood pressure cuff to patient's arm.
2. Have your partner unfold the trousers and lay them flat on a long backboard and place the backboard beside the patient.

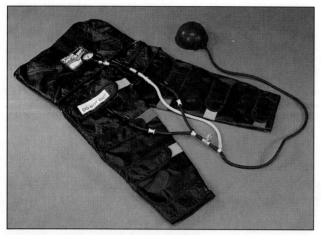

Adult garment and inflation pedal.

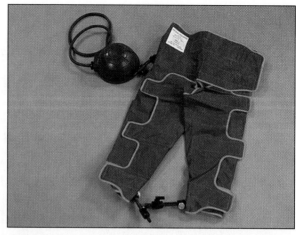

Pediatric garment.

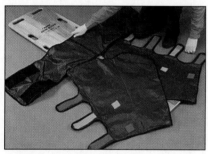

1. Unfold the garment and lay it flat. It should be smoothed of wrinkles.

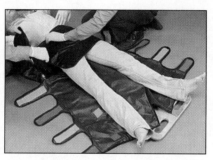

2. Log roll the patient onto the garment, or slip it under him. The upper edge of the garment must be just below the rib cage.

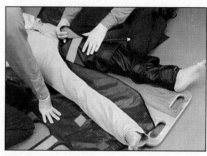

3. Check for a distal pulse and enclose the left leg, securing the Velcro straps.

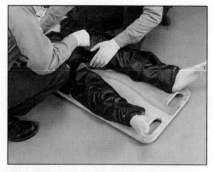

4. Check for a distal pulse and enclose the right leg, securing the Velcro straps.

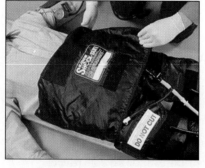

5. Enclose the abdomen and pelvis, securing the Velcro straps.

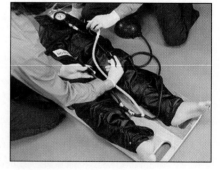

6. Check the tubes leading to the compartments and the pump.

Note: Patient's clothing remains on for demonstration purposes. In actual use, clothing should be removed. Anti-shock garment can be placed over traction splint.

Figure A-1 *Application of an antishock garment.*

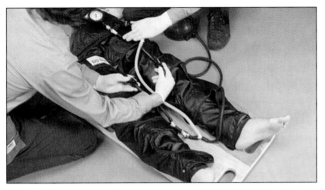

7. Open the stopcocks to the legs and close the abdominal compartment stopcock.

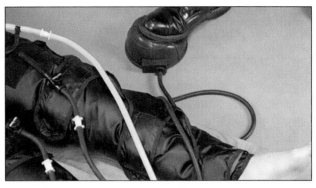

8. Use the foot pedal to inflate the lower compartments simultaneously, or the required lower extremity compartment. Inflate until air exhausts through the relief valves, the Velcro makes a crackling noise, or the patient's systolic blood pressure is stable at 100–110 to 90–100 mmHg or higher.

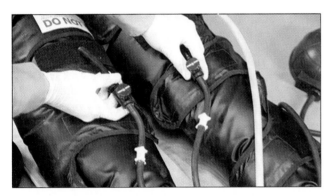

9. Close the stopcocks.

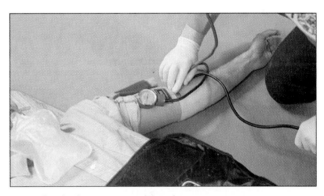

10. Check the patient's blood pressure.

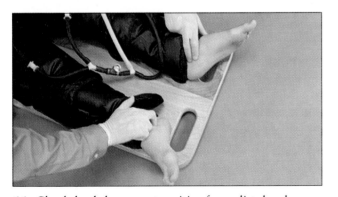

11. Check both lower extremities for a distal pulse.

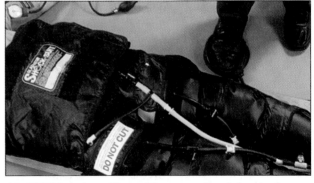

12. If BP is below 90 mmHg, open the abdominal stopcock and inflate abdominal compartment. Close stopcock.

Figure A-1 *Application of an antishock garment. (Cont.)*

3. Maintain mobility of the spine by log-rolling the patient (check the back quickly as you do this) onto the backboard. The top of the antishock garment should be just below the lowest rib.

4. Wrap the trousers around the left leg and fasten the Velcro® strips.

5. Wrap the trousers around the right leg and fasten the Velcro® strips.

6. Wrap the abdominal compartment around the abdomen and fasten the Velcro® strips. Be sure the top of the garment is below the bottom ribs.

7. Attach the tubes from the foot pump to the connections on the trousers.

PROCEDURE FOR INFLATION OF TROUSERS

1. Recheck and record the vital signs.

2. Inflate the leg compartments while monitoring the blood pressure. If the blood pressure is not in the range 90 to 100 mm Hg, inflate the abdominal compartment.

3. When the patient's blood pressure reaches 90 to 100 mm Hg, turn the stopcocks to hold the pressure.

4. Remember, it is not the pressure in the trousers you are monitoring but the patient's blood pressure.

5. Continue monitoring the patient's blood pressure, adding pressure to the trousers as needed.

DEFLATION OF TROUSERS: Before deflation occurs, two large-bore I.V.s must be inserted and sufficient volume of fluids and/or blood given to replace the volume lost from hemorrhage. The antishock garment is usually deflated only at the hospital. The only reason to deflate them in the field is if they cause difficulty with breathing (pulmonary edema).

1. Record the patient's vital signs.

2. From Medical Direction, obtain permission to deflate the trousers.

3. Slowly deflate the abdominal compartment while monitoring the patient's blood pressure.

4. If the blood pressure drops 5 mm Hg or more, you must stop deflation and infuse more fluid or blood until the vital signs stabilize again (this usually requires at least 200 cc).

5. Proceed from the abdominal compartment to the right leg and then left leg with your deflation, continuously monitoring the blood pressure and stopping to infuse fluid when a drop of 5 mm Hg occurs.

6. If the patient experiences a sudden precipitous drop in blood pressure while you are deflating, stop and reinflate the garment.

APPLICATION OF ANTISHOCK TROUSERS TO A PATIENT REQUIRING A TRACTION SPLINT:

1. Have your partner hold traction on the fractured leg.

2. Unfold the trousers and lay them flat on a long spineboard.

3. Log-roll the patient, holding traction on the injured leg and keeping the neck stabilized.

4. Slide the spineboard and the patient so that the top of the trousers is just below the lowest rib. If the patient is already on a spineboard, you may simply unfold the trousers and slide them under the patient while maintaining traction on the injured leg.

5. Wrap the trousers around the injured leg and fasten the Velcro® strips.

6. Wrap the trousers around the other leg and fasten the Velcro® strips.

7. Wrap the abdominal compartment around the abdomen and fasten the Velcro® strips. Be sure that the top of the garment is below the bottom ribs.

8. Apply a traction splint (Thomas, Hare, Sager, of Klippel) over the trousers. Attach the straps and apply traction.

9. Inflate the trousers in the usual sequence.

OPTIONAL SKILL 2: ESOPHAGEAL GASTRIC TUBE AIRWAY

OBJECTIVES

Upon completion of this skill station you should be able to:

1. Explain seven essential points about the use of this airway.
2. Correctly insert the esophageal gastric tube airway (EGTA).

Introduced in the early 1970s, Blind-insertion airway devices (BIADs) were designed for use by EMS personnel who were not trained to intubate the trachea. All of these devices (EOA, EGTA, PtL®, and Combitube®) are designed to be inserted into the pharynx without the need for a laryngoscope to visualize where the tube is going. All of these devices have a tube with an inflatable cuff that is designed to seal the esophagus thus preventing vomiting and aspiration of stomach contents as well as preventing gastric distention during bag-valve-mask or demand-valve-mask ventilation. It was also thought that by sealing the esophagus more air would enter the lungs and ventilation would be improved. These devices have their own dangers and require careful evaluation to be sure that they are in the correct position. None of the BIADs are equal to the endotracheal tube which has become the invasive airway of choice for advanced EMS providers.

Esophageal obturator airways (EOA) are designed to be inserted into the esophagus at a level beyond the carina, a cuff is then inflated to reduce the likelihood of gastric distension or regurgitation during bag-valve-mask or demand-valve-mask ventilation. Controversy surrounding the use of the EOA surfaced when some studies suggested that it did not provide as adequate ventilation as originally thought. A more recent design, the esophageal gastric tube airway, should replace the older EOA. This design allows for the placement of a nasogastric tube through the lumen of the obturator for decompression of the stomach. In addition, ventilation occurs directly into the oropharynx rather than through the holes of the obturator.

You must remember seven essential points about the EGTA:

1. Use only in patients who are unresponsive and without protective reflexes.

2. Do *not* use in patients with upper airway or facial trauma where bleeding into the oropharynx is a problem. Do *not* use in any patient with injury to the esophagus (e.g., caustic ingestions) or in children who are below the age of 15 and of average height and weight.

3. You must ensure an adequate mask seal; this means appropriate lifting forward of the jaw, with every attempt to avoid movement of the head and neck.

4. Pay careful attention to proper placement. *Unrecognized intratracheal* placement is a lethal complication that produces complete airway obstruction. Such an occurrence is not always easy to detect, and the results are catastrophic. One of the great disadvantages of this airway is the fact that you can determine correct placement only by auscultation and observation of chest movement—both may be quite unreliable in the prehospital setting.

5. You must insert gently and without force.

6. If the patient becomes conscious, you must remove the EGTA as it will cause retching and vomiting.

7. The EGTA is only recommended when endotracheal intubation is impossible or unsuccessful.

TECHNIQUE

The airway is relatively easily inserted and must never be forced. In the supine patient the following procedure is followed:

1. Ventilate with mouth to mask or bag-valve mask and suction the pharynx prior to insertion of the airway.

2. After liberal lubrication, slide the airway, with mask attached, into the oropharynx while the tongue and jaw are pulled forward.

3. Advance the airway along the tongue and into the esophagus. Take care to observe the neck. "Tenting" of the skin in the area of the pyriform fossa or anterior displacement of the laryngeal prominence indicates that misplacement has occurred and indicates that you should reposition by pulling back and reinserting the airway.

4. Gently insert the airway so that the mask now rests easily on the face; then seal the mask firmly on the face as you pull the jaw forward to ensure a patent airway (see Figures A-2 and A-3).

5. Prior to inflating the cuff, attempt ventilation with a mouth-to-mask or bag-valve device. If you see the chest rise, hear breath sounds, and feel good compliance, inflate the cuff of the airway with 35 cc of air.

6. Following inflation, auscultate the lung fields again and feel the chest wall as well as observing for chest wall movement. The epigastrium should not distend.

If there is any doubt about placement of the airway, remove it and reinsert. If the patient becomes conscious, you must remove the EGTA. Extubation is likely to cause vomiting; be prepared to suction the pharynx and turn the backboard.

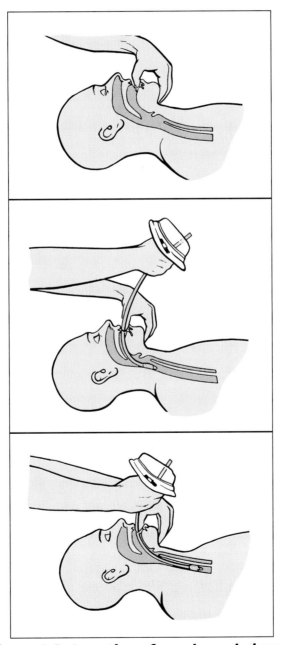

Figure A-2 *Insertion of esophageal airway.*

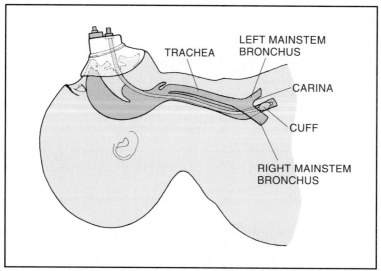

Figure A-3 *Final position of EGTA.*

OPTIONAL SKILL 3: PHARYNGOTRACHEAL LUMEN AIRWAY

OBJECTIVES

Upon completion of this skill station you should be able to:

1. Explain the five essential points about use of this airway.
2. Correctly insert the pharyngotracheal lumen airway (PtL®).

Introduced in the early 1970s, Blind-insertion airway devices (BIADs) were designed for use by EMS personnel who were not trained to intubate the trachea. All of these devices (EOA, EGTA, PtL®, and Combitube®) are designed to be inserted into the pharynx without the need for a laryngoscope to visualize where the tube is going. All of these devices have a tube with an inflatable cuff that is designed to seal the esophagus thus preventing vomiting and aspiration of stomach contents as well as preventing gastric distention during bag-valve-mask or demand-valve-mask ventilation. It was also thought that by sealing the esophagus more air would enter the lungs and ventilation would be improved. These devices have their own dangers and require careful evaluation to be sure that they are in the correct position. None of the BIADs are equal to the endotracheal tube which has become the invasive airway of choice for advanced EMS providers.

The PtL® consists of a smaller-diameter long tube inside of a short large-diameter tube (see Figure A-4). The longer tube goes either into the trachea or the esophagus, while the shorter tube opens into the lower pharynx. Each tube has a cuff; the longer tube's cuff seals the esophagus or trachea, and the shorter tube's cuff seals the oropharynx so that there is no air leak when you ventilate the patient. You insert the PtL® blindly into the pharynx, and then you must carefully determine whether the longer tube is in the esoph-

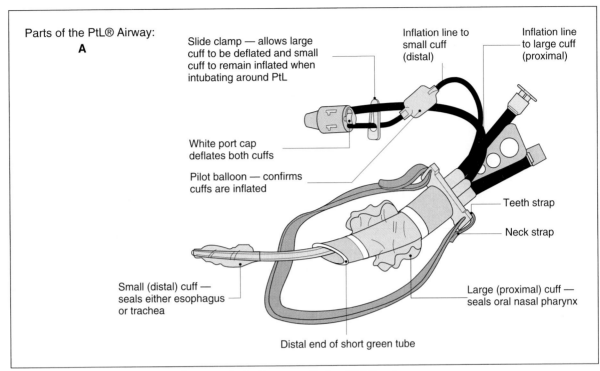

Parts of the PtL® Airway:
A

Slide clamp — allows large cuff to be deflated and small cuff to remain inflated when intubating around PtL

Inflation line to small cuff (distal)

Inflation line to large cuff (proximal)

White port cap deflates both cuffs

Pilot balloon — confirms cuffs are inflated

Teeth strap

Neck strap

Small (distal) cuff — seals either esophagus or trachea

Large (proximal) cuff — seals oral nasal pharynx

Distal end of short green tube

Figure A-4 *Parts of the PtL® airway.*

agus or the trachea. If the long tube is in the trachea, you ventilate through it. If the tube is in the esophagus, you ventilate through the larger tube in the pharynx. The PtL® has advantages over the EGTA in that you don't require extra hands to keep a seal with a face mask and also the cuff the pharynx prevents blood and mucous from entering the airway from above.

You must remember five essential points about the PtL®:

1. Use only in patients who are unresponsive and without protective reflexes.

2. Do *not* use in any patient with injury to the esophagus (e.g., caustic ingestions) or in children who are below the age of 15 and of average height and weight.

3. Pay careful attention to proper placement. *Unrecognized intratracheal* placement of the long tube is a lethal complication that produces complete airway obstruction. Such an occurrence is not always easy to detect, and the results are catastrophic. Like the EGTA, one of the great disadvantages of this airway is the fact that you can determine correct placement only by auscultation and observation of chest movement—both may be quite unreliable in the prehospital setting.

4. You must Insert gently and without force.

5. If the patient regains consciousness, you must remove the PtL® as it will cause retching and vomiting.

TECHNIQUE

The airway is relatively easily inserted and must never be forced. In the supine patient the following procedure is followed:

1. Ventilate with mouth-to-mask or bag-valve mask and suction the pharynx prior to insertion of the airway.

2. Prepare the airway by checking to be sure that both cuffs are fully deflated, that the long no. 3 tube (see Figure A-5) has a bend in the middle, and that the white cap is securely in place over the deflation port located under the no. 1 inflation valve.

3. After liberal lubrication, slide the airway into the oropharynx while the tongue and jaw are pulled forward.

4. Holding the PtL® in your free hand so that it curves in the same direction as the natural curvature of the pharynx, advance the airway behind the tongue until the teeth strap contacts the lips and teeth. On very small patients you may have to withdraw the airway so that the teeth strap is up to an inch from the teeth. Conversely, on very large patients you may have to insert the teeth strap into the mouth, past the teeth.

5. Immediately inflate both cuffs. Make sure that the white cap is in place over the deflation port located under the inflation valve. Deliver a sustained ventilation into the inflation valve. You can detect failure of the cuffs to inflate properly by failure of the external pilot balloon to inflate or by hearing or feeling air escape from the patient's mouth and nose. This usually means that one of the cuffs is torn and the airway must be removed and replaced. When you determine that the cuffs are inflating, continue inflation until you get a good seal.

6. Immediately determine whether the long no. 3 tube is in the esophagus or the trachea. First ventilate through the short no. 2 tube. If you see the chest rise, hear breath sounds, feel good compliance, and hear no breath sounds over the epigastrium, the long no. 3 tube is in the esophagus and you should continue ventilating through the no. 2 tube.

7. If you do not see the chest rise, hear breath sounds, and feel good compliance when the no. 2 tube is ventilated, the no. 3 tube is probably in the trachea. In this case, remove the stylet from the no. 3 tube and ventilate through the no. 3 tube. If you see the chest rise, hear breath sounds, feel good compliance, and hear no breath sounds over the epigastrium, the no. 3 tube is in the trachea and you should continue ventilating through the no. 3 tube.

8. When you are sure that the patient is being adequately ventilated, carry the neck strap over the patent's head and tighten it in place. Continually monitor the appearance of the pilot balloon during ventilation. Loss of pressure in the balloon signals a loss of pressure in the cuffs. If you suspect a cuff is leaking, increase pressure by blowing into the no. 1 inflation valve or replace the airway.

Like the EGTA, if the patient becomes conscious, you must remove the PtL®. Remove the white cap from the deflation port to simultaneously deflate both cuffs. Extubation is likely to cause vomiting; be prepared to suction the pharynx and turn the backboard.

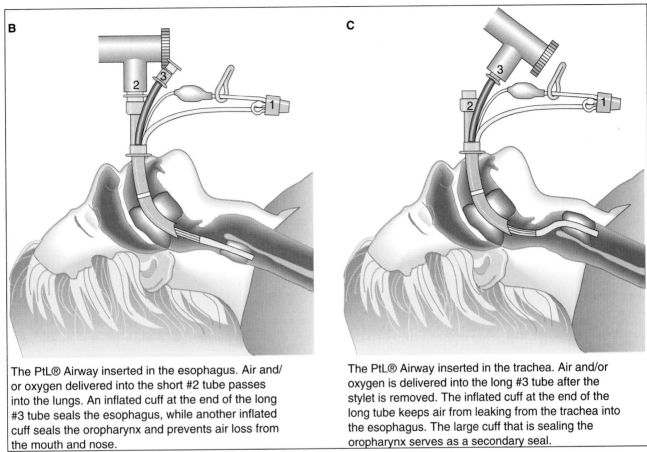

The PtL® Airway inserted in the esophagus. Air and/or oxygen delivered into the short #2 tube passes into the lungs. An inflated cuff at the end of the long #3 tube seals the esophagus, while another inflated cuff seals the oropharynx and prevents air loss from the mouth and nose.

The PtL® Airway inserted in the trachea. Air and/or oxygen is delivered into the long #3 tube after the stylet is removed. The inflated cuff at the end of the long tube keeps air from leaking from the trachea into the esophagus. The large cuff that is sealing the oropharynx serves as a secondary seal.

Figure A-5 *The PtL® in place in (a) the esophagus or (b) the trachea.*

OPTIONAL SKILL 4: ESOPHAGEAL TRACHEAL COMBITUBE

OBJECTIVES

Upon completion of this skill station you should be able to:

1. Explain the five essential points about use of this airway.
2. Correctly insert the Combitube.

Introduced in the early 1970s, Blind-insertion airway devices (BIADs) were designed for use by EMS personnel who were not trained to intubate the trachea. All of these devices (EOA, EGTA, PtL®, and Combitube®) are designed to be inserted into the pharynx without the need for a laryngoscope to visualize where the tube is going. All of these devices have a tube with an inflatable cuff that is designed to seal the esophagus thus preventing vomiting and aspiration of stomach contents as well as preventing gastric distention during bag-valve-mask or demand-valve-mask ventilation. It was also thought that by sealing the esophagus more air would enter the lungs and ventilation would be improved. These devices have their own dangers and require careful evaluation to be sure that they are in the correct position. None of the BIADs are equal to the endotracheal tube which has become the invasive airway of choice for advanced EMS providers.

The Combitube® is like the PtL® airway in that it has a double lumen. However, in the Combitube® the two lumens are separated by a partition rather than one being inside of the other (see Figure A-6). One tube is sealed at the distal end and there are perforations in the area of the tube that would be in the pharynx. When the long tube is in the esophagus, the patient is ventilated through this short tube. The long tube is open at the distal end and it has a cuff that is blown up to seal the esophagus or the trachea, depending on which it has entered. When inserted, if the long tube goes into the esophagus, the cuff is inflated and the patient is ventilated through the short tube. If the long tube goes into the trachea, the cuff is inflated and the patient is ventilated through the long tube. Like the PtL® airway, this device has a pharyngeal balloon that seals the pharynx and prevents blood and mucous from entering the airway from above. The Combitube® is somewhat quicker and easier to insert than the PtL® airway but, as with the other BIADs, you must be sure that you are ventilating the lungs and not the stomach.

You must remember five essential points about the Combitube®:

1. Use only in patients who are unresponsive and without protective reflexes.

2. Do not use in any patient with injury to the esophagus (e.g., caustic ingestions) or in children who are below the age of 15 and of average height and weight.

3. Pay careful attention to proper placement. Unrecognized intratracheal placement of the long tube is a lethal complication that produces complete airway obstruction. Such an occurrence is not always easy to detect, and the results are catastrophic. Like the EGTA & PtL®, one of the great disadvantages of this airway is the fact that you can determine correct placement only by auscultation and observation of chest movement—both may be quite unreliable in the prehospital setting.

4. You must Insert gently and without force.

5. If the patient regains consciousness, you must remove the Combitube® as it will cause retching and vomiting.

TECHNIQUE

1. Insert the tube blindly, watching for the two black rings on the Combitube® that are used for measuring the depth of insertion. These rings should be positioned between the teeth and the lips (see Figure A-6).

2. Use the large syringe to inflate the pharyngeal cuff with 100 cc of air. When inflated, the Combitube® will seat itself in the posterior pharynx behind the hard palate.

3. Use the small syringe to fill the distal cuff with 10 -15 cc of air.

4. The long tube will usually go into the esophagus. Ventilate through the esophageal connector. It is the external tube that is the longer of the two and is marked #1. As with the PtL® airway, you must see the chest rise, hear breath sounds, feel good compliance, and hear

no breath sounds over the epigastrium in order to be sure that the long tube is in the esophagus.

5. If you do not see the chest rise, hear breath sounds, feel good compliance, and you hear breath sounds over the epigastrium, the tube has been placed in the trachea. In this case, change the ventilator to the shorter tracheal connector, which is marked #2. Again you must check to see the chest rise, hear breath sounds, feel

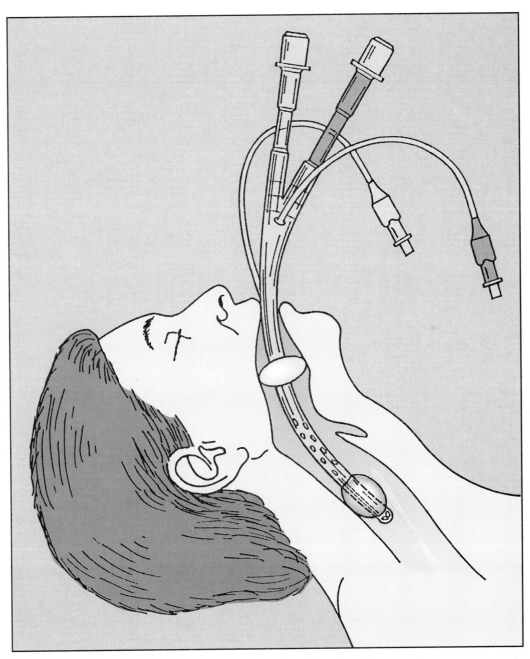

Figure A-6 *The Combitube® in place in the esophagus.*

good compliance, and hear no breath sounds over the epigastrium
in order to be sure that you are ventilating the lungs.

Like the EGTA & PtL®, if the patient becomes conscious, you must remove the Combitube®. Extubation is likely to cause vomiting; be prepared to suction the pharynx and turn the backboard.

Appendix B
Radio Communications

Corey M. Slovis, M.D., F.A.C.P., F.A.C.E.P.

It is imperative that you provide your hospital base station physician with an accurate, succinct, on-scene assessment. This can be very difficult, as there are potentially thousands of bits of information that could be relayed. In the field, you do not have the luxury of giving a long and complete history and physical to the physician at the other end of the radio. The purpose of radio communication is not to give all available information to the physician but to transmit only the information needed for appropriate care. Due to responsibilities to patients already in the emergency department, the physician receiving the call would like to spend a minimum of time on the radio.

When speaking over the radio, no matter how emergent the situation, you should speak clearly and avoid speaking rapidly in an emotional, high-pitched voice. However, using a slow monotone voice in reporting a cardiac arrest would be inappropriate as well. You should try to convey the urgency of the situation in a professional manner. The radio microphone should be held a few inches from your mouth to allow accurate voice transmission but not so far (greater than 6 inches) as to allow interference from other noises at the scene.

The following format for communications is designed to maximize the efficient transfer of information. It may also be used for calls not involving trauma.

FOUR-PHASE COMMUNICATION POLICY

The BTLS communications policy is divided into four parts. The first of these phases is devoted to the EMS unit confirming radio contact with a specific hospital or base station.

PHASE I: CONTACT PHASE

STEP 1—IDENTIFICATION: In attempting to establish radio contact, you should state what EMS service is calling, the unit's level of function (e.g., basic, paramedic), and the unit's identification number. For example, "This is County Advanced Unit 501 calling County Hospital." It is important for you to identify your level of function so the physician knows which procedures and medications to consider. The EMS service should be identified, because different services operating in the same area may function with different protocols. The EMS unit's own identification number needs to be included for potential recontacting and for retrospective tape audit purposes. As different hospitals may have the same radio frequency, the specific facility being called should be stated each time contact is initiated.

STEP 2—FACILITY RESPONSE: The base station or receiving hospital should now respond by identifying the facility, which person is on the radio, and to what EMS unit they are responding. An example might be: "This is Dr. Thomas Smith at County Hospital. Go ahead County Advanced Unit 501." By restating the EMS unit's service and number, confusion will be minimized when multiple units are involved with a single receiving facility. It is recommended that hospital-based radio operators identify themselves. This is important because often the initial response is not by a physician. It is just as important that physicians identify themselves so that you may record who is giving you orders.

PHASE II: IN-THE-FIELD REPORT

The second phase of communications is the most important. Here you should give all important primary survey information and request appropriate orders. This phase of communications is divided into the six steps that follow.

STEP 3—REIDENTIFICATION: Once contact has been confirmed, the in-the-field report begins by you reidentifying the EMS service, its level of function, and unit number. This information may not yet have been recorded or even heard by the physician who has probably just arrived at the radio console.

STEP 4—CHIEF COMPLAINT/ON-SCENE REPORT: After you have identified your level of function and unit number, the next sentence should provide the physician with the most complete picture of the patient possible. This sentence should include the patient's approximate age, sex, complaint, and/or mechanism of injury. Having information such as the victim's approximate age and sex allows the physician to get a mental picture of the patient. Similarly, by knowing the chief complaint and/or type of injury, the physician has an idea of the type of emergency call with which he or she will be handling. An example of this part of communication might be: "We are on the scene of a 23-year-old female involved in an MVA. She is now complaining of chest pain" or "We are on the scene with a 23-year-old female who has a gunshot wound to the chest." The patient's medications, additional complaints, or more complete description of injuries should not be given at this time.

STEP 5—LIFE-SAVING RESUSCITATION: If any emergency maneuvers or lifesaving therapy has been performed during the primary survey, it should be reported next. Thus, if an airway maneuver has been performed or CPR started, it should be reported at this point. Examples of this include "The patient's sucking chest wound has been sealed" or "We have begun CPR and defibrillated the patient." Results of a fingerstick glucose, if already performed on a comatose patient, should be reported during this phase.

STEP 6—VITAL SIGNS/PRIMARY SURVEY ABNORMALITIES: In the next sentence, you should give vital signs and/or primary survey abnormalities. In stable patients with a normal primary survey, a complete set of vital signs are blood pressure, pulse, respiratory rate, and skin temperature (if pertinent). A typical communication might be: "The patient has a normal primary survey with vital signs of: blood pressure 130/90, pulse 90, respiration 16." If, however, there is an abnormal primary survey, a full set of vital signs would not be reported. In this type of unstable patient, problems with airway, breathing, cardiovascular stability, and screening neurologic exam would be reported to the physician. In this so-called "load-and-go" type of call, no additional physical findings, historical facts, or medication usage would be reported at this time. A typical communication would be: "Primary survey as follows: no palpable pulses present, respiration is 40, chest exam reveals a sucking chest wound; patient is confused and combative."

STEP 7—ESTIMATED TIME OF ARRIVAL: You should now state how much time it will take to get to the hospital from the present location. If you are en route, this should be reported. If however, significant additional time is required to extricate or load the patient into the EMS vehicle, this should be specifically stated. Examples of the estimated time of arrival

(ETA) phase of communication include: "We are en route to your location, our ETA is less than 4 minutes" or "We are still on-scene and will require 10 to 15 minutes before we begin transport to the hospital."

STEP 8—REQUEST FOR ORDERS: Prior to relinquishing radio control to the base station, you should state what orders are desired, that no orders are desired, or that the base station physician's help is needed to determine what to do for the patient. Examples of these respective situations include: "Requesting that the PASG be inflated to maintain blood pressure," or "No orders requested," or "Base station, how do you advise?"

PHASE III: BASE STATION–CONTROLLED ACTIVITY

In this phase of communication you are no longer in charge of the radio. You should now respond to the physician's approval or denial of orders. In other cases there may be talk back and forth between you and the physician.

STEP 9—PHYSICIAN'S RESPONSE: It is now up to the physician to determine how to proceed with management of the patient. The physician may merely agree with your request by stating, "Go ahead with your requested therapy" or might completely disagree: "Orders denied, transport the patient as soon a possible." With complicated patients, the physician may need more information than you have transmitted. This is *not* a criticism of the rescuer's radio abilities, but merely as need for the physician to obtain additional information. For example, "Are the patient's neck veins flat or distended?" or "Does the patient seem to improve in the Trendelenburg position?" You should be prepared to answer routine questions readily and to perform requested maneuvers.

STEP 10—YOUR RESPONSE: You should confirm any given orders by repeating them. If the base station has given orders that are either incomplete or with which you disagree, it is now appropriate to give additional history or request an order. Examples of these problems include: "Be advised the patient has a long history of cardiac problems and is on multiple medications" or "Base station, did you copy that the patient is hypotensive and that we are requesting permission to inflate the PASG?" If you cannot answer the questions, tell the physician. Examples of this type of exchange would be: "We don't have any available information on down-time" or "We are unable to attempt this, the patient is still trapped inside the vehicle."

PHASE IV: SIGN-OFF

The final phase of EMS–base station communications is the sign-off. You should make it very clear that the unit is leaving the medical frequency and returning to dispatch frequency.

STEP 11—EMS UNIT SIGN-OFF: You should now advise the base station that you are ending communications. Although everyone seems to favor a different phrase to end with, each EMS service should agree on a common sign-off phrase. The use of a time signal at the end of a comment is recommended but is optional. Acceptable closings include: "Unit 501 is clear" or "Unit 501 is out at 13:59 hours."

Avoid using code numbers, as many physicians do not understand them or may use similar codes for different purposes; thus "Unit 501 is 10-8 your location code 3" is not recommended, nor is "501, 10-8, 1359."

STEP 12—BASE STATION CLOSING: The base station physician should similarly end communication with the same agreed-upon phrase: for example, "County Hospital clear."

Keep a copy of the Table B-1 by the EMS radio in the hospital. *You should try to concentrate on transmitting the most information with the least amount of words.*

PHASE I:	*ESTABLISHING CONTACT*
1.	INITIATION OF CALL EMS SERVICE LEVEL OF FUNCTION (BASIC, PARAMEDIC, ETC.) UNIT NUMBER MEDICAL CONTROL FACILITY BEING CONTACTED
2.	RECEIVING FACILITY RESPONSE NAME OF FACILITY NAME AND TITLE OF RADIO OPERATOR RENAMING OF CALLING EMS SERVICE
PHASE II:	*IN-THE-FIELD REPORT*
3.	REIDENTIFICATION EMS SERVICE LEVEL OF FUNCTION (BASIC, PARAMEDIC, ETC.) UNIT NUMBER
4.	CHIEF COMPLAINT/ON-SCENE REPORT *ONE* BRIEF SENTENCE INCLUDES AGE, SEX, COMPLAINT, AND/OR MECHANISM OF INJURY
5.	LIFE-SAVING RESUSCITATION PATIENT'S RESPONSE TO LIFE-SAVING MANEUVERS
6.	VITAL SIGNS/PRIMARY SURVEY ABNORMALITIES VITAL SIGNS IN STABLE PATIENT OR PRIMARY SURVEY IN UNSTABLE PATIENT
7.	ETA STATE ETA
8.	REQUEST FOR ORDERS STATE WHAT IS DESIRED OR STATE "NO ORDERS REQUESTED"
PHASE III:	*HOSPITAL-CONTROLLED ACTIVITY*
9.	PHYSICIAN RESPONSE AGREE OR DENY OR STATE DESIRED ORDERS REQUEST FOR ADDITIONAL HISTORY AND/OR INFORMATION
10.	RESCUER RESPONSE CLARIFICATION OR RESPONSE TO REQUESTED MANEUVER OR THERAPY
PHASE IV:	*SIGN-OFF*
11.	EMS UNIT SIGN-OFF
12.	BASE STATION SIGN-OFF

Table B-1 *BTLS Communications Format*

DO'S
THINK ABOUT YOUR REPORT BEFORE MAKING RADIO CONTACT.
BE BRIEF AND CONCISE.
TALK CLEARLY.
RELATE ONLY THE KEY POINTS OF THE HISTORY—DON'T GIVE EVERY SINGLE FACT YOU'VE LEARNED ABOUT THE PATIENT.
STATE THE PATIENT'S PRIMARY PROBLEM AND WHAT YOU ARE REQUESTING EARLY IN THE CALL.
ASK QUESTIONS IF YOU ARE UNSURE OF THE BASE STATION'S REPLY.
ASK FOR CLARIFICATION ON THERAPIES YOU THINK ARE WRONG OR DANGEROUS.
CALL YOUR SUPERVISOR FOR "UNRESOLVABLE" PROBLEMS.
DON'TS
DON'T MAKE A SPEECH.
DON'T RAMBLE.
DON'T USE JARGON, CODES, OR ABBREVIATIONS.
DON'T SIGNIFICANTLY ALTER HOW YOU NORMALLY TALK.
DON'T ASSUME ANYTHING.
NEVER GIVE A THERAPY YOU THINK IS DANGEROUS.
DON'T MAKE UNPROFESSIONAL COMMENTS THAT WILL EMBARRASS YOU WHEN THE TAPE IS REPLAYED.
DON'T ARGUE OVER THE RADIO.

Table B-2 *Do's and Don'ts of Successful Radio Communications*

Appendix C

Documentation: The Written Report

Arlo F. Weltge, M.D., F.A.C.E.P.

With the recognition of the important and increasing role of the prehospital care provider has come deserved respect. However, with this recognition comes the expectation of a standard of care and resultant liability when the care does not meet that standard.

This appendix will show how to create a document that chronicles the medical care given, communicates medical information, and provides a permanent record that can be used as evidence that the standard of care was delivered.

THE WRITTEN REPORT

The EMS system written report can vary dramatically from being primarily a billing form to an excellent narrative medical record. In most EMS systems the written report will usually provide enough space for medical documentation to be adequate for the majority of transports, since most runs do not require much more than a simple transport.

It is important to use the system written report effectively. There should be enough space for a chief complaint, simple history and assessment, and space for other comments. All written reports should be filled out completely. Even though the transport may have been "simple," failure to document vital signs, complete check-off boxes for the history and physical, and enter times, events, and other "simple" information may reflect poorly on the care delivered if the report is ever reviewed.

If the system report does not provide adequate space for a reasonable history and assessment, or if the case is more difficult, for example, requiring intervention, long transport times, or involving potential patient complications, it may be necessary to include a continuation sheet. The continuation sheet can be a simple form. It does require some basic identification, including the patient's name, date, identification of the EMS system, and the run identification number. The report should be written at or near the time of the run, and the original must be signed and kept as a regular part of the system's medical records and attached to the regular written report. A simple form is shown in Figure C-1.

A simple continuation sheet can be used for almost any situation or problem. The written, or narrative report, using the continuation sheet, requires much more effort, however, since there are not a host of "fill-in-the-blank" or "check-off" boxes when writing the report. To document a complex case adequately using the continuation sheet, you need to be familiar with the general form or sequence of a written narrative report. The form is dictated by convention (or otherwise known as a generally agreed-upon habit or standard in the medical community). Effective documentation requires using this convention, as well as skill and practice to yield a useful record.

The written report should be brief, yet, like the verbal report, relevant and focused. There are times when the clinical problem is confusing and the report must be more lengthy,

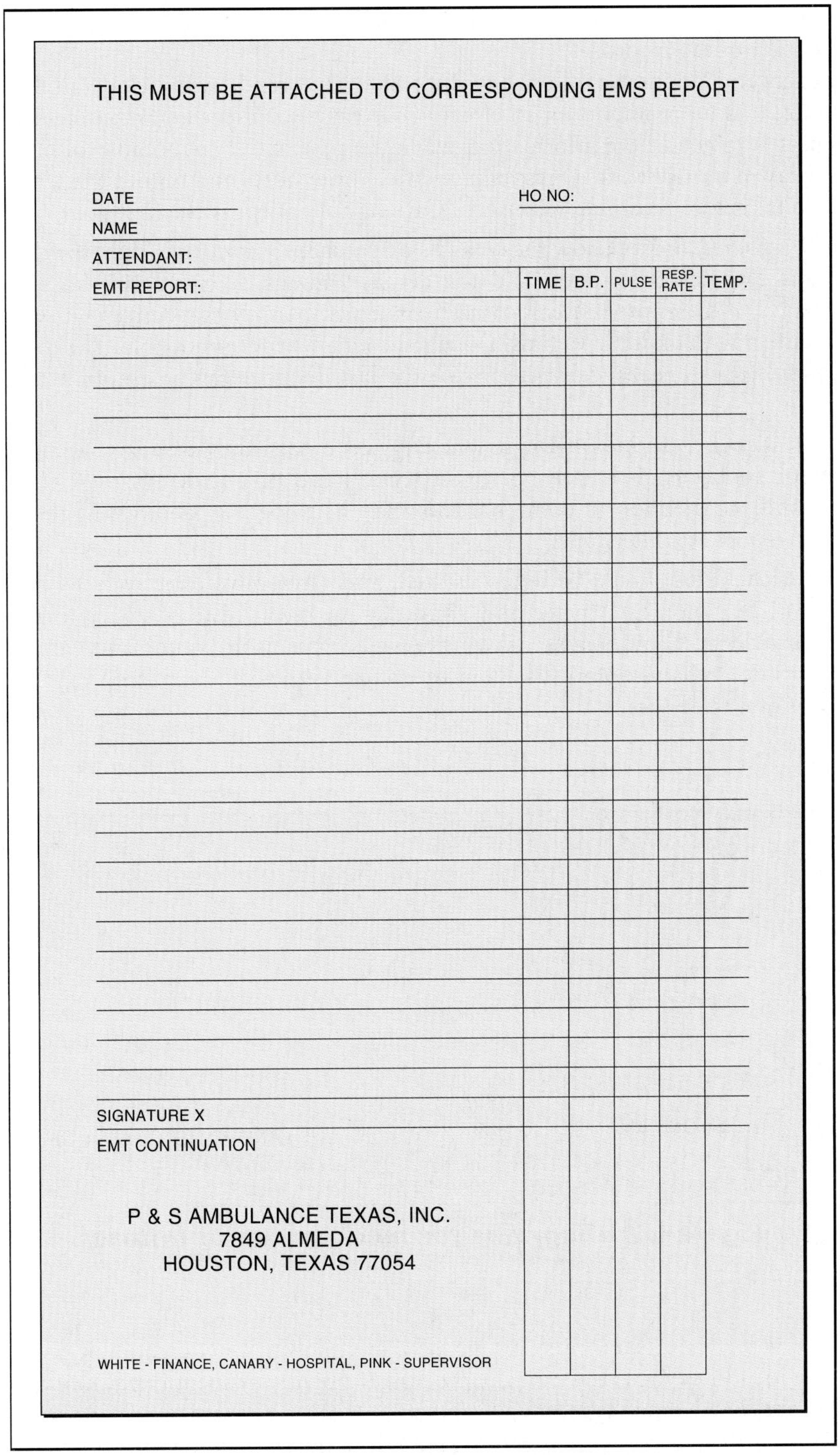

THIS MUST BE ATTACHED TO CORRESPONDING EMS REPORT

DATE _____   HO NO: _____

NAME _____

ATTENDANT: _____

EMT REPORT:	TIME	B.P.	PULSE	RESP. RATE	TEMP.

SIGNATURE X

EMT CONTINUATION

P & S AMBULANCE TEXAS, INC.
7849 ALMEDA
HOUSTON, TEXAS 77054

WHITE - FINANCE, CANARY - HOSPITAL, PINK - SUPERVISOR

Figure C-1 *Example of a continuation sheet.*

but length does not necessarily reflect accuracy or relevancy. The report should document relevant events and discrepancies, and should be written so another reader can reconstruct the events. The report should also justify the action, even if one's impression at the time was wrong. A "mistake" may have been entirely justified given the circumstances at the time, but that mistake can be justified only if the circumstances are clearly and honestly documented as part of the record.

The report contains the following information, but rarely will include all the information. In fact, it is more important to effectively treat the patient and document that treatment than it is to get all the information while the patient suffers because of lack of treatment or delay in transport. It is reasonable to take brief notes and fill out the written report at the hospital before returning to service. Care of the patient is the first goal.

1. *Run Call:* Note how the call was dispatched, particularly if there is discrepancy between the dispatch description and the actual findings. It is helpful, for example, to explain delays in transport if a call came in as a sick party when actually it was a motor vehicle accident with multiple victims. Document time whenever possible. The dispatch time is important because, realistically, it may be the last documented time until arriving at the hospital.

2. *Scene Description:* Document any scene hazards that delay or affect patient treatment or transport. It is easy to forget scene hazards, but delays may affect patient outcomes and the mention of scene hazards may help jog the memory of the run when reading the report at a later time.

The mechanisms should be noted as well, and often most effectively by stick figures (see Figure C-2). You are often the only source of the mechanism of injury for subsequent treatment providers. Clear, simple drawings of mechanisms are quick and easy, useful for communicating mechanism and suspicion of occult injuries, and can help jog the memory of the event at a later time.

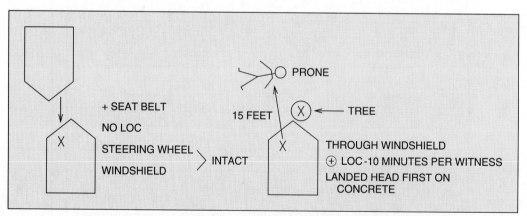

Figure C-2 *Diagrams for mechanisms of injuries.*

3. *Chief Complaint:* Record age, sex, mechanism, chief complaint or injury, and time. These identifiers focus the thought process. If previously mentioned, mechanism does not have to be documented here.

4. *History of the Present Illness/Injury or Symptoms:* Record relevant positives and negatives. Document any relevant history that you obtain from the patient. If the history does not come from the patient but from another witness, note the source and the specific information from that person, especially when it conflicts with other history.

Additional useful information includes the patient's recollection of the events immediately prior to the accident (e.g., did the patient faint first and then fall?), prior injuries to the same location (e.g., fractured the same leg last year), and any treatment prior to your arrival (e.g., patient pulled from car by bystanders).

5. *Past Medical History:* Record previous illness, medications, recent surgery, allergies, and when the patient last ate. You are usually not responsible for getting a complete medical history. However, in acutely sick and injured victims, you may be the last person able to get this information before the patient loses consciousness. Again, treating the patient is the most important priority, but a little bit of useful information may save a lot of complications.

Other information that can be useful may include relevant family history (any diseases that run in the family) and social history (use of alcohol, tobacco, or other drugs).

This should be documented as the SAMPLE history:

> S—symptoms
>
> A—allergies
>
> M—medications
>
> P—past medical history (other illnesses)
>
> L—last meal
>
> E—events preceding accident

6. *Physical Exam:* Record appearance, vital signs, level of consciousness, primary survey, and secondary survey. A general statement of the appearance helps focus the reader on urgencies (e.g., the patient appeared alert and in no distress, or appeared in extreme pain and was ashen and short of breath). The level of consciousness should be documented with the vital signs. This is best done using stimulus and response (responds to voice/pain with moan, decerebrate posturing). The best method is to note the stimulus that provokes a response or the AVPU method:

> A—alert
>
> V—responds to verbal stimuli
>
> P—responds to pain
>
> U—unresponsive

Document that a complete exam was done. Simply stating the body part (back, abdomen, upper extremity) with a zero or slash afterward can be used to indicate the part was examined and there were no significant findings.

One of the easiest and best ways to document the exam in a seriously injured patient is to sequentially note the findings and procedures as one did the primary and secondary survey. It can be helpful to write "Primary Survey," note findings, describe the resuscitation, then start the rest of the exam with "Secondary Survey." By doing this, anyone reviewing the record should immediately recognize that you are oriented to trauma assessment, and by assumption, have performed an organized primary survey.

One picture is worth a thousand words and may aid the memory at a later date. Diagrams of injuries for locations or for severity (like cuts) should be simple yet contain enough detail to locate site of injury, that is, identify if it is right or left, volar (palmar) or dorsal, part of an extremity, or front or back trunk (see Figure C-3).

7. *Procedures (Indication, Procedure, Result):* Document the need, describe the procedure, and note the time and patient response when performing an invasive procedure. Any procedure potentially can have a harmful effect, sometimes delayed, so all procedures should be documented You should document the need, the confirming evidence, the procedure, and the effect—even if the effect is a negative result.

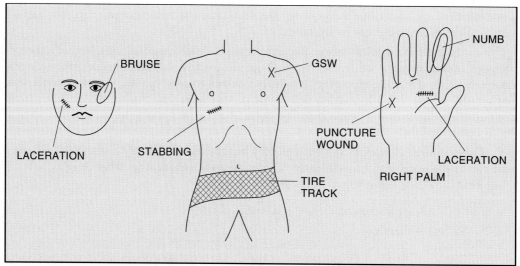

Figure C-3 *Diagrams of injuries.*

Example

Properly Documented Prehospital Procedure

The patient had a laceration of the right upper arm with evidence of excessive blood loss. The patient was pale, sweaty, and confused. Blood pressure was 40mmHg systolic. The bleeding was controlled by direct pressure and the PASG was applied and inflated. The patient's blood pressure increased to 80/50 and he became more alert.

8. *Reassessment Survey (recheck, changes, condition on arrival):* Documenting the initial findings establishes a baseline, but reassessment during long transports, changes while the patient is still in your care, and condition on or just prior to arrival should be recorded as necessary to establish that decompensation did not occur while in your care. It is important to remember that as soon as the patient arrives, other people will perform an exam and record their findings. Any discrepancies or findings documented in their report will be presumed to have occurred while in your care unless documented by you as having existed prior to your intervention. The burden for documentation is then on you to show that complications did not occur while in transport but at the scene prior to your arrival. This is not to suggest that patients will not decompensate while in your care, but you should notice such decompensation and document that you responded to it.

9. *Impression:* Your impression may be included to summarize the significant findings. However, care must be taken not to overdiagnose. A tender forearm does not necessarily mean fracture any more than shortness of breath must mean a tension pneumothorax. Impressions should be as "generic" as possible, noting the actual finding, such as pain or bruising (not the diagnosis, such as fracture or "pulmonary contusion") and include relevant information such as distal pulse. Suspicions should be noted:

Shortness of breath, decreased breath sounds on right, and tender right chest. Tender right forearm, possible fracture, sensation/pulse intact

10. *Documenting the Priorities:* The detailed description is designed for the occasion when events allow time for gathering of the information and completion of the secondary survey. There are times when urgent priorities limit the evaluation to treating the immediate complications and the exam never gets past the primary survey. Care of the patient is the first priority. Often the best way to document this is to describe the sequence as it occurs, using the primary and secondary surveys.

Example

Documenting the Priorities (Just the Facts)

Call: Single MVC.

Scene: One victim in roadway, car head-on into pole, patient through windshield supine in roadway.

Diagram: See Figure C-2.

Primary assessment: Midtwenties, unresponsive male, ashen, grunting respiration with contusions to face, neck, and anterior chest. Rapid, thready carotid pulse, absent radial pulse, sucking wound right chest. Abdomen distended, pelvis stable, extremities appeared to have no major injuries.

C-Spine controlled manually, no change in respiration with jaw thrust, chest wound covered. Patient log-rolled onto long board, no obvious back injuries. Loaded and transported.

Reassessment: Patient's right pupil fixed and dilated, left midposition. Respirations remained rapid and shallow. Patient given oxygen and hyperventilated by BVM. Arrived at city hospital in three minutes, patient still with rapid thready carotid pulse.

See Figure C-4.

SUMMARY OF THE NARRATIVE REPORT

1. Run call
2. Scene description
3. Chief complaint
4. History
5. Past medical history
6. Physical exam
7. Procedures
8. Reassessment
9. Impression
10. Priorities

IMPROVING DOCUMENTATION SKILLS

Documentation reflects on the quality of clinical practice. Like clinical care, one can improve skills by practice, as well as by observing the better qualities of others. Some of the following are suggestions to help improve the quality of documentation.

Practice documentation with critique. Have somebody else try and reconstruct the events based on your narrative and evaluate what comments were useful, and what comments were left out. Sometimes the most obvious events are the easiest to forget to document.

Read other's narrative reports and try to reconstruct the events.

Practice anticipating problems and criticisms. A fractured bone needs to have distal pulse and sensation checked and documented. Invasive procedures, complications, unusual events, or anticipated patient complaints can be noted and justification written. Many complications of invasive procedures, such as infections, may not be discovered for days or weeks. Anticipation of these delayed complications can be an important part of the documentation process.

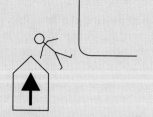

CALL: INJURED PARTY 10:15 A.M.

SCENE: AUTO-PEDESTRIAN   DIAGRAM:
        SINGLE PATIENT KNOCKED DOWN (NOT THROWN
ANY DISTANCE) AND PULLED FROM THE STREET PRIOR
TO ARRIVAL BY BYSTANDERS. PATIENT LAYING ON
SIDEWALK ON ARRIVAL.

CC: MID-TEENS MALE COMPLAINING OF PAIN IN THE HEAD AND NECK.

HISTORY:
        PATIENT: DENIES LOSS OF CONSCIOUSNESS. COMPLAINS OF HEAD AND NECK AND
LEFT HIP, BUT NO OTHER INJURIES. DENIES PAIN IN ARMS, LEGS, OR BACK.

        MOTHER: BRIGHT RED HAIR AND LIPSTICK – VERY EXCITED – STATES PATIENT IS
"ALLERGIC TO "EVERYTHING," DID NOT SEE ACCIDENT.

        DRIVER: STATES PATIENT STEPPED OUT AND KNOCKED DOWN – NOT THROWN –
AND NOT KNOCKED OUT.

PMH: PATIENT: NO MEDIAL PROBLEMS, NO MEDICATIONS OR SURGERY, AND NEVER
BEEN HOSPITALIZED. THINKS HE IS ALLERGIC TO PENICILLIN AND CODEINE.

EXAM: ALERT MALE, SCARED BUT NOT CONFUSED.
        BP 110/70 P 98
HEAD — HEMATOMA RIGHT OCCIPUT, FACE NONTENDER PUPILS EQUAL REACTIVE
NECK — TENDER RIGHT SIDE C-COLLAR AND PLACED ON BACKBOARD
CHEST — NONTENDER BREATH SOUNDS EQUAL
ABD — NONTENDER SOFT
BACK — 0
UP/LOW EXT—00 + DISTAL PULSE AND MOVEMENT

PATIENT TRANSPORTED CODE I TO CITY GENERAL WITH C-COLLAR AND BACKBOARD.

10:25 EN ROUTE — ALERT REPT VS: BP 118/70 P 70

10:30 ARRIVED — PATIENT ALERT, VS UNCHANGED, MOVING ALL EXTREMITIES

IMPRESSION: AUTO-PEDESTRIAN WITH INJURIES HEAD AND LEFT HIP, AND PAIN IN
NECK. NO LOSS OF CONSCIOUSNESS.

Figure C-4 *Example of a completed narrative report.*

Write to remind yourself. If there are specific events unique to this run, or which will help you distinguish this run from other similar runs, note it in the record.

Be professional. People's lives depend on your care. Your records should reflect that you take your responsibility seriously. The medical record is not a place for humorous or derogatory comments. Use caution when describing the patient. Do not use words that could indicate your care was prejudiced by the patient's presentation. Words such as "the patient was hysterical" would be better written as "the patient was very excited and upset."

Be concise. Longer is not necessarily better. If it is of interest, write it down, but get to the point and write what is important.

Review your own records. Can you reconstruct the events and were complications anticipated? Would this record be a friend in court?

Practice quality care including caring for the patient. A patient is a potential adversary or advocate. The excitement of the minute often results in a brusque attitude. Ask yourself if you would have been happy with the way you were treated if you had been the patient.

IMPORTANT POINTS ABOUT THE WRITTEN REPORT

The written report should be kept as a regular part of the patient's record and be considered a legal document. There are some basic rules to follow:

1. Keep the report legible

2. If there are blanks, fill them in. Empty boxes imply that the question was not asked. Open spaces leave the implication that information might be added after the fact.

3. Never alter a medical record. If there is an error on the record, draw a single line through the error and make a note that it was an error and why.

4. The record should be written in a timely manner. Events fade and memory can be challenged. Write the chart as soon as possible after the event. If there is some delay, note the reason.

5. Always be honest on the chart. Never record observations not made. Never try to cover up actions. (We can't always be right, but we must always be honest.) The record, your primary source of support, may be discredited if any of your observations are shown not to be accurate.

6. Always make any changes or addititons to the chart clearly distinguished, timed, and dated. Changes after the fact may be used against you if the appearance is that you were trying to alter the record in your favor. Such alterations give the apearance of lying.

7. What do you do if there is a complication or bad result and you did not record pertinent information on the run report? The best method is to sit down immediately and write, as accurately as possible, the sequence of events using whatever records are available and to the best of your memory. This is not as useful as a document transcribed at the time, but an accurate record even after the fact can be useful at a late date in reconstructing the events.

Appendix D

Trauma Care in the Cold

Jere F. Baldwin,* M.D., F.A.C.E.P., F.A.A.F.P.

*Special warm thanks to Craig Lewis, David Akin, and Shiloh Lightfoot of Fairbanks, Alaska, for their invaluable assistance with this appendix.

On a given evening during the winter of 1994 it was reported that 24 of the United States and all of the Canadian provinces had temperatures below freezing. Thus, for many prehospital EMS providers, special thought needs to be given to the application of BTLS in the cold environment. This appendix will address some of the problems encountered in applying the principles of BTLS in the cold. Although basic principles in the management of the hypothermic trauma patient (core temperature more than 95 degrees Fahrenheit or 35 degrees Celsius) are presented, this material does not pretend to be a treatise on hypothermia.

COLD WEATHER AND THE SIX STAGES OF AN AMBULANCE CALL

Of six stages of an ambulance call that are reviewed in Chapter 2, the *predispatch stage* is the most important in the successful application of the principles of BTLS in the cold environment. Effective cold weather response is heavily dependent on adequate preparation before the emergency. EMS providers living in cold environments have already learned the importance of proper clothing, including hand and foot wear. Likewise, EMS systems operating in cold environments have already learned the importance of maintaining the rescue vehicle, including special tires and the use of engine warming blocks. EMS systems also must develop a system so that the equipment remains at an appropriate temperature for immediate use. Obviously, the best solution is to keep the rescue vehicle in a heated garage.

The *travel to the scene stage* often takes on additional meaning in the winter. The shortest route, because of travel conditions, may not be the quickest or the safest. Several EMS systems have recognized that more than one mode of travel is needed. This may include any combination of helicopter, ambulance, snowmobile or even dog sled.

The *travel to the hospital stage* may be long and arduous for you during winter rescue. The distances may be greater, the travel may be slower, and the vehicle more likely to break down or become stuck. Some EMS systems in North America have developed relay and backup systems for the patient. These relay systems facilitate the transfer of the patient to the nearest appropriate facility by the most appropriate mode of travel. The backup systems include a buddy system to ensure that there is someone aware of the location of the ambulance who can intervene in the event of a breakdown or a loss of communication.

SCENE SURVEY

On-scene trauma assessment in the cold environment starts with the *scene survey*. The hazards may not be apparent; for example, the slippery walk or road under foot or the hidden power line. The total number of victims may not be apparent; you must look for clues to more victims. The essential equipment may need to be slightly different, hydraulic equipment does not work efficiently, batteries last 25% as long, flares last half as long. The phenomena of icy fog and the suspended vehicle exhaust from the rescue vehicles themselves cause decreased visibility. You must constantly reevaluate the safety of the scene, and you need the ability and backup equipment to react appropriately.

Determine the mechanism of injury. Look for clues to hypothermia. Even in a relatively warm 50 degree (10 degrees Celsius) environment, the patient could have hypothermia. Consider this possibility in the aged patient, the stroke victim, or the septic patient who has been lying on the bathroom floor for hours, or the intoxicated patient who has been lying at the foot of the basement stairs for hours. In the outside environment, wet clothing and the wind chill can cause rapid hypothermia in the trauma victim.

PRIMARY TRAUMA SURVEY

The primary trauma survey is even more critical in the cold environment. Evaluation of the airway, C-spine control, and documentation of initial level of consciousness is the same. However, you must consider that the decreased level of consciousness is a result of hypothermia in addition to any trauma or shock. The evaluation of breathing is the same; however, a decreased rate and depth of respiration may be due to hypothermia in addition to head injury or intoxication from alcohol or drugs. The treatment of an inadequate respiratory effort is the same: adequate ventilation with 100% oxygen. If your patient has head injury or shock, hyperventilate with 100% oxygen. If the patient has *isolated hypothermia* ventilate with *warm* humidified oxygen. In this case do not hyperventilate since you should avoid respiratory alkalosis.

The evaluation of the circulation has the same importance as described in Chapter 2; however, the cold environment may make it more difficult to evaluate. Note the rate and quality of the carotid pulse and compare it to the radial pulse. This may take longer than usual because of the vasoconstriction caused by the exposure or because the pulse is slowed by the hypothermic state. It is important not to start chest compressions on the hypothermic patient who simply has a slow weak pulse; the compressions could induce ventricular fibrillation. The examination of the skin color and condition may be nonproductive. Because of the peripheral vasoconstriction, the skin may be pale and cool even when the patient is not hypothermic.

The patient in a cold environment, especially the patient who is thought to be hypothermic, cannot be exposed for a complete examination of the chest, abdomen, pelvis, and extremities. Palpate the patient's chest with your bare hand (covered only with a latex glove) under all the layers of clothing. Palpate for tenderness, instability, and crepitation (TIC) as well as for deformity, abrasions, penetrations, paradoxical movement, burns, lacerations, and swelling. Feel for adequate and symmetric chest wall rise. Your hand is also evaluating the patient's temperature. If the anterior chest underneath the clothing feels in any way cool, then the patient may be hypothermic. You may at this point decide that the patient is suffering from hypothermia in addition to the other injuries you may have found. *Handle the hypothermic patient very gently to prevent a lethal cardiac arrhythmia.* Even if the patient is hypothermic, you must complete the primary survey. Auscultate the lungs, and examine the neck, abdomen, pelvis, and extremities as well as possible. No more than 2 minutes should be spent doing the primary survey in the cold environment, in part to conserve body heat and prevent further heat loss.

CRITICAL INTERVENTIONS AND TRANSPORT DECISION

When the primary survey is complete, enough information is available to decide if the patient is critical or stable. If you find that the patient falls into the "load-and-go" category outlined in Chapter 2, perform critical interventions and package the patient on a wooden or plastic backboard (not metal) and immediately load into an ambulance for transport. If the patient appears stable but is in a cold environment, or if it is cool but the victim is also wet, consider this a "load-and-go" situation. Gently transfer the patient to the warm ambulance for the secondary survey, additional critical care and the reassessment exams. Close the ambulance door quickly to prevent any further heat loss from the vehicle so you can remove the patient's wet clothes soon after loading.

SECONDARY TRAUMA SURVEY

When the weather is cold, you should perform the secondary survey in the ambulance. Remove wet and cold clothing. Down clothing probably should not be cut off in the usual fashion since the heater in the ambulance will blow the feathers into the patient's wounds and the EMS equipment. Begin to rewarm the patient by both passive external rewarming with dry blankets in the warm ambulance and by core rewarming with warm (100 degrees Fahrenheit) humidified oxygen. This is usually an adequate method of rewarming for the patient with mild hypothermia (core temperature of 90 degrees Fahrenheit or greater). Do not massage or put hot compresses on the cold extremities. This may block the shivering reflex and may cause an "afterdrop" in core temperature. Rapid warming of the skin abolishes the vasoconstriction allowing the cold blood in the extremities to return to the core causing a further lowering ("afterdrop") of temperature. Perform the secondary survey as described in Chapter 2.

CRITICAL CARE AND REASSESSMENT EXAM

Critical care is usually performed in the ambulance during transfer. Not only is this advantageous for the patient, but also your warm hands are better able to provide the care. Provide the patient with warm humidified oxygen in the ambulance; the plastic humidifier bottle can be filled with saline warmed to about 45–55 degrees Celsius (80–100 degrees Fahrenheit). But in 1994 there are no warming units that operate on the DC voltage of the ambulance. You can carry heated saline or water in a thermos. Perform frequent reassessment surveys during transport. Especially watch the pulse, blood pressure, and the cardiac rhythm. The mildly hypothermic patient will often have muscle artifact (sometimes from the shivering), there may be sinus bradycardia, there may be a J or Osborne wave immediately after the QRS complex, or there may be atrial fibrillation. At 82.4 degrees Fahrenheit (28 degrees Celsius) core body temperature, there may be ventricular fibrillation that is unresponsive to defibrillation, and below 69.8 degrees (21 degrees Celsius), there may be asystole. The abdomen needs to be examined frequently. Your initial assessment may miss an abdominal catastrophe in the hypothermic patient. You should also frequently check and record the neurologic exam.

CONTACTING MEDICAL DIRECTION

If your patient is hypothermic, it is extremely important to contact Medical Direction early. Even though it may take considerable time to arrive at the nearest appropriate medical facility, the facility needs time to assemble the proper trauma team or to arrange for more expeditious transfer to another facility. Medical Direction needs to know how long the patient was exposed to the cold and what is the patient's core body temperature. Remember that axillary and skin temperatures are not closely correlated with core body temperature in the cold environment. The oral temperature is inaccurate at temperatures below 96 degrees. A tympanic membrane thermometer is the most practical method to take an accurate core temperature in the ambulance.

SUMMARY

The application of the principles of BTLS in the cold is challenging and rewarding. You need a thorough understanding of the principles of BTLS, and a knowledge of the conditions and limitations imposed by the cold environment. You must also always be aware of the possibility of your patient being hypothermic. The signs and symptoms of hypothermia are listed in Figure D-1. This chapter has described how the presence of a cold environment and/or the existence of hypothermia changes the application of the principles of BTLS.

NEUROMUSCULAR SYSTEM

AMNESIA, DYSARTHRIA, POOR JUDGMENT (34 DEGREES CELSIUS)
LOSS OF COORDINATION APPEARING "DRUNK" (33 DEGREES CELSIUS)
SHIVERING CEASES (32 DEGREES CELSIUS)
PROGRESSIVE DECREASE IN LEVEL OF CONSCIOUSNESS (29 DEGREES CELSIUS)
PUPILS DILATED (29 DEGREES CELSIUS)
LOSS OF DEEP TENDON REFLEXES (27 DEGREES CELSIUS)

GASTROINTESTINAL SYSTEM

ILEUS

RESPIRATORY SYSTEM

INITIAL HYPERVENTILATION (34 DEGREES CELSIUS)
PROGRESSIVE DECREASE IN RATE AND DEPTH OF RESPIRATION (<34 DEGREES CELSIUS)
NONCARDIAC PULMONARY EDEMA (25 DEGREES CELSIUS)

CARDIOVASCULAR SYSTEM

SINUS BRADYCARDIA
ATRIAL FIBRILLATION (30 DEGREES CELSIUS)
PROGRESSIVE DECREASE IN BLOOD PRESSURE (29 DEGREES CELSIUS)
PROGRESSIVE DECREASE IN PULSE (29 DEGREES CELSIUS)
VENTRICULAR IRRITABILITY (28 DEGREES CELSIUS)
HYPOTENSION (24 DEGREES CELSIUS)

KIDNEYS, BLOOD, ELECTROLYTES

COLD DIURESIS LEADING TO HYPOVOLEMIA AND HEMOCONCENTRATION
LACTIC ACIDOSIS AND HYPERGLYCEMIA

Figure D-1 *Signs and symptoms of hypothermia.*

BIBLIOGRAPHY

1. Auerback, P. S., and E. C. Geehr, *Management of Wilderness and Environmental Emergencies*, 2nd ed. St. Louis, MO: C. V. Mosby, 1989.

2. Hector, M. G. "Treatment of Accidental Hypothermia" *American Family Physician*, Vol. 45, no. 2 (1992), pp. 785–792.

Appendix E

Role of the Air Medical Helicopter

Russell B. Bieniek, M.D., F.A.C.E.P.

Air medical helicopters were used extensively to transport injured servicemen during the military conflicts of Korea and Vietnam. On October 12, 1972, Flight for Life, the first hospital-based civilian air medical helicopter service went into operation at St. Anthony Hospital in Denver, Colorado. In the years following this, similar programs were established at multiple hospitals and various other organizations across the United States. In 1993, there were approximately 178 air medical helicopter programs, utilizing 231 helicopters and transporting 125,000 patients per year. The structure and role of these air medical programs vary tremendously, as does their integration with the local EMS system and involvement in trauma care.

The sponsoring agency and organizational structure of an air medical service encompass a wide range of models. They may be military or other government service—federal, state, or local—that may be independent or work in cooperation with local medical care providers to provide rescue and/or transportation of injured patients. The crews may be on-call and/or the helicopter may need to be reconfigured or additional equipment brought on board. The other end of the spectrum is the fully dedicated medical helicopter that flies only critically injured or ill patients, where the aircraft's interior is specifically designed and configured, always medically staffed and consistently available for a medical mission.

The role may be one of primary interfacility transport (hospital to hospital), scene transport (field to hospital), or as is most frequently the case, a combination of the two with varying percentages of each type. The involvement that an air medical service may have in the local EMS community may depend on its percentage of scene involvement.

The type of patient a service transports is usually a mixture of medical classes. However, it may be only a specific specialty type. Examples of the various types are neonatal, pediatric, cardiac, maternal, medical, and trauma. The service may transport all patients, they may limit their transports to specific types of patients, or they may have specific teams that accompany each medical class of patients. The medical crew on board also varies with the specific program. A survey in 1993 showed that 98% of air medical helicopter programs utilized two medical attendants and 2% utilized one. The two medical crew members' credentials varied widely. They may be at the level of an emergency medical technician (EMT, various levels), respiratory therapist, paramedic, nurse, and/or physician. The two attendant crews are comprised as follows: 71% RN/paramedic, 21% RN/RN, 3% RN/physician, 2% RN/other, and 3% other/combinations. (See *The Journal of Air Medical Transport*, reference 3.) The makeup of the crew may also be determined by the type of medical mission to which the helicopter is dedicated.

If an air medical service is available in your region, it is important that you become acquainted with them and know in advance what type of cases on which they will be utilized. You will also need to know how to access them and involve them in your system to improve patient care.

Multiple factors influence the availability of an air medical helicopter. These are scheduled maintenance, mechanical, weather, and being committed on a previous mission. This resource can be very beneficial to the EMS service and the patient, but there shouldn't be dependence on it. They may not be able to respond or have to cancel en route. Contingency plans must always be in place.

Regarding safety, there needs to be prior education and training with the air medical service. This education would entail learning proper communications between ground and air, picking and describing a safe landing zone, and coordinating unloading and loading of the aircraft. In the uncommon, but possible, event of an accident, correct knowledge of the helicopter's equipment and access could be vital to crew and ground personnel. Safety must always be the first concern, as in your BTLS training: "Is the scene safe?"

THE AIR MEDICAL HELICOPTER AND THE TRAUMA PATIENT

Caring for the trauma patient can be extremely challenging; however, quite rewarding to you and patient if all the components are in place and things are done properly. As an established component and resource to an EMS service, the air medical helicopter can improve patient outcome by providing assistance in two areas. The first is speed of transportation; the second is the introduction of a higher level of clinical expertise, equipment, or procedures at the scene or en route to the hospital.

Helicopters obviously are able to transport patients quicker than ground units over long distances. This involves their ability to travel at high speeds and in a straight line. Also they do not have to fight road conditions, either environmental or traffic. This decreases the exposure of the general public or the caregivers themselves to the potential dangers of an ambulance rushing through busy streets with other traffic and pedestrians.

In many areas of the United States, the only care available at an accident scene is basic life support (BLS). An air medical helicopter would then be able to provide advanced life support (ALS) assessment and care at the scene and en route to the hospital. Often even in areas where ALS is available, the air medical crew may be able to provide additional expertise, skills, and/or equipment. Some of these may include, but not be limited to, needle or surgical cricothyroidotomy, needle or tube thoracostomy, intraosseus needle insertion, pericardiocentesis, and various medications for such things as sedation and chemical paralysis of the head-injured patient for control of the airway and to assist in controlling increased intracranial pressure. Additional equipment might include pulse oximetry, end-tidal CO_2 monitors, positive pressure ventilators, and Doppler-assisted blood pressure monitoring devices, to mention a few. Many services also carry packed red blood cells for initiation in the field. The air medical service personnel also usually handle a higher volume of critically injured trauma patients than the average provider in a rural ground system, so they may exhibit greater familiarity and comfort in working with these patients.

For interfacility transports, the patient is evaluated by the nursing and physician staff at the referring hospital, who determine whether the patient requires additional evaluation and/or treatment at a facility with more resources available to handle the serious trauma patient. The air medical helicopter provides the vehicle, crew, and speed necessary for accomplishing a continuum of the critical care environment.

BTLS AND AIR MEDICAL HELICOPTER

Basic trauma life support (BTLS) provides for a common language that can be used through the continuum of care for the seriously injured trauma patient. This would require coordinated education and training in a region and possibly could be an educational program offered by the air medical service. Trauma patients would then be assessed rapidly, accurately, and completely in the field by the prehospital providers, and the decision scheme that is developed for the region on utilizing the air medical service could be partly based on the results of this assessment, other specific trauma scores, types of injuries, and mechanism of injury. The air medical service would then understand the assessment and initial treatment that was done prior to their arrival, and the report could be accomplished quickly. The helicopter medical crew can then quickly do their BTLS assessment and begin transport with further treatments if necessary.

You must constantly evaluate your skills at doing a rapid assessment of the trauma patient. When you turn your patient over to another service for transport such as an air medical service, you will not get immediate feedback regarding the outcome of the patient, as you do when you deliver the patient to the hospital yourself. The air medical service may serve as a link between you and the hospital to assist in obtaining this important information. When cases are reviewed, the BTLS assessment and initial management can be used as a standard to compare with the actual care given.

SUMMARY

Air medical helicopter services are one of many special tools available to you and the hospital. As with all tools there needs to be initial and continued education and training to insure proper and safe usage. This will improve the resources in your service area and help achieve everyone's common goal of improved patient outcome.

BIBLIOGRAPHY

1. "Mid-Year Report and Fleet Survey." *The Journal of Air Medical Transport,* Vol. 11, no. 7 (1992).

2. "1993 Program Survey." *The Journal of Air Medical Transport,* Vol. 12, no. 9 (1993), p. 306.

3. Walters, E. "Program Profile, 20 Years of Service." *The Journal of Air Medical Transport,* Vol. 11, no. 9 (1992).

Appendix F

Trauma Scoring in the Prehospital Care Setting

Leah J. Heimbach, J.D., R.N., NREMT-P

Trauma scoring systems consist of assigning a numerical rating or score to various clinical signs, such as vital signs or response to pain. They are used to assess the severity of injury and are especially valuable in assessment of the multiple-injured trauma patient. Trauma scoring systems have important uses in trauma systems at all levels, including the hospital setting and the prehospital setting and in overall health care system analysis. There are several methods of scoring severity of injury in trauma patients, including the *Glasgow Coma Scale* and the *Revised Trauma Score* (see Table F-1 and F-2).

In the hospital setting, trauma scoring systems have several uses, including

1. Standardizing triage between health care facilities (deciding when it is appropriate to transfer a patient to a trauma center)

2. Allocating medical resources

3. Evaluating the health care facility's overall effectiveness in providing patient care

4. Conducting audits (making sure that patients who are predicted to survive their traumatic event actually do survive)

5. Predicting morbidity and mortality of patients based on a particular trauma score

Although prehospital care providers should *never* delay transport to complete a trauma score, trauma scoring systems can provide an objective and standardized way for you to triage patients appropriately (including whether a patient should go to a trauma center) and to communicate injury severity, using a common language, to other members of the health care team. Trauma scores recorded in the field are also useful in EMS systems analysis and research. This analysis can then be used to develop protocols for prehospital care to meet the needs of a specific EMS region. The BTLS patient assessment includes a neurological assessment, using the AVPU method (alert, responds to verbal stimulus, responds to painful stimulus, and unresponsive), and identifies parameters to determine whether or not the patient is a "load and go." Communicating this information along with a list of the patient's injuries to the receiving hospital will allow the hospital personnel to gather the necessary resources to optimize care.

The use of trauma scores in the prehospital setting can be confusing at a time when patient assessment, injury management, and communication to the receiving hospital need to be concise. It is recommended that you report the following information to the receiving facility:

1. Age, sex, and chief complaint

2. Mechanism of injury

3. Level of consciousness

4. What parameters lead to the "load-and-go" decision

5. A list of the patient's injuries
6. What treatment was rendered
7. The patient's response to treatment

EYE OPENING		MOTOR RESPONSE	
SPONTANEOUS	4	OBEYS COMMAND	6
TO VOICE	3	LOCALIZES PAIN	5
TO PAIN	2	WITHDRAW (PAIN)	4
NONE	1	FLEXION (PAIN)	3
		EXTENSION (PAIN)	2
VERBAL RESPONSE		NONE	1
ORIENTED	5		
CONFUSED	4		
INAPPROPRIATE WORDS	3		
INCOMPREHENSIBLE WORDS	2		
NONE	1		

Table F-1 *Glascow Coma Scale*

SCORE	SCORE	CONTRIBUTION TO REVISED TRAUMA
TOTAL GLASCOW	13-15	4
COMA SCORE	9-12	3
(SEE COMPONENTS BELOW)	6–8	2
	4–5	1
	3	0
EYE OPENING SPONTANEOUS = 4 TO VOICE = 3 TO PAIN = 2 NONE = 1		
VERBAL RESPONSE ORIENTED = 5 CONFUSED = 4 INAPPROPRIATE WORDS = 3 INCOMPREHENSIBLE WORDS = 2 NONE = 1		
MOTOR RESPONSE OBEYS COMMAND = 6 LOCALIZES PAIN = 5 WITHDRAW (PAIN) = 4 FLEXION (PAIN) = 3 EXTENSION (PAIN) = 2 NONE = 1		
SYSTOLIC BP (MM HG)	>89	4
	76–89	3
	50–75	2
	1–49	1
	NONE	0
RESPIRATIONS (PER MINUTE)	10—29	4
	>29	3
	6–9	2
	1–5	1
	NONE	0

Table F-2 *Revised Trauma Score*

NOTE: IF TOTAL SCORE IS 11 OR LESS, THE PATIENT SHOULD BE TAKEN TO A TRAUMA CENTER.

Many EMS regions will require the use of some type of trauma score system in the prehospital setting to facilitate patient care and/or to promote prehospital research. Examples of some of the current trauma scores that are utilized in the prehospital and hospital setting follows, including one that has been modified for use in pediatric trauma patients (see Table F-3).

	+2	+1	-1
WEIGHT	>44 LB (>20 KG)	22–44 LB (10–20 KG)	<22 LB (<10 KG)
AIRWAY	NORMAL	ORAL OR NASAL AIRWAY	INTUBATED OR TRACHEOSTOMY
BLOOD PRESSURE	PULSE AT WRIST	CAROTID OR FEMORAL PULSE PALPABLE	NO PALPABLE PULSES
LEVEL OF CONSCIOUSNESS	COMPLETELY AWAKE	OBTUNDED OR ANY DECREASED LOC	COMATOSE
SKIN	NO EVIDENCE OF TRAUMA	ABRASION OR MINOR INJURY	PENETRATION OR MAJOR AVULSION OR LACERATION
FRACTURE	NONE	CLOSED FRACTURE	OPEN OR MULTIPLE FRACTURES

Table F-3 *Pediatric Trauma Score*
NOTE: IF TOTAL SCORE IS 8 OR LESS, THE CHILD SHOULD BE TAKEN TO A TRAUMA CENTER

BIBLIOGRAPHY

1. Champion, H. R., and others. "A Revision of the Trauma Score." *Journal of Trauma* Vol. 29: (1989), p. 623.
2. Tepas, T. A., "Pediatric Trauma Score." *Journal of Pediatric Surgery* Vol. 22: (1987), p. 14.

Appendix G

Drowning, Barotrauma, and Decompression Injury

James H. Creel, Jr., M.D., F.A.C.E.P., and John E. Campbell, M.D., F.A.C.E.P

DROWNING

Approximately 7000 people drown annually, making drowning the third leading cause of accidental death in the United States. Freshwater drownings are more common than salt-water drownings, and there are more immersion accidents in pools than in lakes, ponds, and rivers. The peak incidence occurs in the warm months and most commonly involves teenagers and children under the age of 4.

Drowning is death from suffocation after submersion in the water. There are two basic mechanisms:

1. Breath holding, which leads to aspiration of water and wet lungs

2. Laryngospasm with glottic closure and dry lungs

Both these mechanisms lead to profound hypoxia and death. With the aspiration of at least 22 cc per kilogram of seawater (which is hypertonic to the plasma), fluid is drawn into the alveoli from the circulation. Aspiration of at least 22 cc per kilogram of freshwater (which is hypotonic to the plasma) causes fluid to be absorbed across the alveoli into the circulation. These are of no concern in the prehospital phase. Survival of the victim depends on your rapid evaluation and management of the ABCs.

Initiate management as soon as possible. Be aware of surfing/ diving mechanisms that indicate potential occult C-spine injury. Protect the cervical spine during rescue of the patient. In water, CPR is generally ineffective. Remove the patient to a stable surface as soon as possible; then initiate CPR and appropriate protocol. In cases where hypothermia is responsible for the near-drowning, it appears to provide the brain, heart, and lungs some degree of protection (diving reflex) by slowing the metabolism. Therefore, no one is dead until warm and dead; do not stop CPR.

BAROTRAUMA

Barotrauma refers to injuries due to the mechanical effects of pressure on the body. We all live "under pressure" since the weight of the air in which we live exerts force on our body. At sea level the weight of air pressing on the body equals 14.7 pounds per square inch (psi). Since solids and liquids are not compressible, they are not usually affected by pressure changes. The study of barotrauma is the study of the effect of pressure on gas-filled organs of the body. Gas-filled organs are ears, sinuses, upper and lower airways, stomach, and intestines.

To understand the effects of pressure changes, you must know some properties of gases. Boyle's law states that the volume of a gas is inversely proportional to the pressure applied to it. This simply means that if you double the pressure on a gas, the volume of the gas will decrease by one-half. If you halve the pressure on a gas the volume will double. The pressure at sea level is called one atmosphere absolute (ATA). If you go up in an airplane (or climb a mountain), you have less atmosphere above you; thus the pressure decreases and the gas inside the body expands. Most commercial airliners fly at about 35,000 feet elevation (one-fifth ATA or gas volume 5 times normal) but are pressurized to a cabin pressure equal to 5,000 to 8,000 feet elevation (two-thirds to three-fourths ATA) so that gas expands to only about 1.2 to 1.4 times its original volume. Airline passengers notice no change except for "popping" of the ears as the expanding gas in the middle ears vents off through the eustachian tubes into the pharynx.

Water is much heavier than air. When one descends into salt water there is a change of one atmosphere for every 33 feet of depth (34 ft for fresh water). This means that at 33 feet of depth the body is subjected to two ATA and gas in the body has been compressed to one-half of its original volume. Because of the pressures involved, divers are exposed to certain potential injuries during both descent and ascent.

TRAUMA OF DESCENT: "MIDDLE EAR SQUEEZE"

Since there is a large pressure change during the first few feet of a dive, skin divers and snorkelers as well as scuba divers are subject to this type of injury. Let's say that a skin diver takes a breath and rapidly descends to a depth of 33 feet, all the gas in your body will decrease in volume by one-half. This includes gas in the lungs, intestines, stomach, sinuses, and middle ears. The elastic lungs, intestines, and stomach will simply decrease in size to match the volume of gas. Problems develop with the middle ears and sinuses if the pressure cannot be equalized. The sinuses (air pockets in the bones of the face and skull) each have an opening through which air from the pharynx can enter to equalize the pressure. If the openings are blocked, the skin diver will experience pain in the sinuses and may even develop bleeding and inflammation (barosinusitis). Other than the discomfort, this causes no serious problem. Each middle ear has an opening, the eustachian tube, through which air from the pharynx can enter to equalize pressure. If the eustachian tube is blocked (mucosal congestion from allergy, infection, etc.), the pressure will push in on the eardrum and cause intense pain. This begins to be noticeable at a depth of 4–5 feet. If the diver cannot equalize the middle ear pressure and yet continues to descend, the pressure will eventually rupture the eardrum and flood the middle ear with cold water (even the warm waters of the Caribbean are 20 degrees below body temperature). Cold water in the middle ear causes dizziness, nausea, vomiting, and disorientation ("twirly bends"). The result can be panic and drowning or near-drowning. The diver surface rapidly and develop air embolism or neurologic decompression sickness. Vomiting under water can cause aspiration and drowning.

Barotitis media (middle ear squeeze) requires no prehospital treatment. The pressure is relieved when the diver returns to the surface. If there is hearing loss or continued ear pain, the diver should see a physician for treatment of ruptured eardrum or bleeding into the middle ear. The conditions that you are more likely to have to manage are the near-drowning cases caused by the disorientation from water in the middle ears.

TRAUMA OF ASCENT

Injuries from expanding gas can occur as divers ascend. These injuries are much more common in scuba divers since such injuries usually either require some time to develop (longer than a skin diver can hold his breath) or require the breathing of compressed air.

1. *Reverse Middle Ear Squeeze:* If a eustachian tube becomes blocked during a dive, the gas in the middle ear will expand and cause pain during ascent. If there is enough expansion, the eardrum can rupture, with all the symptoms and dangers mentioned previously.

2. *Gastrointestinal Barotrauma:* If the diver swallows air while breathing compressed air or if the diver has previously eaten gas-forming foods (e.g., beans), he/she may accumulate a significant amount of stomach or intestinal gas during a dive. If he/she was at a depth of 66 feet, the gas will expand to three times its original volume during ascent. If he/she is unable to expel this gas, he/she will develop abdominal pain and occasionally even collapse and develop a shocklike state.

3. *Pulmonary Overpressurization Syndromes (Burst Lung):* These occur only in divers who have been breathing compressed air. During a dive the lungs are completely filled with air, which is at a pressure equal to the depth at which the diver is swimming. If a diver panics and surfaces without exhaling, the rapidly expanding gas will overinflate the lungs and cause one of the three overpressurization syndromes listed below. Remember, the total volume of the lungs is about 6 L. An ascent from 33 feet would cause expansion to 12 L; 66 feet, 18 L; and 100 feet, 24 L. It is easy to see how delicate alveoli can be ruptured by this expansion. The expanding air will dissect into the interstitial space, pleural space, pulmonary venules, or a combination of the three.

a. *Air in the Interstitial Space.* This is the most common form of pulmonary overpressurization syndrome. As millions of tiny air bubbles escape into the interstitial tissue, they may dissect into the mediastinum and up into the subcutaneous tissue of the neck. Symptoms may develop immediately upon surfacing or may not develop for several hours. The diver may have increasing hoarseness, chest pain, subcutaneous emphysema in the neck, and difficulty breathing and swallowing. Any diver with these symptoms should get oxygen (no positive pressure ventilations unless the diver is apneic) and transport to the hospital. While interstitial air does not require treatment with a recompression chamber (hyperbaric chamber), these patients often develop air embolism or decompression sickness. They should be observed in a facility that is capable of providing recompression treatment if necessary.

b. *Air in the Pleural Space.* If the alveoli rupture into the pleural space a pneumothorax and possibly a hemothorax will develop. The amount of pneumothorax will depend on how much air escaped into the pleural space and how far the diver surfaced after the air entered the pleural space. A 10% pneumothorax at 33 feet will be a 20% pneumothorax at the surface. A 20 to 30% pneumothorax at 33 feet may be a tension pneumothorax at the surface. The symptoms will be the same as for interstitial air except the diver will now have decreased breath sounds and hyperresonance to percussion on the affected side (may be on both sides). A tension pneumothorax will also have distended neck veins and shock (and possibly tracheal deviation—a late sign). These patients may require a needle decompression if they have a tension pneumothorax. Otherwise give 100% oxygen and transport immediately.

c. *Air Embolism.* The most serious syndrome of overpressurization is pulmonary air embolism. If the overdistended alveoli rupture into the pulmonary venules, the millions of tiny air bubbles can return to the left side of the heart and then up the carotid arteries to the small arterioles of the brain. These bubbles, composed mostly of nitrogen, obstruct the arterioles and produce symptoms similar to a stroke. The symptoms produced depend on which vessels are obstructed. There will usually be loss of consciousness and focal neurological signs. The symptoms almost always occur *immediately* when the diver surfaces. This is a very important point in differentiating air embolism from decompression sickness (which usually takes hours to develop). The patient should be placed in Trendelenburg's position (30 degrees head down) on the left side, given 100% oxygen, and transported to a facility that can provide recompression treatment. The left-side, head-down position prevents further embolism of air to the brain and helps distend the vessels, thus allowing small bubbles to pass through and return to the lungs where they can be eliminated. This is one instance where you should not hyperventilate or give positive pressure ventilations. Hyperventilation causes vasoconstriction, which will trap the bubbles. Positive pressure ventilation may force more air into the veins, worsening the injury (if the patient is not breathing you must give positive pressure ventilation). This patient must have immediate recompression in a recompression chamber no matter how much time has passed since the injury and no matter how far away the recompression chamber may be. In a recompression chamber, the pressure is raised to 6 ATA, which will decrease the size of the bubbles to 1/6 of their previous volume. This may allow them to pass through the capillaries back to the lungs to be expelled. Air embolism may rarely affect the coronary arteries causing myocardial infarction, dysrhythmias, or cardiac arrest.

DECOMPRESSION ILLNESS

Decompression illness is caused by another property of gases. Henry's law states that the amount of gas disssolved in a liquid is directly proportional to the pressure applied. This means that twice as much gas would be dissolved in a liquid at 33 feet as at sea level. It also means that gas dissolved in a liquid at 33 feet will come out of solution as that liquid ascends. This is analogous to a sealed bottle of carbonated beverage that has no bubbles as long as it is sealed but bubbles the instant the cap is removed and the pressure is released.

Nitrogen, which accounts for about 80% of the volume of inspired air, is an inert gas that dissolves in blood and fat. When a diver is under water, nitrogen dissolves in the blood and fat tissue. This nitrogen is released as he surfaces so he must surface slowly enough to allow this nitrogen to be expelled through the lungs. The U.S. Navy has developed a set of tables of no-decompression limits that give general guidelines about how long one can stay at a certain depth without going through stage decompression during ascent. There are also standard air decompression tables for those dives that exceed the no-decompression limit. Theoretically, if one follows the recommendations of the tables, nitrogen bubbles will not form in the blood during ascent. This may not always be true because the tables were developed from studying U.S. Navy divers, who are uniformly young, healthy, well-conditioned men who were diving in salt water. Today, 3 million recreational scuba divers and 300,000 new divers are certified each year. Sport divers are not uniformly young, healthy, or conditioned. They are often older, poorly conditioned, and not always healthy. A special problem is obesity. Fat absorbs about five times as much nitrogen as blood or other tissue, so obese divers require longer decompression times or shorter dives. Sport divers should be *very* conservative when using diving tables, especially when diving in fresh water or in lakes above sea level. The greatest danger occurs when a diver who has been submerged for a significant period of time has a diving accident, panics, and surfaces rapidly. Nitrogen bubbles will form in his blood and tissue just as carbon dioxide bubbles form in champagne. This is a different injury from barotrauma or pulmonary overpressurization syndrome and may exist along with any of the barotrauma syndromes. It is frequently seen in divers in near-drowning situations. The symptoms are almost always delayed for minutes to hours after a dive. As a general rule, symptoms that develop within 10 minutes of surfacing are caused by air embolism until proved otherwise. Symptoms developing after 10 minutes are decompression illness until proved otherwise. A special case is the vacationing diver who is asymptomatic after a deep dive and then catches a plane home the same day. This diver may develop symptoms during flight since the cabin pressure is only 2/3 or 3/4 ATA. These symptoms may not appear until the diver has returned home far inland from the site of the dive. All emergency providers should have some knowledge of diving injuries.

TYPE I DECOMPRESSION ILLNESS

1. *Cutaneous ("skin bends"):* Millions of tiny nitrogen bubbles may form in the microvasculature of the skin. This causes a generalized itching rash that may be red and inflamed or mottled with a central purple discoloration. It is called "marbleised skin." This condition requires no treatment but may be an early sign of more serious decompression sickness, so the patient must be observed. Give the patient 100% oxygen and transport to a facility capable of recompression therapy.

2. *Musculoskeletal ("bends" or "pain-only bends"):* This is the most common presentation of decompression sickness. Over 85% of divers with decompression sickness will present with pain in the joints. The shoulders or knees are affected most commonly, but any joint may be affected. The pain is usually deep and aching, and there may be vague numbness around the affected joint. Characteristically, there are no physical findings and the pain may be eased by pressure such as inflating a blood pressure cuff. These patients require recompression therapy no matter how long it has been since the symptoms started and no matter how far the nearest recompression chamber may be.

TYPE II DECOMPRESSION ILLNESS

These syndromes are more serious and may be life threatening. They are emergencies that require rapid diagnosis and treatment.

1. *Pulmonary ("chokes"):* Nitrogen bubbles forming in the vasculature of the lungs cause symptoms like the interstitial pulmonary overpressurization syndrome. The patient will develop cough, chest pain, difficulty breathing, and sometimes hemoptysis. These symptoms usually develop within an hour of surfacing (50%) but may be delayed for up to six hours and even rarely for 24 to 48 hours. Pulmonary overpressurization syndrome usually appears within a few minutes of surfacing. In either case the patient requires oxygen and recompression therapy. Here again, be careful of positive pressure ventilation, as it may cause gas bubble emboli to the brain.

2. *Neurologic:* Nitrogen bubbles in the nervous system may present with any symptom from personality changes to specific localized neurologic changes. By far the most common symptoms involve the lower spinal cord and often produce weakness or paralysis of the legs and urinary bladder. Bladder problems are so common that historically, urinary catheters were considered essential equipment for divers. These patients must have recompression therapy or irreversible paralysis will occur.

MANAGEMENT OF DIVING INJURIES

HISTORY

1. *Type of Diving and Equipment Used.* This is very important. Remember that skin divers and snorkelers cannot get overpressurization syndrome or decompression sickness, but all divers can drown. The treatment for near-drowning is very different from that for decompression sickness or air embolism.

2. *History of the Dive.* You need to know where the dive occurred, at what depth, how many dives, how long on the bottom, and any in-water decompression. This information is also needed for dives during the preceding two days.

3. *Past Medical History.* Pulmonary problems that predispose to air trapping (asthma or obstructive lung disease) are frequently associated with overpressurization syndrome.

4. *Exactly When the Symptoms First Occurred.* This may be helpful in differentiating air embolism and decompression illness.

5. *Complications of the Dive.* Did the diver run out of air? Was there an attack by marine animals? Did a diving accident occur?

6. *Travel After the Dive.* Traveling at higher altitudes may precipitate decompression sickness.

INITIAL MANAGEMENT

1. Follow standard patient assessment protocol: primary survey, critical interventions and transport decision, secondary survey, and reassessment surveys.

2. If there is any chance of overpressurization syndrome or decompression illness, do not hyperventilate or give positive pressure ventilation. Positive pressure ventilation is indicated only for apneic patients.

3. Check for hypothermia (see Appendix D) in all diving accident victims.

4. Patients with air embolism or neurologic decompression sickness should be placed on their left side in the head-down position.

5. All diving accident patients should get oxygen.

6. Shock and other injuries are treated by routine protocols.

7. If a recompression facility is needed and you need information about the one nearest to your facility, you may obtain assistance 24 hours a day through the National Diving Alert Network at Duke University: (919) 684-8111.

SUMMARY

No matter how far you may live from a large body of water, you may be called upon to manage a patient with near-drowning or diving injuries. When treating the near-drowning patient, the performance of the ABCs is most important in the prehospital phase, but don't forget the possibility of hypothermia. When treating barotrauma, you should not only follow the basic principles of BTLS, but also remember the importance of the history, patient positioning, the possibility of hypothermia, and the dangers of positive pressure ventilation.

BIBLIOGRAPHY

1. S. Jeppeson, *Open Water Sport Diving Manual,* 4th ed., pp. 2, 25–49. Engle-wood, Colo.: Jeppeson Sanderson, 1984.

2. Kizer, K. W. "Dysbarism." In *Emergency Medicine,* ed. J. E. Tintinalli, 3rd ed., pp. 678–688. New York: McGraw-Hill, 1992.

Appendix H

Injury Prevention and the Role of the EMS Provider

Steve Hargarten, M.D., M.P.H., and Janet M. Williams, M.D.

THE INJURY EPIDEMIC

Every day prehospital health care providers serve the public by delivering quality emergency care. The BTLS curriculum has been developed to convey the principles of acute prehospital care of the injured patient, and well-trained prehospital care providers with BTLS skills save many lives of injured patients each year. Unfortunately, over 50% of trauma deaths occur immediately after the injury event. As a result, you often arrive at the scene only to find a patient who has died or is dying and for whom no life-saving measures can be taken. These cases illustrate the importance of recognizing injury as a disease which is preventable. Your role extends far beyond the acute care of the injured patient. The entire EMS community must become active in preventing injury from occurring in the first place.

Though underrecognized, injury is a major public health problem worldwide. In the United States injury is the single greatest killer between the ages of 1 and 44 and is responsible for more years of potential life lost than cancer and heart disease combined. In the United States alone, the cost of injury is estimated to be over $180 billion annually.

Injury has been misconceived by the public as being a result of an unavoidable "act of God," an "accident," due to "bad luck," or resulting from a behavioral problem of the injured individual. In reality, injuries are health problems that behave like classic infectious diseases. They may be characterized by demographic distributions, seasonal variations, epidemic episodes, and risk factors, and they are predictable and preventable. An analogy has been made between the cause of injury and the cause of a disease such as malaria. Table H-1 illustrates how disease causation can be applied to both of these entities.

Traditionally, medical education programs have emphasized the treatment of acute injury and have neglected the concept of injury prevention and control. It is interesting that patients presenting with cardiac symptoms are nearly always asked if they have risk factors such as history of smoking, diabetes, hypertension, hypercholesterolemia, and family history of heart disease. In addition, these patients are counseled as to how to reduce their risk for heart disease. As health care providers, we have a responsibility to do the same for injured patients. Besides playing a vital role in the acute care of injured patients, prehospital care providers have a unique opportunity to assess risk factors for injury, to examine patients in the injury setting, to provide valuable injury information to other medical care providers, and to educate the public on injury prevention. In addition, prehospital care providers often see the "near-miss" patient who survives what could have been a fatal injury event. Such circumstances are an opportune time for prehospital care providers to give injury prevention advice.

DISEASE	HOST	AGENT	VECTOR/ VEHICLE	EXPOSURE EVENT
MALARIA	HUMAN	*P. VIVAX*	MOSQUITO	MOSQUITO BITE
INJURY (HEAD INJURY, FOR EXAMPLE)	HUMAN	KINETIC ENERGY	MOTOR VEHICLE	CRASH

Table H-1 *An Etiologic Comparison of Injury and a Classic Infectious Disease*

WHAT IS AN INJURY?

Injury may be defined as any damage to the human body that results from acute exposure of physical energy or damage that results from an absence of vital entities such as heat and oxygen. There are five basic forms of injurious energy: thermal, mechanical, electrical, radiating, and chemical. Roughly three-fourths of all injuries are caused by exposure to mechanical or kinetic energy during incidents such as motor vehicle crashes, falls, and firearm discharges. Examples of injury resulting from a lack of heat or oxygen are frostbite and drowning respectively. An individual's tolerance for injury depends on factors such as physical size, age, and presence of underlying disease.

Injury has also been defined as a disease that results from the interaction of three components of the epidemiology triangle: the host, agent, and environment (see Figure H-1). The host refers to the human being or victim, the agent is the form of energy involved, and the environment provides the opportunity for the agent (energy) to be transmitted to the host.

The environment may be either protective and prevent injury or unsafe and encourage injury (see Figure H-2).

The mechanism by which the agent or energy is transferred to the host is referred to as the vector. For example, during a motor vehicle crash, the automobile is the vector that may transmit physical (kinetic) energy to the host if the environment is permissive.

Injury may be classified as intentional or unintentional. Intentional injuries include those such as suicide, assault, and homicide. Unintentional injuries include those that are not deliberate or planned, such as falls, motor vehicle crashes, and burns. In some cases, it may be difficult to distinguish intentional from unintentional injury. Injury may also be categorized by the actual type of injury (such as fracture or head injury), by the mechanism or cause of injury (such as motor vehicle crash or fall), or by the population at risk, such as pediatric, black males, or the elderly.

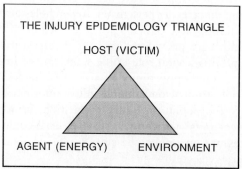

Figure H-1 *The injury epidemiology triangle.*

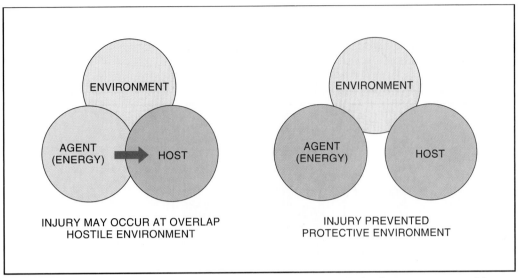

Figure H-2 *The relationship of the environment, injuring agent, and host.*

THE INJURY PROCESS AND WHY INJURIES OCCUR

Injury results when the victim is exposed to energy in amounts that exceed the threshold of human tolerance. In most cases, energy is transmitted as the victim is attempting to perform a specific task or action. The performance of a task refers to how well the individual executes an action, and the task demand is the amount of skill that is required to successfully perform the task. Any time that an individual's performance is below the task demand for the action, there is potential for release of injurious energy (Figure H-3). For example, a drunk driver may lack the skills necessary to drive an automobile and ultimately crash. The crash results in the release of kinetic energy (motion), which may be transmitted to the driver causing injury. In an unprotective environment, the energy is transmitted to the individual and results in an injury.

The environment may also protect the victim from injury in cases where the road conditions are favorable, guard rails are present to prevent driving over an embankment, or the victim is restrained (Figure H-4).

ANALYZING INJURY EVENTS

An injury event can be analyzed by separating it into three phases: the preinjury phase, the injury event, and the postinjury phase. Within each phase, there are host, vehicle, and environmental factors that may contribute to the injury process. Preinjury factors are those that either contribute to or inhibit the potential release of energy prior to the injury event. The injury phase has factors that may enhance or inhibit transmission of energy to the host during the injury event. Postinjury factors tend to contribute to or diminish the severity of injury once it has occurred. Prehospital care providers play a major role in the postinjury phase by providing rapid and high-quality care to injured victims in the field.

The analysis of injury events into the three phases and host, vehicle and environmental factors is referred to as Haddon's matrix. Table H-2 provides an example of an analysis of a motor vehicle crash using Haddon's matrix. This tool is very useful to identify factors contributing to the outcome of an injury event, broaden the discussion for developing prevention strategies, and reveal that most injuries are the product of a large number of causal factors and are not just random happenings.

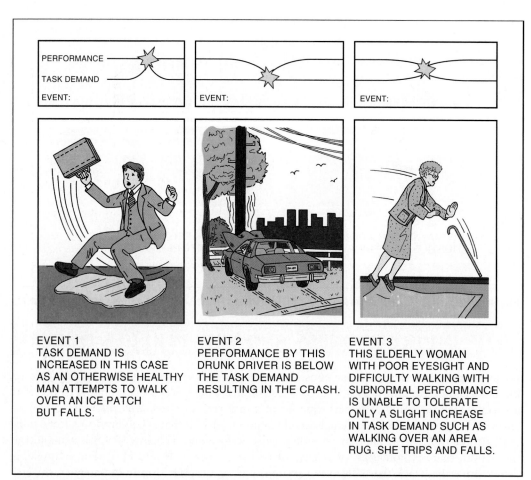

EVENT 1
TASK DEMAND IS
INCREASED IN THIS CASE
AS AN OTHERWISE HEALTHY
MAN ATTEMPTS TO WALK
OVER AN ICE PATCH
BUT FALLS.

EVENT 2
PERFORMANCE BY THIS
DRUNK DRIVER IS BELOW
THE TASK DEMAND
RESULTING IN THE CRASH.

EVENT 3
THIS ELDERLY WOMAN
WITH POOR EYESIGHT AND
DIFFICULTY WALKING WITH
SUBNORMAL PERFORMANCE
IS UNABLE TO TOLERATE
ONLY A SLIGHT INCREASE
IN TASK DEMAND SUCH AS
WALKING OVER AN AREA
RUG. SHE TRIPS AND FALLS.

Figure H-3 *The relationship of performance and task demand in the injury process.*

WHAT IS INJURY PREVENTION AND CONTROL?

Perhaps the most important principle of injury prevention and control is that injury is a disease which is subject to prevention by modifying transmission of energy to the individual. The goal of primary injury prevention is to prevent injury from occurring in the first place. Examples include wearing a seat belt, helmet use by motorcyclists and bicyclists, and the installation of smoke detectors. Strategies that attempt to minimize further injury or death after the initial trauma or injury event has occurred is called secondary injury prevention. Prehospital care providers practice secondary injury prevention, or acute care, by assuring adequate airway, breathing, and circulation as well as C-spine immobilization and rapid transportation to the closest appropriate medical facility.

INJURY SURVEILLANCE

Injury surveillance data forms the foundation of injury control. Accurate and detailed data are needed to determine the incidence of specific injury events, the demographic distributions, the cause of an injury event, and injury risk factors, as well as other factors involved in injury. Prehospital data such as location of the injury site, mechanism of injury, host fac-

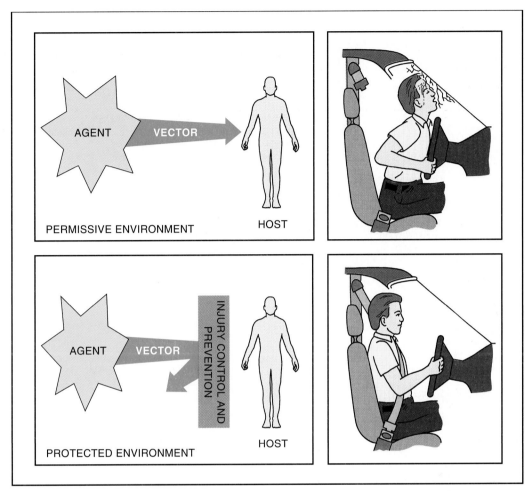

Figure H-4 *The role of injury control and prevention in providing a protective environment.*

tors, agent factors, and environmental factors are required. Prehospital care providers are in a crucial position to document the mechanism of injury in great detail, including information such as the extent of damage to a motor vehicle (starred windshield or deformed steering wheel). Description of the location and conditions of the injury site may also be useful in identifying a dangerous section of road where motor vehicle crashes occur time and again or a hazardous area such as an unsafe playground where injuries occur frequently.

RISK FACTORS

Injuries are not random events. Some populations, such as males, alcoholics, and certain age groups, are at higher risk for injury than others. A risk factor is a variable that makes an individual more likely to be injured. Injuries can be prevented by reducing or eliminating risk factors. An example of a host risk factor that may predispose an individual to injury is the use of drugs or alcohol while driving a motor vehicle. A high-risk group is defined as a subset of the population that has a higher incidence of injury. This group may be exposed to hazards more frequently, may be unable to avoid a hazard, or may have a lower injury threshold. Young males are one well-known group that is at higher risk for being involved in a motor vehicle crash than the general population.

		FACTORS		
PHASES	**HOST**	**VEHICLE**	**PHYSICAL ENVIRONMENT**	**SOCIOCULTURAL ENVIRONMENT**
PRE-EVENT	IMPAIRED CAPACITY DUE TO ALCOHOL, AGE, POOR VISION, FATIGUE, INEXPERIENCE, POOR JUDGMENT	DEFECTIVE PARTS (BRAKES, TIRES); POOR MAINTENANCE, DIRTY WINDSHIELD/ WINDOWS, IMPROPER BRAKE LIGHTS, EASE OF CONTROL, SPEED OF TRAVEL	NARROW ROAD SHOULDER, POOR LIGHTING, ROAD CURVATURE AND GRADIENT, ROAD SURFACE TYPE, WEATHER CONDITIONS, DIVIDED HIGHWAY, VISIBILITYOFHAZARDS, SIGNALIZATION	ATTITUDES ABOUT ALCOHOL, DRUNK DRIVING LAWS, SPEED LIMITS, INJURY PREVENTION PROGRAMS
EVENT	TOLERANCE OF BODY TO ENERGY; INJURY THRESHOLD DUE TO AGING, CHRONIC DISEASE (OSTEOPOROSIS), ETC.; SAFETY BELT USE	PLACEMENT HARDNESS AND SHARPNESS OF CONTACT SURFACES (DASH, STEERING WHEEL), AUTOMATIC RESTRAINTS, VEHICLE SIZE	RECOVERY AREAS, GUARD RAILS, FIXED OBJECTS (TELEPHONE POLES, TREES), MEDIAN BARRIERS, EMBANKMENTS	ATTITUDES ABOUT SEAT BELT USE, ENFORCEMENT OF CHILD SAFETY SEAT LAWS
POSTEVENT	EXTENT OF INJURY SUSTAINED, KNOWLEDGE OF FIRST AID, PHYSICAL CONDITION AND AGE	FUEL SYSTEM INTEGRITY (BURSTING GAS TANK), ENTRAPMENT OF VICTIM	ACCESS TO EMS, QUALITY OF EMS CARE, AVAILABILITY OF EXTRICATION EQUIPMENT, REHABILITATION PROGRAMS	TRAINING OF EMS PERSONNEL, TRAUMA SYSTEM PROGRAMS
RESULTS	PHYSICAL AND MENTAL IMPAIRMENT	COST OF VEHICLE REPAIR	DAMAGE TO ENVIRONMENT	LEGAL COSTS, COSTS TO SOCIETY (LOSS OF LIVES AND INCOME)

Table H-2 *Haddon's Matrix*

PREVENTIVE INTERVENTIONS

Haddon's matrix can be used to identify the factors affecting the extent of injury during specific injury events. Some of the factors may be amenable to prevention strategies or interventions designed to reduce the incidence or severity of injury.

There are three types of interventions: educational, enforcement, and engineering. Interventions may also be classified as either active or passive. An active intervention requires a change in behavior by the individual to be protected. Educational programs such as those that encourage seat belt use or installation of home smoke detectors are examples of active interventions that attempt to persuade individuals to alter their behavior for increased self-protection. These programs may increase public awareness, but are often ignored by those who are at highest risk for injury such as the economically and educationally deprived. Laws against drunk driving and mandatory helmet use by motorcyclists are other examples of active interventions that are aimed at changing an individual's behavior. However, the introduction of a legal intervention does not necessarily imply that it will be enforced by the authorities or adhered to by the public. Unfortunately, alcohol continues to play a part in half of all fatal motor vehicle crashes despite laws against driving under the influence of alcohol. Active education and enforcement interventions are more effective when used together.

Passive interventions provide automatic protection and are generally more effective than active interventions since they do not rely on human behavior change. Modifications in the engineering and design of vehicles and the environment have been very effective in reducing the incidence and severity of injuries. The incorporation of air bags and softer dashboards into automobiles has significantly reduced the incidence and severity of motor vehicle related injuries. Engineering improvements in road design have also been found to be effective countermeasures in preventing motor vehicle crashes.

DESIGNING INTERVENTIONS: When developing injury prevention programs, it is critical to recognize pitfalls for potential failure as well as ingredients for success. Many intervention programs are difficult to initiate, expensive to maintain, and require the use of limited community resources. The following suggestions will be helpful in selecting injury prevention activities:

1. Target efforts toward a problem that occurs frequently or results in severe injury in your community. In some regions, this may be house fires and, for others, motor vehicle crashes.

2. Address the problem injuries that have specific countermeasures that are known to be effective. Focus on limited, concrete solutions to specific injury events and avoid diffuse, general approaches. Examples of directed specific solutions include fire-safe cigarettes, smoke detectors for house fire prevention, and helmets for bicycle-related head injury prevention.

3. Make the intervention as simple as possible to increase public acceptance and minimize the chance of misuse.

4. Develop a critical mass of community awareness through broad-based grass-roots support, legislation, enforcement, and professional action. Prehospital care providers should take advantage of their connections with local and regional community leaders to build coalitions for effective prevention programs.

5. Promote institutionalization of programs that will last beyond the initial volunteer effort or temporary grant funding. Injury prevention programs should be designed to become a permanent component of prehospital care.

Table H-3 provides an example of injury-specific interventions which have been developed and found to be successful.

INJURY EVENT	RISK FACTOR	EXAMPLES OF INJURY-SPECIFIC INTERVENTION
DROWNING	2- TO 5-YEAR-OLD MALES	INSTALL FENCING AROUND POOLS AT LEAST ONE METER HIGH WITH SELF-LOCKING DOOR; WATER MOTION ALARM; SWIMMING LESSONS; PROMINENT "NO DIVING" NOTICES NEAR SHALLOW WATER; EASY ACCESS TO EMS
BICYCLE RELATED	5- TO 12-YEAR-OLD MALES	ENCOURAGE HELMET USE; USE OF SAFETY REFLECTORS; BICYCLE TRAFFIC LANES; RIDER EDUCATION PROGRAMS
POISONING	1- TO 5-YEAR-OLD	PACKAGE MEDICINES IN CHILDPROOF CONTAINERS; INSTALL SAFETY LATCHES IN STORAGE CABINETS
FALLS	ELDERLY WITH POOR VISION AND/OR UNSTABLE GAIT	REMOVE THROW RUGS; USE NIGHTLIGHTS; HAND RAILS ON STAIRS; ACCESS TO ACTIVATE EMS

Table H-3 *Examples of Injury-Specific Interventions*

ROLE OF THE EMS PROVIDER IN INJURY PREVENTION AND CONTROL

There are four areas in which prehospital personnel can make an impact and prevent injuries in their community:

1. *Acute Care/Secondary Injury Prevention of the Injured Patient.* Medically trained personnel, such as BTLS providers, are the initial and vital link in the trauma care system. By providing prompt and appropriate care, many lives are saved each year.

2. *Community Education/Primary Injury Prevention.* As respected and credible members of the community, prehospital care providers have a unique opportunity to practice primary injury prevention since they interact directly with injured patients and their families. Less severely injured patients and their families and friends can be counseled about how the present and any future injury could be prevented. Examples include advising the public to wear helmets when riding bicycles, motorcycles, and all-terrain vehicles, as well as wearing seat belts and using child carseats in automobiles. By assessing the injury site, prehospital personnel identify specific injury prevention strategies for a given family such as how to "childproof" a home or ways to make the home of an elderly person less risky for falls. As community spokespersons, prehospital care providers often interact with groups such as the local Parent Teachers Association and the Rotary Club. In doing so, community leaders will become more aware of the important concepts of injury prevention and work toward developing a safer community.

3. *Public Policy.* Seat belt and fire-safe cigarette legislation are two examples of regulations that have been instituted with the support of EMS personnel. Seat belt legislation has been very effective in increasing the number of people who wear seat belts and decreasing the number of highway deaths. For those states without seat belt laws, EMS personnel can be effective in encouraging the passage of such legislation. Similarly, it was prehospital care providers who found the most common cause of fatal house fires is cigarette smoking. With their support, a fire-safe cigarette has been developed. Prehospital care providers may be the first to recognize a new injury pattern or high-risk group for a specific injury. By reporting this type of information to local and state authorities, injury prevention strategies may be put into place by legislators in hopes of reducing fatal and serious injuries.

4. *Research/Injury Surveillance.* Accurate documentation of the circumstances surrounding injuries such as demographics, location, mechanism of injury, and associated risk factors is important in identifying problem injuries and designing and implementing prevention strategies. Providing reliable information to local community leaders, legislators, and physicians such as the location of the "dangerous intersection," the poorly supervised quarry and the "unsafe" playground can lead to the development of effective injury prevention strategies and a safer community.

SUMMARY

Prehospital care providers are a vital link in the chain of the national injury control effort. Their interaction with the public is an opportunity to practice both primary and secondary injury prevention. As part of the medical community, EMS personnel provide information to emergency physicians and nurses, which is important in the acute care of injured victims as well as information that is useful in injury control research. The injury epidemic can be addressed only through a concerted effort by the medical, community, and legislative organizations.

BIBLIOGRAPHY

1. American College of Emergency Physicians. *Guidelines for Trauma Care Systems.* Dallas, TX: The College, September 16, 1992.

2. Baker, S., B. O'Neill, M. J. Ginsburg, and G. Li. *The Injury Fact Book.* New York: Oxford University Press, 1992.

3. Centers for Disease Control and Prevention. *Injury Control in the 1990s: A National Plan for Action.* Atlanta, GA: The Centers, 1993.

4. Centers for Disease Control and Prevention. *Setting the National Agenda for Injury Control in the 1990s: Position Papers from the Third National Injury Control Conference.* Atlanta, GA: The Centers, 1992.

5. Committee on Trauma Research, Commission on Life Sciences, National Research Council, and the Institute of Medicine. *Injury in America: A Continuing Public Health Problem.* Washington, D.C.: National Academy Press, 1985.

6. Christoffel, T., and S. P. Teret. *Protecting the Public, Legal Issues in Injury Prevention.* New York: Oxford University Press, 1993.

7. Kaalbfleisch, J., and F. Rivera. "Principles in Injury Control: Lessons to Be Learned from Child Safety Seats." *Pediatric Emergency Care* (1989), pp. 131–134

8. Martinez, R. "Injury Control: A Primer for Physicians." *Annals of Emergency Medicine,* Vol. 19 (1990), pp. 72–77.

9. The National Committee for Injury Prevention and Control, *Injury Prevention: Meeting the Challenge.* New York: Oxford University Press 1989.

10. Wilson M. H., and others. *Saving Children, A Guide to Injury Prevention.* New York: Oxford University Press, 1991.

GLOSSARY

abruptio placenta   early separation of the placenta from the uterus.

acidosis   a condition caused by accumulation of acid or loss of base from the body.

adventitia   the layer of loose connective tissue forming the outermost coating of an organ.

aerobic   requiring oxygen.

alkalosis   a pathologic condition resulting from accumulation of base or loss of acid in the body.

anaerobic   lacking oxygen.

anoxia   absence of oxygen supply to the tissue.

asphyxia   a condition due to lack of oxygen, suffocation.

aspirate   taking foreign matter into the lungs during inhalation.

assessment   evaluation of the condition of a patient.

AVPU   a description of the level of consciousness, i.e., A-alert, V-responds to verbal stimuli, P-responds to pain, U-unresponsive.

avulsion   an injury in which a piece of a structure is torn away.

axial loading   compression forces applied along the long axis of the body. *Example:* a fall in which a victim lands on his feet and force is transferred up his legs to his back, causing a compression fracture of a lumbar vertebra.

Battle's sign   swelling and discoloration behind the ear caused by a fracture of the base of the skull.

BIADs   blind insertion airway devices (EOA, EGTA, PtL airway, and Combitube®)

BLS   Burns, Lacerations, Swelling. Can also mean Basic Life Support.

bronchospasm   contraction of the smooth muscle of the bronchi.

BVM (bag-valve mask)   a system of artificial ventilation in which the oxygen inflow fills a bag that is attached to a mask by a one way valve.

capillary blanch or refill   test for impairment of circulation: pressure on tip of the nail will cause the bed to turn white, if it does not turn pink again by the time it takes to say "capillary refill," the circulation is impaired. The test has been found to be unreliable for early shock.

carbonaceous sputum   sputum that is "sooty" or black.

carina   the lowest part of the trachea, where the trachea divides to form the two mainstem bronchi.

catecholamines   a group of chemicals of similar structure that act to increase heart rate and blood pressure.

central cord syndrome   an injury to the spinal cord that produces more loss of sensory and motor function in the arms than the legs.

cerebral perfusion   blood flow to the brain.

C.N.S.   central nervous system, the brain and spinal cord.

Combitube®   a double lumen airway BIAD similar to the PtL airway.

concussion   a jarring injury to the brain resulting in disturbance of brain function.

contracoup   an injury to the brain on the opposite side of the original blow.

contralateral   situated or affecting the opposite side.

constricted   to shrink or contract.

contusion   bruising; the reaction of soft tissue to a direct blow.

copious   large amount.

coup   an injury to the brain on the same side as the original blow.

crepitation   feeling of crackling; the sensation of fragments of broken bones rubbing together.

Cushing reflex   a reflex whereby the body reacts to increased pressure on the brain by raising the blood pressure.

DCAP   Deformities, Contusions, Abrasions, Penetrations

DCAPP   Deformities, Contusions, Abrasions, Penetrations, Paradoxical movement

deceleration   to come to a sudden stop, decreasing speed.

decumbent position   the position assumed when lying down.

denatured   to destroy the usual nature of a substance.

dermis   the inner layer of the skin, containing hair follicles, sweat glands, sebaceous glands, nerve endings and blood vessels.

diaphoresis   to perspire profusely.

diuretic   an agent that promotes the excretion of urine.

doll's eyes   oculocephalic reflex; a test of brainstem function that is never performed in the prehospital setting.

dura   the tough fibrous membrane forming the outermost of the three coverings of the brain.

EGTA   esophageal gastric tube airway; an improved EOA

EOA   esophageal obturator airway.

epidermis   the outermost layer of skin.

epidural   outside the dura; between the dura and the skull.

etiology   the cause of a particular disease.

ET Tube   endotracheal tube.

eviseration   the protruding of internal organs through a wound.

expeditious   quick, speedy.

exsanguinate   to bleed to death.

full thickness   third degree burn.

genioglossus   the muscle that pulls the tongue out of the mouth.

grunting   a deep, gutteral noise made in breathing; a sign of respiratory distress in small children.

Hare splint   a type of traction splint

Heimlich maneuver   a method of dislodging food or other material from the throat of a choking victim.

hemiparesis   partial paralysis affecting one side of the body.

hemoptysis   to spit up blood or blood stained sputum.

hemothorax   the presence of blood in the chest cavity within the pleural space, outside the lung.

hypercarbia   high blood carbon dioxide level.

hyperresonant   giving an increased vibrant sound on percussion, tympanic.

hypertympany   hyperresonant

hyperventilation   increased amount of air entering the lungs, >24 breaths per minute for an adult.

hypovolemic shock   hemmorrhagic shock; shock caused by insuffcient blood or fluid within the body.

hypoxia   a deficiency of oxygen reaching the tissues of the body.

intraabdominal   within the abdomen.

intracranial   within the skull.

intrathoractic   within the chest.

ipsalateral   situated on or affecting the same side.

JVD   jugular vein distention.

kinematics   the phrase of mechanics that deals with possible motions of the body.

Klippel splint   a type of traction splint.

labial angle   corner of the mouth.

lateral decubitus position   position assumed when lying on one's side.

lesion   an injury or abnormal condition of a part.

LOC   level of consciousness.

MAP   mean arterial blood pressure

mean arterial blood pressure   diastolic blood pressure plus 1/3 (systolic minus the diastolic blood pressure).

medial   toward the middle.

mortality   frequency of death or death rate.

MVA   motor vehicle accident.

necrosis   the death of tissue.

neonate   newborn infant.

NP airway   nasopharyngeal airway; an artificial airway positioned in the nasal cavity.

occult injuries   hidden or concealed from view injuries.

osteomyelitis   inflammation or infection or a bone or bones.

pallor   paleness, absence of skin color.

palpate   to examine by touch.

paradoxical motion   the motion of the injured segment of a flail chest, opposite to the normal motion of the chest wall.

parenchymal   the essential elements of an organ.

paresis   slight or incomplete paralysis.

paresthesia   abnormal sensation; a "tingling" sensation

partial thickness burn   a burn that does not injure the full thickness of the skin. A first degree burn involves only the epidermal layer. A second degree burn involves the epidermis and part of the dermis.

patent   open

pathophysiology   the basic processes of the disease.

perfusion   the passage of blood or fluid through the vessels of an organ.

Pharyngotracheal Lumen Airway   a double lumen BIAD that can be inserted into the esophagus or trachea.

pia mater   innermost of the three layers of tissue that envelop the brain.

placenta previa   an abnormal location of the placenta, so that it covers the opening of the uterus (cervical os).

PMS   Pulse, Motor, Sensory.

pneumothorax   the presence of air within the chest cavity in the pleural space, but outside the lung (collapsed lung).

potential space   a space that does not exist except under abnormal circumstances. *Example:* Normally the lungs completely fill the chest cavity so that the pleural space (between the lungs and the chest wall) is only a potential space. If the pleural space contains blood it is a hemothorax.

PtL Airway   *see* Pharyngotracheal Lumen Airway

pulse pressure   the sensation given by the heart contraction to the palpating finger on an artery.

raccoon's eyes   swelling and discoloration around both eyes; a late sign of basilar skull fracture.

respiratory reserve   lung tissue over and above the body's need to provide oxygenation for the body.

RTSS   radio telephone switch station; a type of radio that accesses the telephone lines.

Sager splint   a type of traction splint.

scaphoid   shaped like a boat. When used to describe the abdomen, scaphoid means sunken in.

scuba diver   a diver who is able to remain under water by breathing compressed air from a breathing apparatus needing no connection with the surface. "Scuba" stands for self-contained underwater breathing apparatus.

sheering forces   forces that occur in such a direction to cause tearing of an organ.

sibling   brother or sister.

skin diver   a diver who holds his breath when swimming under water. He uses no artificial breathing methods.

snoring   to breathe in a hoarse, rough noise, usually with the mouth open.

snorkeler   a diver who uses a short tube (snorkel) in order to float on the surface and observe underwater life. When diving, a snorkeler must hold his breath.

spontaneous pneumothorax   collapsed lung caused by the rupture of a congenitally weak area on the surface of the lung.

stridor   breathing that has a high-pitched, harsh noise; a sign of impending airway obstruction.

stroke volume   the amount of blood pumped by the heart in one beat.

subcutaneous emphysema   the presence of air in soft tissues, giving a very characteristic crackling sensation on palpation; the "rice krispies" feeling.

tachypnea   adult respiratory rate of 24 or more.

tamponade   compression of a part of the anatomy, as the compression of heart by pericardial fluid.

tension pneumothorax   a condition in which air continuously leaks out of the lung into the pleural space, increasing pressure within the space with every breath the patient takes.

Thomas splint   a type of traction splint.

TIC   Tenderness, Instability, Crepitation.

tidal volume   the amount of air that is inspired and expired during one respiratory cycle.

traction   the action of drawing or pulling on an object.

trajectory   the direction a missle takes in flight or in a body.

transected   to cut transversely.

Trendelenburg position   patient supine with lower body elevated about 30 degrees.

vallecula   the space between the base of the tongue and the epiglottis.

venous pressure   pressure of the blood in the veins.

viscera   any large interior organ in any one of the three great cavities of the body, especially the abdomen.

volatile   a substance that evaporates rapidly at room temperature when exposed to air.

wheezing   whistling sounds made in breathing; a sign of spasm or narrowing of the bronchi.

INDEX